A Handbook

of Chinese

Hematology

A Handbook
of Chinese
Hematology

Simon Becker

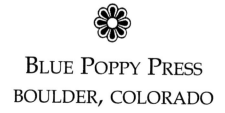

BLUE POPPY PRESS
BOULDER, COLORADO

Published by:

BLUE POPPY PRESS
A Subsidiary of Blue Poppy Enterprises, Inc.
3450 Penrose Place, Suite 110
BOULDER, CO 80301

First Edition, July, 2000

ISBN 1-891845-16-0
LC 00-131750

COPYRIGHT 2000 © BLUE POPPY PRESS

The information in this book is given in good faith. However, the authors and the publishers cannot be held responsible for any error or omission. Nor can they be held in any way responsible for treatment given on the basis of information contained in this book. The publishers make this information available to readers for scholarly and research purposes only.

The publishers do not advocate nor endorse self-medication by laypersons. Chinese medicine is a professional medicine. Laypersons interested in availing themselves of the treatments described in this book should seek out a qualified professional practitioner of Chinese medicine.

COMP Designation: Original work using a standard translational terminology for Chinese medical technical terms

10 9 8 7 6 5 4 3 2 1

Printed at Johnson's Printing in Boulder, CO
on acid-free, elementally chlorine-free paper.

Preface

In the summer of 1997, I traveled to Harbin, China, to complete an internship at the Heilongjiang University of Chinese Medicine. After only a short time, I became good friends with a number of Chinese students of Chinese medicine. One of these friends was the son of the head of the Chinese medical hematology department. Thus, after observing the treatment of children for two months, I began interning with Dr. Sun Wei-zheng, head of the hematology department at the First Hospital affiliated with the Heilongjiang University of Chinese Medicine.

At that time, my knowledge of hematological diseases was minimal. I had studied the biomedical pathology of the different anemias, leukemia, lymphoma, purpura, etc., but I had never seen any material in the English language Chinese medical literature about such diseases and I had never concerned myself with their Chinese medical treatment.

While studying and working with Dr. Sun, I quickly came to realize that Chinese medical hematology is a very specialized field within Chinese internal medicine (*nei ke*). In fact, it is no less specialized than the better known specialities of gynecology (*fu ke*), pediatrics (*er ke*), and geriatrics (*lao nian ke*). Working day after day with Dr. Sun, I also realized that Chinese hematology requires diligent dedication to study and master. Happily, to offset the hard work necessary to gain competence in this specialty, I discovered that Chinese medicine treats most hematological diseases quite successfully. Because of the successes I witnessed in Dr. Sun's clinic and because there were (till now) no English language treatment manuals or textbooks on this subject, I systematically began, with Dr. Sun's blessing and help, collecting information on modern Chinese hematology. This book is the fruit of that research. Therefore, the information in this book comes from four main sources: 1) Dr. Sun's teaching, 2) my own clinical experience, 3) relatively recent articles on various hematological conditions and research appearing in professional Chinese medical journals, and 4) a number of Chinese language books on or including sections on Chinese hematology.

This book has been written for all practitioners of Chinese medicine who A) treat any one of the many different diseases discussed in this book, B) wish to learn more about the disease mechanisms and current standards of care in the People's Republic of China for hematological diseases, and C) use Chinese medicinals in the treatment of disease in general. I hope that this first text on modern Chinese hematology serves as an encouragement to and template for including this subject in the curricula of Chinese medical schools in the West. This would help ensure that graduating students are familiar with the Chinese medical treatment of at least the most common hematological diseases. In addition, I hope this book may open the ears and minds of progressive MDs specializing in the field of hematology and that it helps make them aware that Chinese medicine is a viable and cost-effective complement to many current Western medical treatments for hematological diseases.

Even in the People's Republic of China, Chinese medical hematology is a relatively new area of specialization which is undergoing further intensive research even as I write this Preface. As more Chinese hematology books and articles become available, the information contained in this book will inevitably have to be updated. However, I am confident that, at least for now, this book is a thoroughly researched and relatively comprehensive collection of the most current information available on hematological diseases in the professional Chinese medical literature.

Although my experience in treating hematological diseases, both in China and the U.S., suggests that Chinese medicine does offer an effective alternative and complement to standard Western medical care, it should also be noted at the outset that many blood diseases require Western medical care. Therefore, Western Chinese medical practitioners attempting to treat hematological diseases do need to know something about the Western medical etiology, epidemiology, pathophysiology, diagnosis, and treatment of these conditions. However, because this book is written specifically for practitioners of Chinese medicine and not for MDs, the Western medical sections on different diseases contained in this book are, compared to Western medical hematology texts, somewhat simplified and not completely comprehensive. For more complete and comprehensive Western medical materials on any or all of the hematological diseases contained in this book, readers are referred to the bibliography at the back.

As the reader will see, when it comes to treatment modalities, this book is almost exclusively a Chinese medicinal book. In other words, I do not list any acupuncture treatments for individual hematologic diseases. This is not because I am prejudiced against acupuncture and am in favor of Chinese medicinals. It is rather because acupuncture is simply not considered the professional standard of care for the treatment of hematological diseases in the People's Republic of China. I also have not indicated any specific dosage amounts for the ingredients in the formulas listed under specific patterns of specific hematological diseases. The reason for this seeming omission is that I believe practitioners should never prescribe medicinals they have not studied and for which they do not already know the standard dosage parameters. Similar to adding and subtracting medicinals to formulas and not simply using standard textbook prescriptions, the amounts of individual medicinals within a formula need to be adjusted according to the patient's individual pattern and condition. Hence, I believe that giving dosages for formulas in a textbook like this is potentially misleading and definitely unrealistic. Anyone attempting to use this treatment manual in clinical practice is expected to have completed their professional entry level education in Chinese materia medica and Chinese formulas and prescriptions. Those who have should have no trouble choosing appropriate dosages on an *ad hoc* basis.

When encountering less common Chinese medicinals, I consulted four different materia medica. First I tried to find the medicinals in Bensky & Gamble's *Chinese Herbal Medicine: Materia Medica*. If I was unable to find them there, I a) went to my other three sources and b) added a footnote explaining the medicinals' properties, channel entries, and functions. If I was unable to find the medicinals in the other two English language sources I consulted, *i.e.*, Charles Belanger's *The Chinese Herb Selection Guide* and Hong-yen Hsu's *Oriental Materia Medica: A Concise Guide*, I looked them up in the *Zhong Yao Da Ci Dian (A Great Dictionary of Chinese Medicinals)*. When I had to consult this last source, keeping in mind that descriptions of these medicinals are not otherwise available in the English language, I did add this source's recommended dosage parameters besides listing the medicinal's properties, channel entries, and functions.

As stated above, much of the Chinese medical information in this book is based on translations from Chinese language sources. As a translator, I have chosen to use Nigel Wiseman's terminology as it appears in *English-Chinese Chinese-English Dictionary of Chinese Medicine* (Hunan Science & Technology Press, Changsha, 1995) as my standard. I find the use of a standard translational terminology monumentally important when studying, translating, and writing about Chinese medicine. Only by using a standard translational terminology (referenced to both Chinese characters and Pinyin romanization) can one insure that every reader will understand the same Chinese medical concept as the writer or speaker intended. Using such a standard translational terminology is, in my opinion, the only way of insuring that everybody is talking about the same thing when discussing professional issues such as case histories, pattern differentiation, and treatment principles.

Prior to 1998, Wiseman's terminology existed only as a glossary (even though it was called a dictionary), and one of the complaints against adopting this terminology was that most English language speakers had no idea what Wiseman's terms meant in real-life clinical practice. Happily, Wiseman and Feng's new *A Practical Dictionary of Chinese Medicine* (Paradigm Publications, Brookline, MA, 1998) now exists to give those definitions and explanations. I personally find it of little importance if one agrees or disagrees with every term choice of Wiseman's terminology (although one needs to realize that Wiseman is a linguist and that his word choice is not simply random). The important thing is that Wiseman's glossaries and dictionaries make it possible for anyone interested to identify what Chinese word corresponds to which of Wiseman's term choices. If one disagrees with any of Wiseman *et al.*'s choices[1], all one has to do is footnote any such divergence and then one can use whatever term they prefer. For n

---

[1] In fact, Wiseman is only the focus person for a diverse group of Chinese and English linguists, translators, and Chinese medical practitioners who are continuing to debate and refine this standard terminology. Some of the Westerners engaged in this process besides Nigel Wiseman (either past or present) include Andrew Ellis, Jim Cleaver, the late Paul Zmiewski, Craig Mitchell, Bob Flaws, Bob Felt, and Ken Rose, to name a few.

instance, within this book, several terms are used which are different to Wiseman's suggestions because of the publisher's own, in-house standards. However, in each case, there is a footnote explaining that divergence. Otherwise, all technical Chinese medical terminology does conform to Wiseman's standard.

Chinese medicinal formula names are based on Blue Poppy Press's house style of translating formula names verbatim, as far as possible, using Wiseman's terms for the translation of individual words but not his entire formula name suggestions. Likewise, the Latin for the medicinal identifications is based on Blue Poppy's house style as opposed to Wiseman's inverted Latin word order. A list of the medicinal identifications Blue Poppy Press commonly uses can be found in the Free Articles section of Blue Poppy's Web site at: www.bluepoppy.com. And finally, acupuncture point identifications also follow Blue Poppy Press precedents. This means that first the point names are given in Pinyin romanization with alpha-numeric notation followed in parentheses. These alpha-numeric abbreviations follow the World Health Organization's Standard Acupuncture Point Nomenclature except that Lu = lung, St = stomach, Sp = spleen, Ht = heart, Bl = bladder, Ki = kidney, Per = pericardium, TB = triple burner, Liv = liver, GV = governing vessel, and CV = conception vessel. Therefore, Lu 1 = the WHO's LU 1, St 1 = the WHO's ST 1, etc.

The compilation of the information in this book would not have been possible without the assistance of a number of people who took time away from their busy schedules to help this fledgling writer, and I am grateful to each and every person who helped me gather this information. First and foremost, I would like to thank my Chinese teacher, Dr. Sun Wei-zheng, who, besides introducing me to this subject, taught me all the basics of Chinese hematology and sent me invaluable journal articles. I would also like to thank his son Sun Jing-hui, and his friend, Shi Jing. Besides helping me read medical Chinese and taking me to Chinese medical bookstores to shop for appropriate books, these two spent hours scanning the tables of contents of hundreds of Chinese medical journals and mailed me their findings. I further received a number of important books from my Chinese friend, Tang Nai-pei, an MD in China whose friendship I greatly enjoyed while residing in Harbin. Other contributors of information whom I would like to thank are Bob Flaws and Shawn Oldham. Great thanks also go to Blue Poppy Press and Bob Flaws specifically for supporting this project and giving crucial advice about the strategy of writing this book. Lastly, I am indebted to my wife, fellow acupuncturist, Young-Ju Becker-Shin, who tirelessly supported and encouraged me throughout this endeavor.

Simon Becker
Asheville, NC
February 2000

Table of Contents

Introduction

This book is a clinical manual for the treatment of Western hematological diseases with Chinese medicine. Hematology refers to the study of the blood, and, in clinical practice, it means the treatment of blood diseases. The treatments based on pattern discrimination[1] in this book reflect current standards of care in the People's Republic of China. However, before immediately going on to those treatments, it is important for Western readers to understand that the word "blood" in this context does not refer to the Chinese concept of the blood but only to its Western medical counterpart. Therefore, this book is not a treatment manual on Chinese medical blood diseases, and patients complaining of such Western hematological conditions as anemia, leukemia, or purpura may have absolutely nothing wrong with the Chinese medical concept of their blood. For example, the main clinical symptom of anemia is fatigue, a qi vacuity symptom, not a Chinese blood vacuity symptom. Thus, just because a patient has been diagnosed with anemia (literally meaning "lack of blood"), the Chinese medical practitioner should take care not to assume that this patient also presents a Chinese medical pattern of blood vacuity. Therefore, although this book begins from the point of view of Western medical disease diagnosis, its treatments are based on Chinese medical pattern discrimination, and, the better one understands the Chinese medical prescriptive methodology, the more successful one will be in employing the treatments contained in this book.

The Chinese prescriptive methodology

Standard professional Chinese medicine is characterized by its primarily basing treatment on pattern discrimination (*bian zheng lun zhi*). Therefore, the fundamental first step in the treatment of any hematologic disease listed in this book is correct pattern differentiation. Chinese medical patterns are differentiated by applying the four Chinese medical techniques of examination. These four are inspection, listening/smelling, inquiry, and palpation. The data thus collected is next analyzed according to one or a combination of several Chinese medical systems of pattern discrimination (*e.g.*, five phase pattern discrimination, eight principle pattern differentiation, viscera and bowel pattern discrimination, disease cause pattern discrimination, etc.).

Once the pattern has been differentiated, it is important to take one more step prior to attempting to formulate a treatment plan. This is formulating the correct treatment

---

[1] Wiseman's preferred term is pattern identification for *bian zheng*. However, Blue Poppy Press's house standard is pattern discrimination.

principles. The treatment principles are the logical extension of an accurate pattern discrimination. For example, if the patient's pattern is determined to be spleen vacuity with qi and blood dual vacuity, then the treatment principles must be to fortify the spleen, boost the qi, and supplement blood. Treatment principles dictate the treatment necessary in order to restore balance to the imbalance implied in the name of the patient's pattern. Therefore, the treatment principles guide and simplify the selection of treatment formulas and medicinals. All one has to do is follow the treatment principles in selecting a medicinal or acupuncture prescription. Such a medicinal formula can be selected from two sources: 1) one can find a formula under the corresponding pattern for the specific hematologic disease at hand, or 2) one can select an appropriate formula from a repertoire of the 50-100 formulas every practitioner of Chinese medicine is expected to have memorized.

In addition, after the formula has been selected, it is usually of great importance that this formula not be administered in its standard form as found in the consulted textbook. In real-life clinical practice, unmodified textbook formulas rarely are a perfect fit for individual patients. Medicinals which are not necessary need to be deleted. Similarly, medicinals lacking from the original formula but indicated for a certain patient must be added. Only then can treatment be truly effective.

Thus, for every practitioner of standard professional Chinese medicine, the above three steps—1) pattern discrimination, 2) statement of treatment principles, and 3) medicinal or acupuncture prescription—are of great importance. One should never skip any of these three steps if one wants to treat disease effectively with Chinese medicine. Even more importantly, one should never prescribe a formula simply on the premises of a disease diagnosis alone. In standard professional Chinese medicine, diseases need to be further broken down into individual patterns, and formulas must be prescribed for the pattern the individual patient presents.

Unfortunately, the concept of treatment principles is often disregarded as an excessive and unnecessary step in the Western practice of Chinese medicine. However, the correct formulation of treatment principles is fundamentally important in order to arrive at the correct medicinal or acupuncture prescription. Bob Flaws has very accurately referred to treatment principles as funnels:

> The treatment principles are the funnel or bridge which guide one from the pattern discrimination to the choice of formula or acupuncture points. If one leaves out this crucial step in the TCM methodology, one may veer off the mark when it comes to composing the treatment plan. If one habitually writes down the treatment principles after

each pattern discrimination, this will greatly help one to hone their TCM methodology and make their prescribing all the more precise.[2]

If one follows all of the above steps and has a good understanding of basic Chinese medical theory, then one can effectively treat hematologic diseases. In my experience, it is the skipping of one or more of the above steps which makes Chinese medicine confusing and formulas inaccurate and, therefore, ultimately ineffective. In Western clinical practice, it is not always easy to stick to Chinese medical methodology and come up with an unbiased Chinese medical disease diagnosis, pattern discrimination, and treatment principles at the same time as being bombarded by Western medical terms and concepts. However, I believe that this is the most important underlying prerequisite for successful treatment with Chinese medicine.

The role of Western laboratory tests in modern professional Chinese medicine

Although the Chinese medical treatment of Western hematologic diseases is based on Chinese medical pattern discrimination, the Western medical diagnosis of these diseases is based almost exclusively on laboratory tests. Hence every patient with a pre-established Western hematologic disease diagnosis will be accompanied by one or more laboratory reports. Therefore, it is also important to understand that no single Western laboratory marker indicates any single Chinese medical pattern. For example, every patient with idiopathic thrombocytopenic purpura (ITP) will always manifest a decreased platelet count. Thus we can say that a decreased platelet count is pathognomonic of ITP. However, this count is not very important in terms of Chinese medical diagnosis or treatment (except, of course, for determining the severity of the disease). Two ITP patients with the same platelet count may present radically different Chinese medical patterns, while another two ITP patients with different platelet counts may present with identical Chinese patterns. Therefore, regardless of the lab test showing a decreased platelet count and, therefore, establishing a disease diagnosis of ITP, the practitioner of Chinese medicine still must differentiate the individual patient's pattern. Since treatment in Chinese medicine is based primarily on the patient's pattern, there are many different Chinese medicinal formulas for this disease depending on its different patterns, and the prescription of these various formulas has little if nothing to do with the patient's platelet count.

Nevertheless, modern lab tests do have their value in the clinical practice of Chinese medicine. First, they can be used as a tool for monitoring progress. Subtle changes of

---

[2]   Flaws, Bob, "Treatment Principles as Funnels," Free Articles, www.bluepoppy.com

blood values at a microscopic level often manifest before large changes in symptomatology occur. For many patients suffering from blood diseases, Chinese medicinals must be taken long-term. Therefore, improvements which can be measured with modern laboratory tests serve as an additional encouragement for patients and demonstrate to the practitioner beyond any doubt that the pattern differentiation is valid, the prescription accurate, and the treatment strategy correct. Furthermore, for patients suffering from depressed blood values (either white or red blood cells or platelets) but who are not acutely ill, lab tests can monitor the improvement and stabilization of the condition while patients are taking Chinese medicinals.

Secondly, in certain instances, lab tests can be used to modify medicinal prescriptions. Book I, Chapter 2, titled, "Chinese Medicinals in the Treatment of Blood Diseases," describes many Chinese medicinals' Western pharmacodynamics. For instance, nowadays, the combination of Caulis Milletiae Seu Spatholobi (*Ji Xue Teng*) and Radix Salviae Miltiorrhizae (*Dan Shen*) is indicated for decreased white blood cell count. Therefore, a lab test showing that the leukocyte count is depressed could prompt practitioners to add the above combination to their prescription.

It is important, however, that lab tests not be used to create the prescription in the first place. As stated above, the prescription should always be based on the treatment principles which themselves logically derive from the pattern discrimination. Additions of medicinals based on lab tests are only effective if they also fit the pattern and fit the overall composition of the prescription. For example, even though the combination of Radix Rubrus Paeoniae Lactiflorae (*Chi Shao*), uncooked Radix Rehmanniae (*Sheng Di*), and Cortex Radicis Moutan (*Dan Pi*) has been shown through modern research to stop bleeding, they are the wrong medicinals for a patient suffering from ITP bleeding due to spleen-kidney dual vacuity. These three medicinals are all cold in nature and stop bleeding by cooling the blood, and this is categorically the wrong strategy for dealing with bleeding due to spleen-kidney dual vacuity. Instead, spleen-fortifying, kidney-warming, and neutral-natured hemostatic medicinals, such as Herba Agrimoniae Pilosae (*Xian He Cao*), Radix Morindae Officinalis (*Ba Ji Tian*), and Rhizoma Atractylodis Macrocephalae (*Bai Zhu*), are indicated.

Therefore, to recapitulate, the classification of diseases in this book follows the modern Western biomedical classification of hematological diseases. However, no one hematological disease in Western medicine corresponds to a single blood disease in Chinese medicine.[3] Western and Chinese medicine are two different models of health and disease. The Western biomedical concept of blood is not the same as the Chinese

---

[3]   In point of fact, there really is no category of blood diseases in Chinese medicine. *Xue zheng,* the closest analogue, literally means "blood condition," but figuratively means bleeding or hemorrhagic disorders.

medical concept of blood. Therefore, in order to treat a hematological disease with Chinese medicine, one needs to practice the Chinese medical prescriptive methodology. This means that one needs to first discriminate the patient's pattern using the four examinations, then formulate treatment principles according to the differentiated pattern, and finally compose a medicinal formula according to the treatment principles while also keeping in mind modern pharmacological research. It is this step-by-step prescriptive methodology which helps guarantee success in Chinese medicine.

Book I:

Theory & Principles
of Modern Chinese Hematology

1
Basic Western Medical Theory of Hematological Diseases

In order to understand Book II which deals with the Chinese medical treatment of many different hematological diseases, this chapter discusses the Western biomedical theory of blood physiology, blood pathology, diagnostic measures, and standard biomedical treatment methods. An understanding of these biomedical parameters in the treatment of blood diseases with Chinese medicine is important because hematological diseases manifest on the microscopic level of blood and are thus diagnosed in Western medicine primarily through modern biomedical laboratory testing. In addition, many blood diseases are of a relatively serious nature and require not only Chinese medicine but also Western medical intervention, such as pharmaceutical drugs and laboratory monitoring, for successful management.

This chapter is broken down into four parts: 1) the physiology of the blood, 2) pathology of the blood, 3) the Western medical diagnosis of blood diseases, and 4) the biomedical treatment of blood diseases. As a complete exploration of all these fields lies beyond the scope of this book, only the most important information from each is given below, and the reader is strongly encouraged to study the physiology and pathology of the blood and its related diseases in detail from other sources (see Bibliography).

Physiology of the blood

Blood is a complex connective tissue in which living blood cells, called formed elements, are suspended in a non-living fluid matrix, the plasma. Plasma accounts for about 55% of whole blood; red blood cells (RBCs) for about 45%; and white blood cells (WBCs) and platelets account for less than 1%. Under normal circumstances, blood constitutes approximately 8% of total body weight, and its volume is about 5-6 liters in healthy adult males and 4-5 liters in healthy adult females. Blood has three main functions:

1) Distribution
Blood distributes oxygen from the lungs and nutrients from the digestive tract throughout the whole body. It also transports metabolic waste products to sites from which they can

be eliminated. And last, it transports hormones from the endocrine organs to their target sites.

2) Regulation

The blood regulates the minute balance which needs to exist in the body for all physiological events to take place. Blood regulates temperature through absorption and distribution of body heat, maintains a normal pH balance by carrying many buffer molecules, and controls an adequate fluid volume by regulating fluid loss from the blood stream into tissue spaces, thus maintaining a fluid level which supports efficient blood circulation to all parts of the body.

3) Protection

The blood's protective function includes 1) the prevention of blood loss by initiating a clotting cascade which stops bleeding after vessel rupture and 2) the housing and distribution of a large part of the immune system. Within the blood, antibodies, complement proteins[1], and white blood cells help defend the body against bacteria, viruses, and toxins.

Erythrocytes (Red Blood Cells)[2]

Erythrocytes (RBCs) are very unique cells. Their main function is to load oxygen in the lungs and carry it to body tissues and to load carbon dioxide in the tissues and transport it to the lungs for elimination from the body. To optimize their function, red blood cells are constructed very differently from other cells. They completely lack a nucleus and have only few organelles. They generate adenosine triphosphate (ATP) by an anaerobic mechanism and, therefore, do not consume any of the oxygen they carry. Furthermore, because red blood cells need to squeeze through the tiny capillaries, they are very

---

[1] The complement system refers to a group of 20 plasma proteins which, besides being a source of vasoactive mediators, also help in host defense against bacterial infections. Two activation pathways can be differentiated: the classical and the alternative pathway. The classical pathway needs antigen-antibody complexes for activation and is therefore activated slower than the alternative pathway which only requires derivative products of infectious organisms or foreign materials for activation. Regardless of activation requirements, however, the end result that follows activation is the same for both pathways: the complement proteins form a mem biologically active anaphylatoxins brane attack complex which induces cell lysis and generate.

[2] Erythrocyte is a compound term of erythro- and -cyte. Erythro stems from the Greek word *erythros* which means red. Cyte stems from the Greek word *kytos* meaning cell. Erythrocytes are called red blood cells because they appear either bright red or dark red depending on their state of oxygenation.

flexible. This flexibility results from an abundance of spectrin, a fibrous cytoskeletal protein attached to the cytoplasmic side of the erythrocyte's plasma membrane. Their structure is also unique. Shaped like a biconcave disc with a depressed center, they resemble a doughnut. This provides a large surface area relative to their volume, and, because no point within the cytoplasm is far from the cell's surface, the disc structure is ideal for gas exchange.

Erythrocytes accomplish their function of carrying oxygen from the lungs to the body tissues by reversibly binding oxygen to their hemoglobin. Hemoglobin is made up of four strands of the globin protein—two alpha and two beta. Each of these globin strands contains a red pigment called heme in its center. Oxygen then binds to the heme pigment to form oxyhemoglobin which is bright red in color. When the red blood cell has reached its target tissue, oxygen dissociates from the heme pigment, and the hemoglobin becomes deoxyhemoglobin and turns dark red in color.

Every erythrocyte contains about 250 million hemoglobin molecules. As seen above, every hemoglobin molecule can carry four oxygen molecules. Therefore, a single red blood cell can carry about one billion molecules of oxygen. About 20% of the carbon dioxide transported in the blood combines with hemoglobin. However, carbon dioxide binds to the amino acids of globin and not to the heme group and thus forms carbaminohemoglobin. This process happens more readily in deoxyhemoglobin.

The production of erythrocytes, or hematopoiesis, occurs in the red bone marrow or myeloid tissue. In children, red bone marrow comprises almost all of the marrow. In adults, however, this tissue is found chiefly in the bones of the axial skeleton and girdles and in the proximal epiphysis of the humerus and femur bones. All formed elements of the blood arise from the same stem cell, the hemocytoblast. Hemocytoblasts can differentiate into either a lymphoid or a myeloid stem cell. Erythrocytes then develop from the myeloid stem cell. Even though all the formed elements arise from just a single stem cell, once they are committed to a certain cell path, they cannot change. This is due to membrane receptors which bind to the respective stimulating hormones. For erythrocytes, this hormone is erythropoietin.

Erythrocytes have a life span of 100-120 days. After this period, because they lack a nucleus and cannot divide or synthesize protein, they become increasingly rigid and fragile. This makes them susceptible to entrapment, especially in the smaller circulatory channels of the spleen. In order to balance this die-off of old cells, the body produces red blood cells at the incredible speed of about two million cells per second. The kidney and, to a much lesser extent, the liver are the organs secreting erythropoietin. A small amount of this hormone circulates in the blood at all times and sustains red blood cell production at a basal rate. However, when kidney cells become hypoxic due to either declining numbers of red blood cells (such as due to excessive loss or destruction), reduced availability of oxygen to the blood (such as in high altitudes), or increased tissue demands for oxygen (such as during exercises), the release of erythropoietin is increased. Erythropoietin then stimulates the myeloid tissue which manufactures more red blood cells. Conversely, if there are too many red blood cells or there is too much oxygen, erythropoietin production is decreased. The male sex hormone testosterone also enhances the erythropoietin-generating function of the kidneys. In contrast, female hormones do not. This may be at least a partial reason for the higher RBC count and hemoglobin levels in men.

The synthesis of erythrocytes requires the usual nutrients and structural materials proteins, lipids, and carbohydrates. However, sufficient iron and B-complex vitamins are also very important. Vitamin B_{12} and folic acid are essential for DNA synthesis and, because of the rapid cell division in the erythropoietic process, even minimal deficiencies of these nutrients lead to abnormal erythrocyte production.

Leukocytes (White Blood Cells) [3]

Leukocytes are a group of five different cell types which protect the body from bacteria, viruses, fungi, toxins, and tumor cells. Whereas the erythrocytes are anucleate cells and never leave the blood vessels, leukocytes are complete cells with nuclei and the usual organelles, and they are not necessarily confined to the vessel system only. Through a process called diapedesis, these cells can leave the capillary vessels and mount an inflammatory or immune response where needed.

All leukocytes, just like erythrocytes, are descendants of the hemocytoblast. As stated above, the hemocytoblast divides into the myeloid stem cell and the lymphoid stem cell. The myeloid stem cell gives rise to the granulocytic neutrophil, basophil, and eosinophil and to the agranulocytic monocyte. The lymphoid stem cell is the precursor of the agranulocytic lymphocyte.

Similar to erythropoiesis, leukopoiesis (*i.e.*, the production of white blood cells) is regulated by hormones. Collectively known as colony-stimulating factors or CSFs, these hematopoietic hormones prompt the white blood cell precursors to divide and mature and also enhance the protective potency of the mature leukocytes. Macrophages and T-lymphocytes are the most important sources of CSFs.

---

[3] Similar to erythrocyte, leukocyte is a compound term of leuko- and -cyte. Leuko stems from the Greek work *leukos* meaning white. Cyte again comes from the Greek work *kytos*, cell. Leukocytes are so named because their cell body appears colorless under the microscope.

Neutrophils are the most abundant of all leukocytes and make up between 40-70% (4000-10,000) of the total number of white blood cells. They are granulocytic and their nuclei consist of three to six lobes. Because of this nuclear variability, they are often referred to as polymorphonuclear leukocytes or PMNs. Neutrophils are attracted to sites of inflammation through the process of chemotaxis[4] and are active phagocytes.[5] They attack especially bacteria and some fungi, and they can increase explosively during acute bacterial infections such as meningitis or appendicitis.

Eosinophils account for 1-4% (100-400) of all leukocytes. Their most important role is the killing of parasitic worms, such as flatworms and tapeworms. Such parasites are too large for phagocytosis and thus cannot be harmed by neutrophils. Eosinophils gather around these worms and digest them away, effectively killing them. Therefore, an increased eosinophil count is usually indicative of some type of parasitic infestation. However, eosinophils also have the secondary function of inactivating certain inflammatory chemicals released during allergic reactions and are involved in the phagocytosis of foreign proteins and immune complexes involved in allergy attacks.

Basophils are the rarest of all leukocytes and comprise only 0.5% (20-50) of all WBCs. Basophils contain histamine which is released during the inflammatory process. It then acts as a vasodilator so as to increase diapedesis to the affected site and as a chemotactic agent to attract other leukocytes to the inflamed tissue. Mast cells are sometimes referred to as tissue basophils. Mast cells reside in connective tissue and, like basophils, release histamine.

Monocytes are agranulocytic cells and derive from the myeloid stem cell. Their prominence lies at about 4-8% (100-700) and, with an average diameter of $18 : m^3$, they are the largest of the leukocytes. Once the monocytes have migrated into the tissue, they differentiate into highly mobile macrophages with insatiable appetites. As such, they protect the body from chronic infections, such as tuberculosis, and are crucial in the body's defense against viruses and certain intracellular bacterial parasites. As mentioned above, monocytes are also important in the activation of lymphocytes through the release of CSFs.

Lymphocytes are, like monocytes, agranulocytic. However, unlike monocytes, lymphocytes derive from the lymphoid stem cell. The term "lymphocyte" stems from the

---

[4] Chemotaxis refers to the movement of additional white blood cells to an area of inflammation in response to the release of chemical mediators by neutrophils, monocytes, and injured tissues.

[5] Phagocytes are cells that have the ability to ingest and destroy particulate substances such as bacteria, protozoa, cells and cell debris, dust particles, and colloids by ingesting them. The ingestion process is called phagocytosis.

fact that most lymphoid cells reside in the lymphoid tissues, such as the lymph nodes and the spleen. Only a small number circulate in the blood stream. In terms of a percentage of the entire leukocyte count, they make up about 20-40% (1500-3000). Lymphocytes are divided into two main categories: T-lymphocytes and B-lymphocytes. T-cells are responsible for the cell-mediated immune response and are commonly classified into three major populations: effector cells, also called cytotoxic cells, and two types of regulatory cells, helper and suppressor T-cells. A newer classification of T-cells is based on their membrane glycoprotein (such as CD4 or CD8).

B-cells are responsible for the humoral immune response. If an antigen encounters an intact B-cell, antibodies are produced against that particular antigen. Such antibodies then bind to the antigen, forming immune complexes and marking the cell for destruction by other immune cells.

Platelets[6]

The last of the formed elements are the platelets. They, like all other blood cells, arise from the hemocytoblast. Platelets are not cells in a strict sense. Rather, they are cytoplasmic fragments of the extraordinarily large megakaryocytes. Megakaryocytes become as large as they are by not undergoing cytokinesis[7] when they undergo mitosis. Once the cell has reached the megakaryocytic stage, thousands of compartments are formed by invaginating membranes. When the cell then ruptures, the membranes seal around the cytoplasm and form the platelets. Each milliliter of blood contains between 250,000-500,000 platelets. Their formation, similar to the formation of the other formed elements, is regulated by a hormone called thrombopoietin

Platelets are essential for the clotting process that occurs in plasma when blood vessels rupture or their lining is injured. By forming a plug that temporarily seals the break in the vessel wall, platelets play a central role in the hemostatic process. Therefore, a decrease in their number is a frequent cause of severe and spontaneous bleeding. Furthermore, upon activation, platelets release such potent chemicals as thromboxane A_2 (which causes the platelets to degranulate), serotonin (which enhances vascular spasms), and adenosine diphosphate (ADP, a potent aggregating and platelet degranulating agent) and are thus an integral part of the clotting cascade.

---

6   In old times, platelets were referred to as thrombocytes. Thrombocyte is a compound term of thrombo- and -cyte. Thrombo stems from the Greek word *thrombos* which means clot. Cyte again comes from *kytos*, cell. Thus, platelets are named according to their function of being cells which clot blood.

7   Cytokinesis refers to the separation of the cytoplasm into two parts; this occurs during the latter stages of mitosis or cell division.

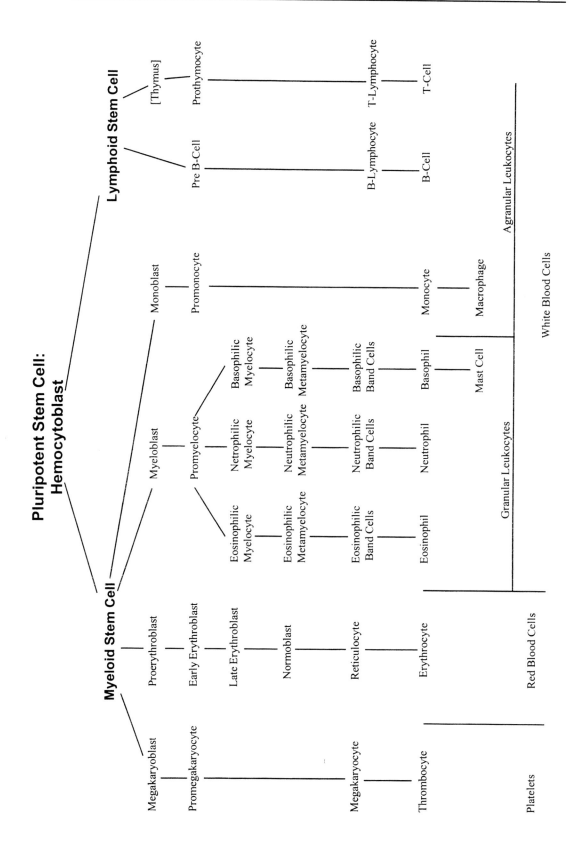

Summary of Formed Elements of the Blood

Cell Type	Description	Number of cells/mm³ (: l) of blood	Duration of development (D) and life span (LS)	Function
Erythrocytes (red blood cells; RBCs)	Biconcave, anucleate disc: salmon-colored; diameter 7-8 : m	4-6 million	**D**: 5-7 days **LS**: 100-120 days	Transport oxygen and carbon dioxide
Leukocytes (white blood cells; WBCs)	Spherical, nucleated cells	4000 - 11,000		
Granulocytes • Neutrophil	Nucleus multilobed; inconspicuous cytoplasmic granules; diameter 10-14 : m	3000 -7000	**D**: 6-9 days **LS**: 6 hrs. to a few days	Phagocytize bacteria
• Eosinophil	Nucleus bilobed; red cytoplasmic granules; diameter 10-14 : m	100-400	**D**: 6-9 days **LS**: 8-12 days	Kill parasitic worms; destroy antigen-antibody complexes; inactivate some inflammatory chemicals of allergy
• Basophil	Nucleus lobed; large blue-purple cytoplasmic granules; diameter 10-12 : m	20-50	**D**: 3-7 days **LS**: ? (a few hours to a few days)	Release histamine and other mediators of inflammation
Agranulocytes • Lymphocyte	Nucleus spherical or indented; pale blue cytoplasm; diameter 5-17 : m	1500-3000	**D**: days to weeks **LS**: hours to years	Mount immune response by direct cell attack or via antibodies
• Monocyte	Nucleus U- or kidney-shaped; gray-blue cytoplasm; diameter 14-24 : m	100-700	**D**: 2-3 days **LS**: months	Phagocytosis; develop into macrophages in tissues
Platelets	Discoid cytoplasmic fragments containing granules; stain deep purple; diameter 2-4 : m	250,000 - 500,000	**D**: 4-5 days **LS**: 5-10 days	Seal small tears in blood vessels; instrumental in blood clotting

Pathology of the blood

Taxonomy

Most hematological disease names state the basic underlying pathology of the condition. Hence, understanding the key terms used in the description of hemopathology is the first step in understanding hematological diseases. The suffix *-penia* means "to lack." Hence, all disease names ending in *-penia*, such as thrombocyto*penia*, neutro*penia*, and leuko*penia*, refer to a lack in the type of cell which precedes the suffix *-penia*. Leukopenia, for example, stands for a lack in *leuko*cytes, *i.e.*, reduced numbers of white blood cells.

The suffix *-penia* must not be confused with the suffix *-emia*, which is present in such common diseases as an*emia* and leuk*emia*. *Emia* is derived from the Greek word *haima* which means blood. In anemia, preceding the word for blood, is the prefix *an-* which is the Greek word for "not." Anemia, therefore, means "no blood" or "not [enough] blood." Leukemia, on the other hand, is composed of the two Greek words *leukos*, white, and *haima*, blood. Therefore, it literally means "white blood," accurately describing the pathological change in leukemia of an explosive increase in white blood cells.

The third most common word in hematological diseases is *purpura*. *Purpura* means "purple" in Latin and is used to describe the purple discoloration caused by bleeding into membranes or subcutaneous tissues. One other important suffix to know is *-osis* which stands for "condition." Hence, thrombocytosis means a condition of thrombocytes and is synonymous to thrombocythemia which means platelet blood, *i.e.*, an excess amount of platelets.

Thus, understanding the key terms *-penia*, *haima*, and *purpura* and combining them with the terms discussed above, such as erythrocytes, leukocyte, and thrombocyte, immediately identifies the basic underlying pathology of blood diseases. For example, the complex term idiopathic thrombocytopenic purpura suddenly starts to have a very clear meaning: idiopathic (no clear cause) thrombocyte (platelet), -penia (lack), purpura (bleeding into membranes and subcutaneous tissues), *i.e.*, a lack of platelets without a clear pathological cause leading to bleeding into membranes and subcutaneous tissues.

Nosology

Hematological diseases can be classified according to erythrocyte disorders, leukocyte disorders, and disorders of hemostasis. This, however, is not the only classification system. Often, these diseases are classified according to functional disorders of the blood and lymphoid organs, neoplastic disorders of the blood and lymphoid organs, and disorders of hemostasis. The first system of classification is employed in the following discussion.

Erythrocyte disorders include a lack of erythrocytes (anemias) and excessive erythrocytes (polycythemia or erythrocytosis). The disorder group "anemia" includes a wide variety of anemias due to very different causes. These causes are addressed in the chapter on anemias in Book II. Contrary to the many varieties of disorders due to a lack of erythrocytes, an excessive amount of erythrocytes, erythrocytosis, only encompasses one main disease, polycythemia vera. Other erythrocytosis conditions may be due to a decreased plasma volume (relative erythrocytosis) or arterial hypoxia leading to an increased production of erythrocytes (secondary erythrocytosis). Polycythemia vera is characterized by an excessive proliferation of erythrocytes and other progenitor cells leading to excessive erythrocytes and an increased hematocrit. Thus, polycythemia may also be classified as a myeloproliferative syndrome and falls into the classification category of neoplastic disorders of the blood and lymphoid organs.

Leukocyte disorders are best divided into two further categories along the lines of the second classification system proposed above: nonmalignant disorders and malignant disorders. Nonmalignant disorders include conditions in which there is either an increased or decreased white blood cell count that is not due to a malignant transformation of a leukocyte progenitor. Such diseases discussed in this book are eosinophilia, infectious mononucleosis, and leukopenia. Malignant disorders of leukocytes include the leukemias and lymphomas which are discussed in more detail in Book II.

Disorders of hemostasis can be divided into three types: 1) platelet disorders, either qualitative or quantitative, 2) coagulation disorders, and 3) vascular disorders. The platelet disorders which are discussed in this text are idiopathic thrombocytopenic purpura (ITP), primary thrombocythemia, and allergic purpura, all quantitative platelet disorders of different pathological origins. Disorders of coagulation describe conditions due to a pathological change in the complicated and extensive coagulation pathway. This text only discusses the coagulative disorder hemophilia. Lastly, the hemostatic disorder of vascular origin discussed in this text is purpura simplex, also called senile purpura.

The following table lists the diseases discussed in this book according to which category of basic pathology they belong. Book II explains the pathology of these individual diseases in greater detail.

Disorders of Erythrocytes (RBCs)		Disorders of Leukocytes (WBCs)		Hemostatic Disorders	
Pathology	Disease	Pathology	Disease	Pathology	Disease
Decrease of RBCs	Anemia	Nonmalignant increase of WBCs	Eosinophilia Infectious Mononucleosis	Quantitative platelet disorder	ITP Primary Thrombo-cythemia Allergic Purpura
Increase of RBCs	Poly-cythemia Vera	Nonmalignant decrease of WBCs	Leukopenia	Coagulation disorder	Hemophilia
		Malignant disorder of WBCs	Leukemias Lymphomas	Vascular disorder	Purpura Simplex

The Western medical diagnosis of blood diseases

Modern biomedical medicine relies almost exclusively on testing to establish its diagnoses. This is no different in hematology. As a matter of fact, because blood is composed of microscopic particles and abnormalities have their origin at such microscopic levels, this is particularly true for blood diseases. Clinical symptoms are always analyzed in conjunction with laboratory test results to determine the disease at hand.

The two most important laboratory examinations are blood examinations and bone marrow examinations, and most blood diseases can be diagnosed by analyzing the results of these two tests. Therefore, below is a summary of the most commonly employed tests in hematology, their explanation, reference values, and possibly critical values.

Bleeding time test

The bleeding time test evaluates the functioning of the vascular and platelet factors associated with hemostasis. Under normal circumstances, after the vascular wall has been injured, the microvessels contract spastically and platelets begin to adhere to the wall of the vessel to plug the hole. An abnormality in either process leads to a prolonged bleeding time.

For this exam, a small, standard superficial incision is made in the forearm, and the time required for the bleeding to stop is recorded. This is referred to as the bleeding time. The most commonly used method is the Ivy bleeding time test.

Reference values: 1-9 minutes (Ivy method)

Possibly critical values: > 12 minutes

Prolonged values occur in the following:

Thrombocytopenia (decreased platelet count), prolonged prothrombin times, disseminated intravascular coagulation (DIC) with consumption of platelets, uremia, coumadin overdose, increased capillary fragility, and ingestion of anti-inflammatory drugs (aspirin).

Blood smear (peripheral blood smear)

During a blood smear test, all three hematologic cell lines (WBCs, RBCs, and platelets) can be examined as to their shape, size, quantity, etc. A smear of peripheral blood is the most informative of all blood tests.

- **RBC size**

    RBC size is used as one of the classification systems of anemias and helps in determining the causes of the anemia.

    Microcytes (small RBC): Iron deficiency, thalassemia, hereditary spherocytosis

    Macrocytes (large RBC): Vitamin B_{12} or folic acid deficiency, reticulocytosis secondary to increased RBC production (erythropoiesis), liver disorders, post-splenectomy anemia

- **RBC shape**

    RBCs are normally shaped like donuts. If they are small and round, they are called spherocytes. If they are crescent or sickle shaped, they are referred to as elliptocytes, and if they are thin and contain less hemoglobin, they are referred to as leptocytes.

- **RBC color**

    Pale (hypochromic) RBCs are indicative of iron deficiency anemia, thalassemia, or cardiac disease. Abnormally colored (hyperchromic) RBCs are commonly due to an increase in hemoglobin concentration which is often caused by dehydration.

- **RBC intercellular structure**

    Normal RBCs do not have a nucleus. If a nucleus is present in RBCs (such RBCs are referred to as normoblasts), increased RBC production is the common cause. Increased RBC production is normal in infants, may be a physiologic reaction of either RBC deficiency (such as in hemolytic anemia, sickle cell crisis, etc.), or hypoxemia (congenital heart disease, congestive heart failure) or may be due to a neoplastic change of the marrow (leukemia).

- **Howell-Jolly bodies**

    These are small and round remnants of nuclear material within the red blood cell. Such nuclear remnants occur after splenectomies and in hemolytic and megaloblastic anemia.

• Heinz bodies

These are small, irregular particles of hemoglobin within the red blood cell. Heinz bodies can be found in such disorders as drug-induced RBC injury, hemoglobinopathies, and hemolytic anemia.

• White blood cells

WBCs are examined for total quantity, differential count, and degree of maturity. An increased number of immature WBCs may indicate leukemia. A decreased WBC count indicates failure of the marrow to produce WBCs, often caused by drugs or due to chronic diseases, neoplasia, or fibrosis of the marrow.

• Platelets

Platelet numbers may be estimated from blood smears by experienced examiners. A decrease in platelet count leads to abnormal coagulation with bleeding diathesis.

Bone marrow biopsy (bone marrow aspiration, bone marrow examination)

Bone marrow biopsy is a microscopic examination of the bone marrow tissue. The bone marrow is the origin of hemopoiesis and an active production along the erythroid, myeloid, and lymphoid cell lines as well as megakaryocyte (platelet) production constitutes a normal finding. The value of bone marrow biopsies/aspirations is that the entire evolution/maturation process of white and red blood cells and platelets can be followed and examined. Generally, a biopsy is preferred to aspiration because it is more accurate.

The following abnormalities are noted:

1) Increased numbers of leukocyte precursors: leukemia or leukemoid drug reaction

2) Decreased numbers of leukocyte precursors: myelofibrosis (fibrosis of the marrow), metastatic neoplasia, agranulocytosis, or sequelae of radiation or chemotherapy. Elderly patients may also manifest with a decreased number of leukocyte precursors.

3) Increased numbers of RBC precursors: polycythemia vera, physiological compensation in hemorrhagic or hemolytic anemia
4) Decreased numbers of RBC precursors: erythroid hypoplasia secondary to chemotherapy, radiation therapy, or administration of other toxic drugs, iron deficiency, marrow replacement by fibrotic tissue or neoplasms

5) Increased numbers of platelet precursors (megakaryocytes): follows acute hemorrhage or some form of chronic myeloid leukemia. This may also occur as a

compensatory mechanism secondary to hypersplenism associated with portal hypertension or other conditions.

6) Decreased megakaryocytes: secondary to radiation therapy, chemotherapy, or other drug therapy; neoplastic or fibrotic marrow infiltrative diseases; aplastic diseases

7) Increased numbers of lymphocyte precursors: chronic infections, viral infections (mononucleosis), lymphocytic leukemia, lymphoma

8) Increased plasma cells (plasmocytes): multiple myelomas, Hodgkin's disease, hypersensitivity states, rheumatic fever, other chronic inflammatory diseases

9) Myeloid to erythroid ratio: the normal ratio of white blood cells (myeloid, M) to red blood cells (erythroid, E) is 3:1. In diseases such as the one listed above, this ratio may change. If the M:E ratio is greater than normal, increased leukocyte precursors are present (leukemia) or erythroid precursors are decreased (erythroid hypoplasia, etc.). If the M:E ratio is below normal, leukocyte precursors are decreased (myelofibrosis, etc.) or erythroid precursors are increased (polycythemia vera, etc.).

A bone marrow biopsy can also determine myelofibrosis (fibrosis of the bone marrow) which usually originates idiopathically or secondary to a drug reaction.

Coagulation factors concentration

This test measures the concentration of specific coagulation factors in the blood. The following factors can be detected: I (fibrinogen), II (prothrombin), V (proaccelerin), VII (proconvertin stable factor), VIII (antihemophilic factor), IX (Christmas factor), X (Stuart factor), XI (plasma thromboplastin antecedent), XII (Hageman factor). The following table lists the conditions that may result in coagulation factor deficiencies:

Condition	Diminished factors
Liver disease	I, II, V, VII, IX, X, XI
Disseminated intravascular coagulation (DIC)	I, V, VIII
Fibrinolysis	I, V, VIII
Congenital deficiency	I, II, V, VII, VIII, IX, X, XI, XII
Heparin administration	II
Warfarin ingestion	II, VII, IX, X, XI
Autoimmune disease	VIII
Vitamin K deficiency or maldigestion	II, VII, IX, X, XI

Complete blood count (CBC)

The CBC is a series of tests of the peripheral blood which provides a tremendous amount of information about the hematologic as well as many other organ systems. The CBC consists of these following tests, all of which will be explained later: red blood cell count, hemoglobin, hematocrit, red blood cell indices, white blood cell count, blood smear, and platelet count.

Folic acid

Folic acid is a B vitamin essential for the proper synthesis of DNA precursors as well as normal functioning of red and white blood cells. Normal levels of folic acid are 5-20mg/mL or 14-34mmol/L.

Decreased levels of folic acid are seen in patients with folic acid deficiency anemia (megaloblastic anemia), hemolytic anemia, malnutrition, malabsorption syndrome, malignancy, liver disease, sprue, and celiac disease. Furthermore, certain drugs, such as anticonvulsants, alcohol, aminopterin, and methotrexate are antagonistic to folic acid.

Elevated levels of folic acid are seen in patients with pernicious anemia.

The folic acid test is often combined with the test for Vitamin B_{12} (folate) and commonly performed on alcoholics to check on their nutritional status.

Glucose-6-phosphate dehydrogenase (G-6-PD)

Glucose-6-phosphate dehydrogenase (G-6-PD) is an enzyme essential in glucose metabolism. In red blood cells, a deficiency of G-6-PD leads to hemoglobin precipitation with changes in the cellular membrane. Such changes may cause hemolysis of varied severity. The disease of G-6-PD deficiency is a sex-linked recessive trait carried on the x chromosome. Two varieties of this disease are noted: the Mediterranean variety (affecting the Sephardic Jews) and a type A variety (affecting the black population). Hemolytic episodes in both varieties are usually elicited by drugs, infections, acidosis, stress, or certain foods (such as fava beans).

Normally, the screening test is negative; sometimes 8.0-8.6 U/g of hemoglobin is present.

Hematocrit (Hct)

The hematocrit is a measure of the percentage of hemoglobin of the total blood volume. Abnormal values go along with pathologies in RBC count and Hgb concentration and indicate an abnormality of the erythrocyte system.

Normal findings:

Male: 42-52%   **Female:** 37- 47% (during pregnancy, > 33%)

In the elderly, values may be slightly decreased

Child: 31-43%   **Infant:** 30-40%   **Newborn:** 44-64%

Hemoglobin (Hgb)

The hemoglobin concentration is a measure of the total amount of hemoglobin in the peripheral blood. As explained in greater detail previously, hemoglobin serves as the vehicle to transport oxygen from the lungs to the tissues and carbon dioxide from the tissues to the lungs. Hemoglobin levels are closely linked to the red blood cell count as well as the hematocrit volume. However, as blood volume may expand through dilution, hemoglobin levels stay constant and thus decrease in dilutional overhydration and increase in dehydration.

Normal hemoglobin values:

Male: 14-18g/dL   **Female:** 12-16g/dL (pregnancy, > 11g/dL)

In the elderly, values may be slightly decreased

Child: 11-16g/dL   **Infant:** 10-15g/dL   **Newborn:** 14-24g/dL

A hemoglobin value less than 5.0 g/dL reflects a possibly critical condition.

Iron level (Fe) & total iron binding capacity (TIBC)

Iron enters the body through food, is absorbed in the small intestine, and is then transported to the plasma. There, it binds with a globulin protein called transferrin and is carried to the bone marrow for incorporation into hemoglobin. The serum iron level is a measurement of the quantity of iron bound to transferrin. The transferrin saturation is the percentage of transferrin still available for the transport of iron. Therefore, the total iron binding capacity is inversely proportional to the transferrin saturation. This relationship can be expressed as follows:

$$\text{transferrin saturation (\%)} = \frac{\text{serum iron level}}{\text{TIBC}} \times 100\%$$

In iron deficiency, serum iron levels are decreased, TIBC increased, and transferrin saturation, therefore, is low. These values are often accompanied by other red blood cell abnormalities, such as microcytic and hypochromic RBCs.

In chronic illness (*e.g.*, infections, neoplasia, and cirrhosis), both serum iron levels and TIBC are decreased and transferrin saturation is, therefore, normal.

During pregnancy, protein levels are high, including transferrin. Because iron requirements are also high, serum iron levels are commonly low, TIBC is high, and transferrin saturation is, therefore, low.

In increased iron intake or increased iron absorption (such as in hemochromatosis), serum iron levels are high, TIBC is stable, and the transferrin saturation is thus very high.

Iron levels vary widely during the course of the day. TIBC, on the other hand, remains relatively stable and the TIBC levels are more a reflection of the liver function (as the liver produces transferrin) and nutrition than of iron metabolism.

Mean platelet volume (MPV)

The mean platelet volume measures the volume of a large amount of platelets. MPV for platelets corresponds to mean corpuscular volume (MCV) for red blood cells (see below).

MPV is a very useful indicator to differentiate the underlying cause of thrombocytopenia. The MPV is large if a decreased platelet count is not due to a problem with the bone marrow. Platelets in this instance are larger because the marrow tries to compensate for the low platelet count and releases younger and larger platelets into the blood circulation. If, however, the marrow function of megakaryocyte production is abnormal (such as in aplastic anemia or chemotherapy-induced myelosuppression), the platelets are small and therefore the MPV is decreased. The normal MPV is $25 : m^3$ in diameter.

Platelet count

The platelet count test is an actual count of the number of platelets (thrombocytes) per cubic millimeter (mm) of blood. A decreased count is termed thrombocytopenia, whereas an increased platelet count is termed thrombocytosis. Because platelet activity is essential to blood clotting, thrombocytopenia leads to prolonged or even spontaneous bleeding, while thrombocytosis leads to vascular thrombosis with subsequent organ infarction.

Normal platelet counts:

Adult: $150,000\text{-}400,000/mm^3$ **Premature infant:** $100,000\text{-}300,000/mm^3$

Newborn: $150,000\text{-}300,000/mm^3$ **Infant:** $200,000\text{-}475,000/mm^3$

Child: $150,000\text{-}400,000/mm^3$

Counts below $100,000/mm^3$ are considered indicative of thrombocytopenia, while counts above $400,000/mm^3$ are considered indicative of thrombocytosis. Spontaneous bleeding rarely occurs as long as platelet counts are above $40,000/mm^3$ but becomes a serious danger when platelet counts fall below 20,000/mm^3. A platelet count above one million/mm^3 is a critical value for severe thrombocytosis.

Reasons for thrombocytopenia are the following:

1) Reduced production of platelets (secondary to bone marrow failure or infiltration by fibrosis, tumor, etc.)

2) Sequestration of platelets (secondary to hypersplenism)

3) Accelerated destruction of platelets (secondary to antibodies, infections, drugs, prosthetic heart valves, etc.)

4) Consumption of platelets (secondary to disseminated intravascular coagulation)

5) Platelet loss through hemorrhage

Thrombocytosis may occur as a compensatory response to severe hemorrhage. Polycythemia vera, leukemia, postsplenectomy syndromes, and various malignant disorders may also be the cause of thrombocytosis.

RBC count

This test counts the circulating red blood cells in one cubic millimeter of peripheral venous blood.

Normal findings:

Adult/elderly: Male: 4.7-6.1 million/mm^3 **Female:** 4.2-5.4 million/mm^3

Infant/child: 3.8-5.5 million/mm^3 **Newborn:** 4.8-7.1 million/mm^3

A decrease in the RBC values more than 10% of the expected normal value leads to the classification of anemia. Low RBC values are caused by hemorrhage, hemolysis, dietary deficiencies, genetic aberration, drugs, marrow fibrosis, chronic illnesses, and renal disease.

An increase in the RBC count may be a physiological response to the body's increased requirement for greater oxygen carrying capacity (high altitude) or a response to a pathologic anoxia (congenital heart disease). However, an increase in the RBC count may also be due to polycythemia vera.

Reticulocyte count

The reticulocyte count test determines bone marrow function and evaluates erythropoietic activity and is a useful test to identify anemias. A reticulocyte is an immature red blood cell, and the reticulocyte count represents a direct measurement of the RBC production by the bone marrow.

Normal findings:

  Adult/elderly/child: 0.5-2%   **Infant:** 0.5-3.1%   **Newborn:** 2.5-6.5%

Pregnancy may cause an increased reticulocyte count.

An increased reticulocyte count indicates the expected compensatory response in anemic patients. A decreased reticulocyte count in anemic patients indicates an inadequate marrow production of RBCs (as in aplastic anemia, iron deficiency, vitamin B_{12} deficiency, etc.). If the reticulocyte count is elevated in patients with normal hemograms, the increased production compensates for hemolysis or hemorrhage.

Reticulocyte index

The reticulocyte index can be calculated as follows:

Reticulocyte index = Reticulocyte count (in %) × Patient's hematocrit/Normal hematocrit

This index determines if the increased reticulocyte count indicates adequate erythropoiesis in patients with anemia and decreased hematocrit.

In a patient with good marrow response to anemia, the reticulocyte index should be 1.0. If it is below 1.0, even though the reticulocyte count is elevated in the patient, the test indicates that the bone marrow response is inadequate to compensate for the anemia (as in iron deficiency, vitamin B_{12} deficiency, or marrow failure).

White blood cell count & differential count

This test has two components. First, the white blood cell count represents the total number of WBCs in one cubic millimeter of peripheral venous blood. Second, the differential count measures the percentage of each type of leukocyte present in the specimen.

Normal findings for both components:

WBC count:

  Adult/child >2 years: 5000-10,000/mm^3

  Child 2 years: 6200-17,000/mm^3 **Newborn:** 9000-30,000/mm^3

Differential count:

  Neutrophils: 55-70%   **Lymphocytes:** 20-40%

  Monocytes: 2-8%   **Eosinophils:** 1-4%   **Basophils:** 0.5-1.0%

An increased total WBC count (leukocytosis) usually indicates infection, inflammation, tissue necrosis, or leukemic neoplasia. Emotional or physical trauma and stress may also increase the WBC count.

A decreased total WBC count (leukopenia) occurs in many forms of bone marrow failure (*i.e.*, following antineoplastic chemotherapy or radiation therapy, marrow infiltrative diseases), overwhelming infections, dietary deficiencies, and autoimmune diseases.

Different types of leukocytes fight different intruders into the body, or different non-selves. An analysis of the abnormalities of the differential diagnosis helps to identify the cause of the abnormality.

The primary function of polymorphonuclear leukocytes (PMLs) or neutrophils is phagocytosis. Thus, acute bacterial infections and trauma stimulate neutrophil production, resulting in an overall increased WBC count with an increased neutrophil count. Neutrophils are also increased in myelocytic leukemia. When neutrophil production is stimulated, the marrow often releases early immature forms of neutrophils into the circulation. These immature forms are called band cells or stab cells, and this process is referred to as a "shift to the left," indicative of an on-going acute bacterial infection.

Lymphocytes can be divided into two types: T-cells and B-cells. Their primary function is to fight chronic bacterial infections and acute viral infections. Lymphocytes are, of course, also increased in lymphocytic leukemia. Note that the differential count does not separate the B and T-cells but rather counts the combination of the two.

Monocytes are similar to neutrophils; they are phagocytes and fight bacteria. However, monocytes are produced more rapidly and can stay in the circulation for a longer period of time than neutrophils. Monocyte levels above the usual 2-8% are indicative of chronic inflammatory disorders, viral infections, tuberculosis, etc.

Basophils and eosinophils are involved in allergic and parasitic reactions. Thus, an increase of eosinophils is indicative of either parasitic infestations, allergic reactions, or eczema. An increase of basophils usually is part of a myeloproliferative disease or leukemia. A decrease of basophils, however, is indicative of acute allergic reactions, stress reactions, or hypothyroidism.

The Western medical treatment of blood diseases

The Western medical treatment of hematological diseases is based upon the underlying pathology. In anemias, this may vary widely. For iron deficiency anemia, for example, iron supplementation is the treatment of choice. However, as explained below in the chapter on iron deficiency anemia, this may not always lead to ideal treatment results since iron absorption in the intestines is just as important as iron intake. For anemias in which an immunologic component is suspected in the pathology, such as in aplastic anemia and certain types of hemolytic anemias, immunosuppressive drugs are commonly used. However, since such immunosuppressive drugs, mostly steroids, are not selective as to which parts of the immune system they suppress, a lowered immunity with a greater chance for infections as well as the negative side effects of steroid therapy have to be expected.

Leukemias are malignancies of white blood cell progenitors and are commonly treated by chemotherapy or radiation therapy. Again, these therapies are not selective and kill even healthy marrow cells. Side effects of such treatments are manifold as pointed out in the section on Chinese medicine and chemotherapy in the chapter on leukemias. Furthermore, such aggressive treatment is not always warranted. Some chronic leukemias, for example, should not be treated with antineoplastic drugs since such treatment does not prolong survival but may be associated with considerable side effects. Similarly, myelosuppressive drugs in polycythemia vera may lead to leukemic transformations of the disease.

Because the white blood cells are the human body's defensive system, a disorder in their production or functioning makes the body much more susceptible to invading pathogens such as viruses, bacteria, and fungi. Therefore, antibiotics are also frequently used in the treatment of hematologic diseases in which the immune system has been affected.

Two other treatments that deserve mention are blood transfusions and bone marrow transplantations. Blood transfusions can provide patients with hemoglobin to carry oxygen as well as platelets to prevent bleeding. Therefore, in severe cases of anemia or thrombocytopenia, transfusions may be a viable, but short-lived, alternative treatment that can save the patient's life.

For diseases whose pathologic abnormality lies at the level of the stem cells, bone marrow transplantation is a possible alternative. Aplastic anemia and certain types of leukemia are both examples of diseases considered for bone marrow transplantation.

Lastly, certain diseases, such as myelodysplastic syndrome and paroxysmal nocturnal hemoglobinuria, do not respond to any current treatment protocol and treatment is still experimental. However, new research is proceeding at incredible speed, and new treatments for some of the diseases listed in this book may appear soon. For instance, this is the case with retinoic acid. Found to be helpful in cell division in a Shanghai hospital in the 1980s, it will most probably soon be a standard in the treatment of acute promyelocytic leukemia.

Having said all this, the treatment of most hematologic diseases with biomedical medicine is less than optimal. Side effects of steroids, antineoplastics, and antibiotics as well as the sometimes poor treatment effects of even the strongest biomedical drugs certainly calls for additional treatment methods. Chinese medicinal therapy presents an effective method of reducing these side effects and enhancing the treatment effects.

2
Chinese Medicinals in the Treatment of Blood Diseases

According to Chinese standards, acupuncture plays a minimal role in the treatment of blood diseases. The standard of care for blood diseases in the People's Republic of China is to administer individually prescribed Chinese medicinals. Therefore, a wide variety of Chinese medicinal formulas are listed in Book II. No dosage amounts are listed for any of the ingredients in these formulas. This is because Chinese formulas need to be tailored to fit each individual patients' needs. Formulas taken from books with ingredient amounts almost never exactly fit a real-life patient's pattern(s). Just as medicinals need to be added and subtracted, dosages must be increased and decreased. This requires an in-depth knowledge of individual Chinese medicinals. Basic information on individual Chinese medicinals, including usual dosage parameters, may be found in Bensky and Gamble's *Chinese Herbal Medicine: Materia Medica* and Hong-yen Hsu's *Oriental Materia Medica: A Concise Guide.*

However, when treating any of the diseases within any of the Chinese medical specialties, it is extremely helpful to know certain facts about medicinals and medicinal combinations which are not commonly known in the West and are not commonly included in the English language materia medica. This also applies to the specialty of hematology. Therefore, prior to studying and applying the medicinal formulas listed in Book II, the reader will benefit by studying the information in this chapter. This will help the practitioner to better understand the compositions and overall functions of formulas applicable in blood diseases and this, in turn, will increase the effectiveness with which such formulas can be modified.

Commonly used & efficacious medicinals for blood diseases

The medicinals listed below have all been shown, through experience, clinical studies, or biomedical research, to be of particular efficacy in the treatment of blood diseases. They are also the most commonly used medicinals in the formulas listed in Book II. The information about these medicinals' functions specifically pertaining to blood diseases comes exclusively from the Chinese literature. It is a compilation of material that I obtained while researching this work. However, the following medicinal descriptions are specific to various blood diseases and are not all-inclusive. Furthermore, some statements are purely empirical opinions of Chinese physicians and may conflict with other information available. Nevertheless, since only the opinions of *lao yi sheng* (old, *i.e.*, experienced, doctors) were considered in creating this book, I believe such claims must have at least some validity.

Supplementing medicinals

Supplementing medicinals are prescribed if the body suffers from a vacuity of qi, blood, yin, or yang. Below, the most effective medicinals for vacuity pattern hematological diseases are listed with an explanation of their functions pertaining to such diseases. Preceding the information about the medicinals is a description of the application and importance of the respective treatment principle *vis à vis* blood diseases.

1. Qi-supplementing medicinals

Qi-supplementing medicinals have a wide application in blood diseases. Qi is the commander of blood and has the functions of engendering the blood, quickening the blood, and containing the blood. Based on the saying, "If yang is engendered, yin grows," it is often very effective clinically to administer qi-boosting medicinals combined with yang-warming medicinals. This promotes blood production and is particularly effective in cases where anemia is accompanied by qi vacuity signs, such as in iron deficiency anemia or megaloblastic anemia.

In addition, because blood flow slows down when qi is vacuous, qi-boosting and blood-quickening medicinals can be combined to increase the speed of blood flow and thus improve blood circulation. In the same way that plants can only grow and live when they receive sufficient water, obtaining sufficient blood supply is of absolute importance for the adequate functioning of the viscera and bowels.

Qi vacuity not containing the blood plays a role in patterns of both recurrent chronic purpuras and hemophilia. In these cases, qi-boosting medicinals are combined with bleeding stopping medicinals so as to control bleeding.

Most qi-boosting medicinals have the function of strengthening the immune system. Qi-boosting medicinals fortify the spleen's function of distilling the finest essence qi from water and grain, thereby optimizing qi production. As long as sufficient qi is produced, the righteous qi is full and evils cannot invade. Therefore, in blood diseases where recurring upper respiratory infections are a problem, qi-boosting medicinals must be added to the formula.

Lastly, qi-boosting medicinals not only improve the organism's ability to cope with low tissue oxygen contents, such as in chronic anemias, but also help in coping with chemotherapeutic agents' debilitating effects on the body.

For all of the above reasons, qi-boosting medicinals are very commonly used in the treatment of blood diseases.

• Radix Panacis Ginseng (*Ren Shen*)

Functions:

1) *Ren Shen* promotes blood production and, therefore, increases not only red blood cells but also hemoglobin and white blood cells. As such, it can be used in the treatment of patients undergoing radiation or chemotherapy during which the hemopoietic system is depressed.

2) *Ren Shen* has an "anti-cardiovascular shock" function and elevates blood pressure. It is, therefore, an important medicinal in the treatment of shock due to acute blood loss with a severe drop in blood pressure.

3) *Ren Shen* excites the adrenocortical system and increases adrenocortical output, thereby effectively treating fatigue and insomnia and enhancing the body's immune response.

4) *Ren Shen* lowers blood sugar, regulates blood cholesterol levels, and reduces hypercholesteremia.

Common Clinical Applications:

1) Boosts the qi and engenders the blood: Combined with such medicinals as Rhizoma Atractylodis Macrocephalae (*Bai Zhu*), Sclerotium Poria Cocos (*Fu Ling*), and Radix Glycyrrhizae Uralensis (*Gan Cao*), *Ren Shen* fortifies the spleen and, therefore, provides a source of blood engenderment. Clinically, this combination is the basic formula for the treatment of anemia due to spleen vacuity. If *Ren Shen* is combined with such yang-invigorating and kidney-supplementing medicinals as Cornu Cervi Parvum (*Lu Rong*) and processed Semen Strychnotis (*Ma Qian Zi*), it effectively treats anemia due to a lack of blood engenderment because of kidney vacuity.

2) Supplements the original qi: Because *Ren Shen* strongly supplements the original qi, it can be used to secure desertion and restore the pulse. In the treatment of acute blood loss, this is based on the saying, "in blood desertion, boost the qi," which itself is based

on the saying, "blood has a form and thus cannot be engendered quickly, qi has no form and thus can be secured rapidly." To secure and boost the qi in desertion patterns, *Ren Shen,* administered in the form of *Du Shen Tang* (Solitary Ginseng Decoction), is the best selection.

From a biomedical point of view, besides the blood pressure elevating function of *Ren Shen,* this medicinal also increases oxygen content in the blood and decreases oxygen consumption in the tissues. Thus, the tissues can better cope with a low oxygen content, and the body has the ability to recover from illness and stress with less available oxygen.

3) Increases leukocyte production: Because *Ren Shen* stimulates the hematopoietic system, the leukocyte count increases. This helps patients to endure radiation or chemotherapy with fewer side effects. As a matter of fact, the combination of *Ren Shen* with Radix Astragali Membranacei (*Huang Qi*) and Fructus Psoraleae Corylifoliae (*Bu Gu Zhi*) not only treats leukopenia but also prevents the arisal of other side effects from radiation or chemotherapy.

4) Enhances immunity: Along with the above stated fact that *Ren Shen* increases leukocytes goes the fact that *Ren Shen* also enhances the immune system. In Chinese medical terms, by boosting the qi of the spleen and lungs, the defensive qi becomes full and evils cannot invade. Thus, *Ren Shen* is used in the treatment of hematological diseases to prevent infections and recover the strength of righteous qi based on the saying, "If the righteous qi is vacuous, evils are exuberant."

5) Boosts the qi and quickens the blood: "When the qi moves, the blood moves." If qi is too vacuous to move blood, static blood accumulates. If *Ren Shen* is combined with blood-quickening medicinals, static blood due to qi vacuity can be effectively treated. The fact that *Ren Shen* enhances blood oxygen and decreases tissue oxygen consumption combined with the fact that blood-quickening medicinals improve the microcirculation and, therefore, tissue oxygenation makes this medicinal combination an extremely useful one in the treatment of a wide variety of blood diseases. If blood supply to the viscera is increased, visceral qi is fortified. This boosts the qi, engenders the blood, and dispels lodged evils.

• Radix Codonopsitis Pilosulae (*Dang Shen*)

Dang Shen is very similar to *Ren Shen.* Accordingly, it can be used to boost the qi, engender the blood, and fortify the immune system. However, *Dang Shen* is much weaker than *Ren Shen.* Therefore, in serious cases, the increased cost of using *Ren Shen* is always warranted.

Large amounts of *Dang Shen* combined with Fructus Zizyphi Spinosae (*Da Zao*) and Massa Fermentata (*Shen Qu*) supplement the spleen, boost the qi, and engender the blood. The use of this combination after or during pediatric hematological diseases, for example, has shown an increase in red blood cells and hemoglobin with an improvement of such symptoms as bodily vacuity and fatigue. *Dang Shen* has also been shown effective in the use for anemia secondary to chronic nephritis.

• Radix Astragali Membranacei (*Huang Qi*)

Huang Qi is one of the most powerful qi-boosting medicinals. It is particularly useful to lift sunken qi and to fortify the spleen, thus improving the spleen's function of blood management and upbearing of the clear. The following are *Huang Qi*'s functions most central to the treatment of hematological diseases:

1) Boosts the qi and engenders the blood: *Huang Qi* combined with either *Dang Shen* or *Ren Shen* strongly supplements the qi so as to engender the blood. Thus, this combination is effectively used for anemia presenting with a qi vacuity pattern. Furthermore, by stimulating the entire hemopoietic system, it also increases white blood cell production and can be used to treat leukopenia.

2) Boosts the qi and quickens the blood: If qi is vacuous and blood seeps outside of the vessels and stagnates in the tissues, *Huang Qi* can be combined with blood-quickening medicinals to resolve stasis and boost qi. When blood flows freely, the viscera and bowels can be nourished and moistened and thus recover their optimal functioning. Clinically, this combination is used for such chronic bleeding diseases as chronic thrombocytopenic purpura, protracted allergic purpura, and hemophilia. If kidney-warming medicinals are added to the combination of *Huang Qi* and blood-quickening, stasis-transforming medicinals, microcirculation of the bone marrow can be improved, thereby increasing the blood engenderment function of the bone marrow. This treatment strategy is suitable for such marrow degenerative diseases as hypo- or aplastic anemia.

3) Boosts the qi and supports the righteous: *Huang Qi* can be combined with Radix Albus Paeoniae Lactiflorae (*Bai Shao*) for the treatment of easy contraction of disease evils. Furthermore, if toxic heat evils have assailed the body, *Huang Qi* can be combined with heat-clearing and toxin-resolving medicinals. Clinically, this is applicable in blood diseases with low white blood cell counts accompanied by infections. If the "evil qi" is radiation or chemotherapy and has damaged the bone marrow's proper hemopoiesis, *Huang Qi* combined with Fructus Psoraleae Corylifoliae (*Bu Gu Zhi*) and processed Radix Polygoni Multiflori (*He Shou Wu*) can be used to prevent bone marrow damage. If the pattern is one of righteous vacuity with evil repletion, one can add Rhizoma Polygonati (*Huang Jing*) to the combination of *Huang Qi* and Radix Albus Paeoniae Lactiflorae (*Bai Shao*). This supports the righteous and expels evils.

• Rhizoma Atractylodis Macrocephalae (*Bai Zhu*)

Bai Zhu boosts the qi and fortifies the spleen. Similar to the qi-boosting medicinals above, by boosting the qi, it also engenders the blood. Therefore, it is suitable for all qi vacuity anemia patterns. Furthermore, by regulating the gastrointestinal's peristaltic and secretory functions, it helps patients with digestive problems to absorb most of the consumed nutrients and is thus an especially essential medicinal for patients who suffer from diseases due to malabsorption of food. Megaloblastic anemia and iron deficiency anemia are two examples.

Also similar to the above medicinals, by boosting the qi, it not only supplements the production of red blood cells but also of white blood cells. This helps to fight infections and to endure radiation and chemotherapies better. Clinical trials have shown the combination of *Bai Zhu, Huang Qi,* and *Bai Shao* to be of particular strength and benefit in treating hematological disease patients suffering from recurrent upper respiratory or other infections.

• Radix Pseudostellariae Heterophyllae (*Tai Zi Shen*)

Tai Zi Shen fortifies the spleen, boosts the qi, and supplements the fluids. In relation to blood diseases, this medicinal is of particular importance as it enhances absorption in the small intestine, thus improving the uptake of important nutrients and micronutrients, such as vitamins, iron, zinc and copper. Therefore, *Tai Zi Shen* is especially suitable in the treatment of iron deficiency anemia. Furthermore, *Tai Zi Shen* also stimulates the bone marrow to increase hemopoiesis.

• Radix Glycyrrhizae (*Gan Cao*)

Gan Cao has a wide variety of functions. It is similar to adrenocorticoids and thus has an anti-inflammatory and anti-allergic function. This function makes this medicinal especially applicable in idiopathic thrombocytopenic purpura (ITP), for which it should be used in large quantities. However, also similar to adrenocorticoids, excessive and prolonged use may lead to water retention.

Gan Cao also resolves spasms of smooth muscle, such as the gastrointestinal tract, resolves toxins, settles cough and eliminates phlegm, regulates the proper functioning of the liver and is inhibitory (in vitro) to staphylococci and *E. coli.*

Furthermore, experience has shown that *Gan Cao* is inhibitory to leukemic cancer cells and should, therefore, be included in all formulas for leukemia.

Because *Gan Cao* also supplements the middle and boosts the qi, it is an important ingredient in the treatment of blood diseases due to a weak spleen and a vacuity of qi. By helping with nutrient absorption and peristaltic function, *Gan Cao* effectively treats many malabsorption diseases.

The combination of Pollen Typhae (*Pu Huang*) with *Gan Cao* in a ratio of 1:3 has been shown to reduce symptoms of thrombocytopenia and to increase the platelet count.

Gan Cao has the function of resolving toxins from hundreds of medicinals. Furthermore, regardless of its use in qi-boosting, yin-enriching, yang-warming, heat-clearing, or toxin-resolving formulas, *Gan Cao* supports the formula's overall function. Thus, with due consideration of its function to retain water, it can be included in almost every hematological disease formula.

• Fructus Zizyphi Jujubae (*Da Zao*)

Da Zao contains 13 types of amino acids and 36 different types of micronutrients. Its traditional functions are to boost the qi, engender the blood, calm the sprit, and harmonize harsh properties of other medicinals. It differs from the above qi-boosting medicinals by having a special affinity for blood supplementation. The addition of *Da Zao* to *Si Jun Zi Tang* (Four Gentlemen Decoction), for example, increases that formula's strength of blood engenderment. Thus, *Da Zao* is an effective medicinal in the treatment of anemias related to spleen vacuity, such as megaloblastic anemia and iron deficiency anemia.

Because *Da Zao* aids intestinal nutrient absorption and is itself rich in micronutrients, such as iron, zinc, and copper, it is an important medicinal in the treatment of many types of anemia, particularly if the pattern corresponds to qi and blood dual vacuity.

Da Zao has the function of decreasing vessel permeability and can, therefore, be used for purpuric diseases, such as allergic purpura and purpura simplex. The combination of Lumbricus (*Di Long*), *Gan Cao,* and *Da Zao* has been shown to be particularly effective in the treatment of allergic purpura. The combination of *Da Zao* with Herba Leonuri Heterophylli (*Yi Mu Cao*) is appropriate for purpura simplex.

2. Blood-supplementing medicinals

Blood is the mother of qi. If blood is insufficient, qi becomes vacuous. Clinically, blood transfusions are regarded as the strongest type of blood supplementation. For less severe anemias, blood-supplementing medicinals are indicated. Furthermore, because blood and qi mutually engender each other, blood-supplementing medicinals typically need to be combined with qi-boosting medicinals. "If the qi is vacuous, the blood becomes insufficient; if the blood is depleted, the qi suffers detriment." The mutual supplementation of qi and blood is, therefore, of great importance.

Likewise, "if static blood is not removed, new blood cannot be engendered." Thus, if blood stasis accompanies blood vacuity, blood-quickening medicinals must be added to the blood-supplementing prescription. From a biomedical point of view, blood-quickening and stasis-transforming medicinals improve the microcirculation throughout the body, and improved microcirculation of the bone marrow leads to increased blood production.

The brain requires constant nourishment by the blood for proper development. Long-term anemia in children may lead to a malnourishment of the brain and hence to decreased intelligence. Therefore, blood-supplementing medicinals are important in even mild cases of pediatric anemia.

• Cooked Radix Rehmanniae (*Shu Di*)

Shu Di is the sovereign medicinal in the most important blood-supplementing formula, *Si Wu Tang* (Four Materials Decoction). *Shu Di* nourishes the blood, engenders essence, and enriches yin and is, therefore, an important and basic medicinal for any type of anemia. According to biomedical research, *Shu Di* contains trace elements of iron, zinc, and copper, all important minerals in blood production. In anemias due to spleen vacuity, *Shu Di* is combined with qi-boosting and spleen-fortifying medicinals. In anemias due to a lack of blood engenderment in the bone marrow, such as aplastic anemia, *Shu Di* typically needs to be combined with yang-warming medicinals. If anemias are accompanied by infections, heat-clearing and toxin-resolving medicinals are combined with *Shu Di*. For anemias manifesting a yin vacuity pattern, *Shu Di* can be combined with other yin-enriching and possibly heat-clearing medicinals, such as Tuber Ophiopogonis Japonici (*Mai Dong*), Rhizoma Polygonati (*Huang Jing*), and Rhizoma Anemarrhenae Asphodeloidis (*Zhi Mu*).

Shu Di is a sticky and slimy medicinal and, therefore, easily hinders the movement and transformation function of the middle burner, leading to an accumulation of dampness. Therefore, it should be combined with Radix Auklandiae Lappae (*Mu Xiang*) and Fructus Amomi (*Sha Ren*). Both of these additions rectify the qi and abduct stagnation, thus moderating and reducing *Shu Di*'s slimy, stagnating side effects.

• Radix Polygoni Multiflori (*He Shou Wu*)

He Shou Wu supplements the essence and blood without being slimy and, therefore, can be taken over prolonged periods of time. Besides supplementing, *He Shou Wu* also frees the flow of the stools and downbears turbidity, thereby eliminating waste products. Thus, it is often regarded as a general anti-aging medicinal.

Regarding blood diseases, *He Shou Wu* is particularly effective for treating leukopenia, aplastic anemia, and nephrotic anemia. Biomedical research has shown that *He Shou Wu* is rich in lecithin, an important component of the red blood cell membrane.

For the treatment of leukopenia or agranulocytopenia, *He Shou Wu* is most effective if combined with Radix Salviae Miltiorrhizae (*Dan Shen*) and Radix Rubiae Cordifoliae (*Qian Cao Gen*). *He Shou Wu* combined with Radix Astragali Membranacei (*Huang Qi*), Herba Epimedii (*Xian Ling Pi*), and Semen Cuscutae Chinensis (*Tu Si Zi*) boosts the qi, warms yang, and engenders the blood and is effective in the treatment of aplastic anemia. Nephrotic anemia is secondary to a decrease in hemopoietin secretion due to damaged kidneys. Anemia resulting from this pathology is treated by combining *He Shou Wu* with Radix Et Rhizoma Rhei (*Da Huang*). *Da Huang* has the function of lowering the blood urea nitrogen level and *He Shou Wu* has the function of stimulating blood production.

In Chinese medicine, the head hair is seen as the surplus of the blood. Because *He Shou Wu* strongly supplements the blood, this medicinal can be used to prevent hair loss while undergoing radiation or chemotherapy. For this, *He Shou Wu* should be combined with Fructus Psoraleae Corylifoliae (*Bu Gu Zhi*), Radix Panacis Ginseng (*Hong Shen*), and Radix Angelicae Sinensis (*Dang Gui*).

• Radix Angelicae Sinensis (*Dang Gui*)
Dang Gui is the minister in *Si Wu Tang* and thus, similar to *Shu Di*, is one of the main medicinals in blood supplementation. However, *Dang Gui* differs from *Shu Di* in that it is said to be a qi within the blood medicinal (whereas *Shu Di* is a blood within the blood medicinal). Thus, *Dang Gui* not only supplements the blood but also quickens the blood and moves the qi, thus stopping pain. It is used to supplement blood vacuity, free the flow of static blood, and moisten dry, desiccated blood.

For these reasons, *Dang Gui* is a main medicinal in the treatment of all types of anemia. However, similar to *He Shou Wu*, it needs to be combined with different medicinals depending on the anemia patient's Chinese pattern discrimination. For spleen vacuity anemia, qi-boosting and spleen-fortifying medicinals need to be added. For anemias due to abnormal bone marrow blood production manifesting a kidney vacuity pattern, kidney-supplementing medicinals need to be added. For nephrotic anemia, *Dang Gui* is combined with *Shou Wu* and *Da Huang*. For anemias with concurrent infections, righteous qi-supporting and evil-eliminating medicinals must be added.

Dang Gui can be combined with Bombyx Batryticatus (*Bai Jiang Can*) and Radix Salviae Miltiorrhizae (*Dan Shen*) for the treatment of leukopenia or agranulocytopenia. This combination has the function of increasing the white blood cell count.

Because *Dang Gui* not only supplements but also quickens the blood, it affects platelet function and can be used in the treatment of thrombocytopenic purpura. In this case, it often must be combined with yin-enriching, blood-cooling, bleeding stopping, and stasis-dispelling medicinals for best effects.

• Radix Albus Paeoniae Lactiflorae (*Bai Shao*)

Bai Shao has the functions of supplementing the blood, resolving tetany, supporting the righteous, and eliminating evils. Thus, it is a commonly used medicinal in hematological diseases.

Bai Shao nourishes the blood and constrains yin. It is the assistant ingredient in *Si Wu Tang*. In order to treat blood vacuity signs, such as sallow yellow facial and skin complexion, dizziness, vexation and agitation, and insomnia, it is combined with Radix Angelicae Sinensis (*Dang Gui*), Radix Polygoni Multiflori (*He Shou Wu*), and Fructus Ligustri Lucidi (*Nu Zhen Zi*).

For the treatment of abdominal pain because of gastrointestinal spasms, *Bai Shao* is combined with Radix Auklandiae Lappae (*Mu Xiang*). This combination resolves tetany and stops pain and is effective for abdominal pain secondary to blood diseases. If spasms affect the four limbs, *Bai Shao* is combined with Periostracum Cicadae (*Chan Tui*).

Prolonged diseases damage the righteous qi. If the righteous qi is vacuous, evils can encroach, and, as long as righteous qi is insufficient, evils cannot be expelled. This situation often manifests clinically as recurrent infections, mostly upper respiratory tract infections, in weak patients. This is a commonly encountered complaint in hematological diseases in which the white blood cells are affected. The combination of *Bai Shao* with Radix Astragali Membranacei (*Huang Qi*) is particularly powerful for treating this presentation. *Bai Shao*'s function of supporting the righteous and dispelling evils was first noted in *Zhu Jie Shang Han Lun (Annotations to On Cold Damage)* where it says: "Sourness contracts and drains; thus *Shao Yao*'s sourness contracts yin and drains evil qi." The combination of *Bai Shao* and *Huang Qi* prevents recurrent infections by supporting the righteous and eliminating evils.

• Gelatinum Corii Asini (*E Jiao*)

E Jiao supplements the blood, enriches yin, and stops bleeding. It is, therefore, an important medicinal in a variety of blood diseases but is particularly effective for the following: yin vacuity type anemias, leukopenia, thrombocytopenic purpura, aplastic or hypoplastic anemias, and a wide variety of bleeding diseases.

Because *E Jiao* enriches yin, it is particularly effective in the treatment of yin vacuity pattern anemia. For this purpose, it is commonly combined with cooked Radix Rehmanniae (*Shu Di*) and Radix Polygoni Multiflori (*He Shou Wu*).

If *E Jiao* is combined with Caulis Milletiae Seu Spatholobi (*Ji Xue Teng*) and Fructus Lycii Chinensis (*Gou Qi Zi*), it strongly increases the white blood cell count and can thus be used in the treatment of agranulocytopenia secondary to chemotherapy.

For hypoplastic or aplastic anemia, *E Jiao* needs to be combined with kidney-supplementing and spleen-fortifying medicinals.

Because *E Jiao* has the function of stopping bleeding, it can be combined with blood-cooling and bleeding stopping medicinals for the treatment of a wide variety of bleeding diseases.

As shown above, *E Jiao* strongly supplements blood and yin and is, therefore, thick and heavy in flavor. Its slimy and sticky nature can be detrimental to the digestive function. In case of spleen and stomach vacuity weakness, only a relatively small amount of *E Jiao* should be used. Further, in such cases, *E Jiao* must be combined with stomach-fortifying and qi-rectifying medicinals so as to reduce its side effects.

3. Yang-supplementing medicinals

"If yang extends, yin grows." Thus, in order to engender yin-blood, yang must be sufficient. The treatment principle of warming yang in order to engender blood is of particular importance for all hypoplastic and aplastic anemias. These types of anemias usually manifest as kidney vacuity pattern anemias. Also, modern research has clearly indicated that yang-warming medicinals activate hemopoiesis.

For anemias presenting with spleen vacuity patterns, warming yang may also be of some importance. The spleen relies on kidney yang. If the spleen becomes vacuous, kidney yang warming medicinals supplement and warm not only the kidneys but also the spleen, thus increasing qi and blood engenderment.

It is heart yang which circulates blood throughout the body. If heart yang is vacuous, blood does not move and becomes static. Furthermore, cold has a congealing and constricting nature and thus hinders the free flow of qi and blood. Warming yang is, therefore, also effective and important for treating static blood if such stasis is due to heart yang vacuity or cold congelation. Heart yang vacuity often manifests with a bound or irregularly interrupted pulse. Warming heart yang and boosting heart qi promotes the blood circulation and thus increases blood supply to all organs. This, in turn, benefits the organ functions.

Because yin and yang are rooted in each other and engender each other, warming yang is often combined with enriching yin. This combination treats the source yin and source yang of the body and is applicable in natural endowment insufficiencies, such as slow development.

• Cornu Parvum Cervi (*Lu Rong*)

Lu Rong supplements the kidneys and boosts the essence, supplements the marrow and engenders blood, and strengthens the sinews and fortifies the bone. *Lu Rong* is, therefore, one of the main medicinals in the treatment of hypo- or aplastic anemias. The combination of *Lu Rong* with Radix Panacis Ginseng (*Ren Shen*) and processed Semen Strychnotis (*Ma Qian Zi*) not only activates the marrow to produce blood but also promotes stem cell differentiation. Thus, these three medicinals should be included in most prescriptions administered to patients suffering from hypo- or aplastic anemias. It is also notable that this combination needs to be taken long-term to provide the patient with the best possible effect.

By stimulating hemopoiesis, *Lu Rong* increases the production of all formed elements in the blood. Therefore, this medicinal, combined with qi-boosting and blood-quickening medicinals, can also be used for leukopenia.

• Herba Epimedii (*Yin Yang Huo*)

Yin Yang Huo is an important medicinal for increasing blood production due to bone marrow abnormalities, *i.e.*, hypo- or aplastic anemias. It works most efficiently if combined with Semen Cuscutae Chinensis (*Tu Si Zi*) and assisted by yin-enriching medicinals. Again, the prolonged use of this combination is an important requirement for treatment success. From a biomedical perspective, *Yin Yang Huo* and *Tu Si Zi* have similar effects to androgenic drugs. However, androgenic drugs have pronounced side effects if taken over a long period of time. This is not the case with Chinese medicinals.

Yin Yang Huo can also be used in cases which present with vacuity weakness of the defensive and recurrent colds or upper respiratory infections. Besides being an excellent medicinal to supplement the kidneys and engender blood, *Yin Yang Huo* has the function of stopping coughing and eliminating phlegm. Pharmaceutical research has further shown that this medicinal inhibits viruses and bacteria. To effectively employ *Yin Yang Huo* in this context, it needs to be combined with Radix Astragali Membranacei (*Huang Qi*) and Radix Albus Paeoniae Lactiflorae (*Bai Shao*).

• **Herba Cistanchis Deserticolae (*Rou Cong Rong*)**

Rou Cong Rong warms the kidneys and strengthens the sinew and bones. Similar to all other yang-supplementing medicinals, it can be used for anemias due to bone marrow abnormalities presenting with a yang vacuity pattern. For these cases, it should be combined with Semen Cuscutae Chinensis (*Tu Si Zi*) and yin-supplementing medicinals.

Rou Cong Rong, combined with cooked Radix Rehmanniae (*Shu Di*) and Carapax Amydae Sinensis (*Bie Jia*) boosts the essence and supplements the marrow. It can thus be used for natural endowment insufficiencies leading to retardation and slow growth and development.

• **Fructus Psoraleae Corylifoliae (*Bu Gu Zhi*)**

When *Bu Gu Zhi* is combined with Semen Cuscutae Chinensis (*Tu Si Zi*), processed Radix Polygoni Multiflori (*He Shou Wu*), and cooked Radix Rehmanniae (*Shu Di*), it enriches yin, reinforces yang, and engenders the blood. This combination is effectively used for hypo- or aplastic anemias and also supports the body and bone marrow while undergoing radiation or chemotherapy.

Bu Gu Zhi combined with Radix Salviae Miltiorrhizae (*Dan Shen*) and Radix Astragali Membranacei (*Huang Qi*) increases the white blood cell count and is effective in the treatment of leuko- or granulocytopenia.

Because *Bu Gu Zhi* is a relatively warm and dry medicinal, it has a propensity to damage yin fluids and is, therefore, prohibited for use in yin vacuity-fire effulgence patterns.

• **Semen Cuscutae Chinensis (*Tu Si Zi*)**

Tu Si Zi is an important medicinal for supplementing the marrow and increasing essence, strengthening the sinews and fortifying the bones. It is particularly good for treating the liver and kidneys. Furthermore, it is level or neutral in nature and moist and not drying or slimy. *Tu Si Zi* both supplements yang and boosts yin. Thus, it is commonly used in the treatment of blood diseases manifesting insufficiencies of the liver and kidneys and is commonly combined with Fructus Lycii Chinensis (*Gou Qi Zi*), Fructus Psoraleae Corylifoliae (*Bu Gu Zhi*) and processed Radix Polygoni Multiflori (*He Shou Wu*).

• **Cordyceps Sinensis (*Dong Chong Xia Cao*)**

Dong Chong Xia Cao warms kidney yang. If it is combined with yin-enriching medicinals, it regulates the balance of yin and yang and improves the functioning of the visceral qi. It is, therefore, particularly appropriate in the treatment of patterns due to yin vacuity-yang detriment. If *Dong Chong Xia Cao* is combined with Bombyx Batryticatus (*Jiang Can*), it quickens the blood and transforms stasis. If it is combined with yin-enriching and blood-supplementing medicinals, it strengthens the visceral qi and engenders the blood. Therefore, it treats chronic anemias due to yin and blood vacuity.

4. Yin-supplementing medicinals

"Yang engenders yin and yin engenders yang." Yin-enriching medicinals provide the source or nourishment for yang-warming medicinals to supplement, boost, and engender the blood. In clinical practice, the combination of yin-enriching and yang-warming medicinals is very common. Only rarely is it appropriate to use simply yang-supplementing medicinals or to use simply yin-enriching medicinals.

Many hematological diseases are marked by bleeding signs. Bleeding is often due to frenetic movement of hot blood. Blood heat may be due to repletion heat or vacuity heat. Yin-enriching medicinals are an important addition to blood-cooling medicinals in the treatment of bleeding due to yin vacuity-fire effulgence with heat leading to frenetic movement of the blood and scorching of the vessels and network vessels.

A wide variety of blood diseases, such as leukemia, aplastic anemia, anemias accompanied by infections, etc., manifest vacuity heat patterns. In order to treat vacuity heat, yin-enriching medicinals need to be combined with heat-clearing medicinals.

• Fructus Lycii Chinensis (*Gou Qi Zi*)

The *Ben Cao Hui Yan (Convergent Speech on the Materia Medica)* says: "...*Gou Qi Zi* fills the qi, supplements the blood, engenders yang, grows yin, downbears fire, and removes wind dampness. It has a magical effect on everything." Biomedical research has demonstrated that *Gou Qi Zi* contains vitamins A, B, and C as well as calcium, phosphorus, and iron. It also actively stimulates blood production and enhances immunity.

Thus, *Gou Qi Zi* is an excellent medicinal in the treatment of all types of anemia. It is particularly effective in the treatment of anemias due to either old age or malnourishment. If *Gou Qi Zi* is combined with qi-boosting medicinals, it can be used for the treatment of leukopenia since this combination increases the white blood cell count. If *Gou Qi Zi* is combined with cooked Radix Rehmanniae (*Shu Di*) and processed Radix Polygoni Multiflori (*He Shou Wu*), it can be used in the treatment of slow and retarded growth and development.

• Fructus Ligustri Lucidi (*Nu Zhen Zi*)

Nu Zhen Zi enriches yin and supplements the liver and kidneys as well as cools and supplements the blood. When combined with qi-boosting medicinals, it can be used in the treatment of blood diseases manifesting with a pattern of blood and yin dual vacuity.

When combined with other blood-cooling and bleeding stopping medicinals, it treats frenetic movement of the blood due to yin vacuity-fire effulgence. When combined with blood-supplementing medicinals, it constrains yin and supplements the blood. If patients suffer from a lack of trace minerals (zinc and iron in particular)[1], the combination of *Nu Zhen Zi* with processed Radix Polygoni Multiflori (*He Shou Wu*), Radix Panacis Ginseng (*Ren Shen*), Rhizoma Atractylodis Macrocephalae (*Bai Zhu*), Sclerotium Poriae Cocos (*Fu Ling*), and Radix Glycyrrhizae (*Gan Cao*) is much preferable to the mere administration of zinc and iron supplements. The combination of *Nu Zhen Zi* and processed Radix Polygoni Multiflori (*He Shou Wu*) is also very effective in promoting hair growth, blackening the hair, and making it lustrous.

• Rhizoma Polygonati Odorati (*Yu Zhu*)
Yu Zhu is a moderate medicinal, and it needs to be taken over prolonged periods of time to be effective. If *Yu Zhu*'s yin-enriching functions are combined with Radix Panacis Ginseng's (*Ren Shen*) qi-boosting function, yin obtains reinforcement from yang and yang obtains reinforcement from yin. Thus, this is an effective combination in the treatment of blood diseases and anemias due to qi vacuity or qi and yin dual vacuity. Furthermore, this combination has the function of strengthening the heart qi. From a biomedical point of view, it improves blood circulation velocity and oxygen carrying capacity. If *Yu Zhu* is combined with *Ren Shen* and blood-supplementing medicinals, qi is boosted, yin is enriched, and blood is engendered. If *Yu Zhu* is combined with *Ren Shen* and blood-cooling and bleeding stopping medicinals, yin is enriched, qi is boosted, and bleeding is stopped. This last combination is effective in the treatment of hematological diseases with recurrent bleeding.

• Rhizoma Polygonati (*Huang Jing*)
Huang Jing has the function of supplementing the middle and boosting the five viscera, replenishing the essence and strengthening sinews and bones. Legend has it that, in ancient China, slave girls who ran away depended on *Huang Jing* for nourishment. Thus, their hunger was alleviated and their life was invigorated. In the treatment of hematological diseases with a prolonged history presenting the patterns of yin vacuity with essence and blood vacuity and fluid insufficiency, *Huang Jing* should be combined with Radix Polygoni Multiflori (*He Shou Wu*), Fructus Lycii Chinensis (*Gou Qi Zi*), and Endothelium Corneum Gigeriae Galli (*Ji Nei Jin*). For the treatment of bleeding due to yin vacuity-fire effulgence, *Huang Jing* can be combined with such blood-cooling and bleeding stopping medicinals as Pollen Typhae (*Pu Huang*) and Radix Sanguisorbae (*Di Yu*). Because *Huang Jing* not only enriches yin but also boosts the qi, it is one of the most important medicinals in the treatment of qi and yin dual vacuity hematological disease patterns. In these cases, it needs to be combined with Radix Codonopsitis

---

[1] Note that anemias with a lack of iron and zinc often manifest with withered, brittle hair.

Pilosulae (*Dang Shen*), Rhizoma Atractylodis Macrocephalae (*Bai Zhu*), and Sclerotium Poriae Cocos (*Fu Ling*).

Because of this medicinal's moderate function, it also needs to be taken over a prolonged period of time for best effect. Furthermore, *Huang Jing* is an enriching and slimy medicinal. If the digestive function is weak or if there is diarrhea, only a small amount should be used, and, in order to moderate its slimy quality, it needs to be combined with medicinals that abduct stagnation and rectify the qi, such as Endothelium Corneum Gigeriae Galli (*Ji Nei Jin*) and Massa Medica Fermentata (*Shen Qu*).

• Tuber Ophiopogonis Japonici (*Mai Men Dong*)

Mai Men Dong is appropriate for the treatment of blood diseases due to yin vacuity-internal heat, heart vexation, thirst due to fluid insufficiency, or dry cough with sticky phlegm due to lung heat. It is often combined with uncooked Radix Rehmanniae (*Sheng Di*) and Radix Scrophulariae Ningpoensis (*Xuan Shen*).

• Herba Ecliptae Prostratae (*Han Lian Cao*)

Han Lian Cao enriches yin, cools the blood, and stops bleeding. Thus, this medicinal is commonly used for all kinds of bleeding illnesses due to yin vacuity-blood heat. It is commonly combined with Rhizoma Imperatae Cylindricae (*Bai Mao Gen*), Herba Cirsii Japonici (*Da Ji*), Herba Cephalanoploris Segeti (*Xiao Ji*), and uncooked Radix Rehmanniae (*Sheng Di*).

• Carapax Amydae Sinensis (*Bie Jia*)

Bie Jia contains animal glue and proteins and is, therefore, a very nutritive substance which enriches yin and supplements the kidneys, boosts the marrow and strengthens the bones. It is particularly suitable in the treatment of anemic patients suffering from natural endowment insufficiency with slow and retarded growth and development. In this case, it is best combined with cooked Radix Rehmanniae (*Shu Di*) and Herba Cistanchis Deserticolae (*Rou Cong Rong*). If *Bie Jia* is combined with uncooked Radix Rehmanniae (*Sheng Di*) and Rhizoma Anemarrhenae Asphodeloidis (*Zhi Mu*), blood diseases due to yin vacuity and blood heat can be treated. For bleeding due to frenetic movement of hot blood, *Bie Jia* should be combined with uncooked Radix Rehmanniae (*Sheng Di*), Pollen Typhae (*Pu Huang*), and Radix Rubiae Cordyfoliae (*Qian Cao Gen*). This combination enriches yin, cools the blood, stops bleeding, and, according to modern biomedical research, increases the number of platelets. Because *Bie Jia* is a hard substance, it must be smashed up first and then cooked for a prolonged period of time.

• Plastrum Testudinis (*Gui Ban*)

Gui Ban softens hardness, enriches yin, and boosts the essence. Depending with which other medicinals it is combined, it is widely used in different hematological diseases. In combination with hardness-softening and nodulation-scattering, blood-quickening and stasis-transforming medicinals, it treats swelling of the liver and spleen. Combined with Spica Prunellae Vulgaris (*Xia Ku Cao*), it can be used for swelling of the lymph nodes. To treat hypoplastic anemias or to treat leukopenia, *Gui Ban* is best combined with yang-supplementing medicinals so that yin is enriched and yang reinforced, thus engendering the blood. *Gui Ban* combined with Radix Astragali Membranacei (*Huang Qi*) and blood-cooling and bleeding stopping medicinals can be used in hemorrhagic conditions due to yin vacuity with blood heat. Because *Gui Ban* also enriches yin and boosts the essence and, therefore, replenishes the marrow, it promotes development and growth. Combined with Rhizoma Acori Graminei (*Shi Chang Pu*) and Fructus Schisandrae Chinensis (*Wu Wei Zi*), it sharpens the hearing and brightens the vision, boosts the intelligence, opens the orifices, and improves the memory.

Other efficacious medicinals in the treatment of blood diseases

The following short descriptions of medicinals or medicinal combinations in relation to certain biomedical or Chinese medical functions have been composed from various little bits and pieces reported in the Chinese literature or stemming from the personal experience of Dr. Sun Wei-zheng from the First Hospital affiliated with the Heilongjiang University of Chinese Medicine. As stated above, these medicinal descriptions are not complete in and of themselves and are only presented as they pertain to the field of hematology. Furthermore, not all the research protocols used for the analysis of the statements below are clear to me and have, therefore, not been verified. However, most of the following are well established and agreed upon functions of individual Chinese medicinals or their combinations. Furthermore, the information comes from articles in respected Chinese medical journals from China as well as from the experience of a respected *lao yi sheng,* Dr. Sun Wei-zheng.

• Bleeding stopping medicinals

Radix Rubiae Cordifoliae (*Qian Cao Gen*), uncooked Pollen Typhae (*Pu Huang*), uncooked Radix Rehmanniae (*Sheng Di*), and Herba Cephalanoploris Segeti (*Xiao Ji*) all have the function of stopping bleeding. Thus, the combination of these four medicinals is particularly effective for bleeding disorders. It has been shown to shorten blood coagulation time and simultaneously reduce platelet aggregation. *Qian Cao Gen* and uncooked *Pu Huang* improve coagulation function while also quickening the blood.

Thus, the combination of these two medicinals enhances hematoma absorption and is particularly important in the treatment of hemophiliacs.

Other medicinals which have the function of increasing platelets and, therefore, help to stop bleeding are Herba Agrimoniae Pilosae (*Xian He Cao*), Radix Pseudoginseng (*San Qi*), and Folium Callicarpae (*Zi Zhu Cao*). *San Qi*, in addition to stopping bleeding, also quickens the blood and, therefore, helps with hematoma absorption and microcirculation activation. When mentioning *San Qi*, it must be added that, according to some Chinese doctors, this medicinal stops bleeding more effectively when it is first stir-fried until yellow and then frozen for 2-3 hours. Its fire qi is thus removed by this freezing.

Da Huang is another medicinal which is especially important in the treatment of blood ejection due to repletion heat in the stomach. *Da Huang* contains tannins and astringes and contracts the blood vessels. It is best combined with Radix Bletillae Striatae (*Bai Ji*) which has the function of stopping bleeding by promoting RBC coagulation and thrombus formation.

Modern research has also found Herba Kummerowiae (*San Ye Ren Zi Cao* or *Ji Yan Cao*) to be particularly effective for stopping urinary bleeding. *Ji Yan Cao* is not a well-known medicinal. It is sweet, bland, and slightly cold in nature. Its functions are to clear heat and resolve toxins, quicken the blood, disinhibit urination, and stop diarrhea. Experience has recently determined that it can be effectively used to treat severe urinary bleeding. It thus is employed in the treatment of PNH and RBCs in the urine due to a variety of kidney diseases as well as bloody urine secondary to bladder cancer. The recommended dose for this medicinal in the treatment of urinary tract bleeding is about 30g per day.

• Leukocyte-increasing medicinals

Some of the prime medicinals for stimulating the production and appropriate functioning of leukocytes are Caulis Milletiae Seu Spatholobi (*Ji Xue Teng*), Radix Salviae Miltiorrhizae (*Dan Shen*), Squama Manitis Pentadactylis (*Chuan Shan Jia*), Radix Astragali Membranacei (*Huang Qi*), and Fructus Zizyphi Jujubae (*Da Zao*). The combination of *Dan Shen* and *Ji Xue Teng* seems to be particularly effective. Furthermore, *Chuan Shan Jia* should always be combined with *Dan Shen* if used for leukocyte-enhancing purposes.

More generally, the combination of blood-quickening and stasis-transforming medicinals has the function of benefitting the immune system.

• Anti-cancer medicinals

Some of the most often used anti-cancer medicinals are Herba Selaginellae (*Juan Bai*), Radix Lithospermi Seu Arnebiae (*Zi Cao*), Semen Strychnotis (*Ma Qian Zi*), Herba Oldenlandiae Diffusae Cum Radice (*Bai Hua She She Cao*), Herba Scutellariae Barbatae (*Ban Zhi Lian*), Spica Prunellae Vulgaris (*Xia Ku Cao*), and Rhizoma Paridis Polyphyllae (*Qi Ye Yi Zhi Hua*). All these medicinals have the traditional function of resolving toxins and clearing heat and the modern function of suppressing the growth of tumorous cells, such as white blood cells in leukemia, red blood cells in polycythemia vera, and other cancer cells.

Juan Bai is an especially useful medicinal. Pharmaceutical research shows that it can prolong survival in tumorous lab rats. *Juan Bai* further has the function of enlarging the fascicular zone of the adrenal cortex. Traditionally seen, this medicinal has the dual function of supporting the righteous and dispelling evil. Thus, it is appropriate in the treatment of cancer patients.

Furthermore, Sclerotium Polyporia Umbellati (*Zhu Ling*), traditionally used to disinhibit urination and expel turbidity, also has the function of suppressing cancer cell growth.

• Blood-quickening medicinals

Scolopendra Subspinipes (*Wu Gong*), Buthus Martensis (*Quan Xie*), and Hirudo Seu Whitmania (*Shui Zhi*)[2] break the blood and transform stasis. From a biomedical point of view, they increase blood velocity and increase blood oxygen concentration. Furthermore, these three medicinals penetrate the blood/brain barrier and can attack and kill leukemic cells located in the brain. Thus, *Wu Gong* and *Quan Xie*'s function of reducing cancerous swellings, *i.e.*, killing cancerous cells, is of particular importance in the treatment of meningeal leukemia.

Another "worm" (*chong*), Agkistrodon Seu Bungarus (*Bai Hua She*), also has a similar function to the three blood/brain barrier crossing medicinals above. Therefore, in the treatment of headaches due to increased cranial pressure, *Bai Hua She* can be combined with *Wu Gong* and Bombyx Batryticatus (*Jiang Can*). This combination extinguishes and courses wind and stops tetany, quickens the blood and frees the flow of the network vessels, transforms stasis and removes impediment.

Another combination of medicinals which can cross the blood brain barrier and attack leukemic cells within the brain is Radix Salviae Miltiorrhizae (*Dan Shen*), Rhizoma

---

[2] This medicinal should not be cooked. Typically, it is administered as a powder. Cooking destroys its effective proteinS.

Curcumae Zeodoariae (*E Zhu*), Caulis Milletiae Seu Spatholobi (*Ji Xue Teng*), Radix Rubrus Paeoniae Lactiflorae (*Chi Shao*), and Radix Ligustici Wallichii (*Chuan Xiong*). The combination of these medicinals with the five "insects" mentioned above has the function of breaking the blood and transforming stasis, dispersing conglomeration and scattering nodulation. Thus, the blood circulation of the entire body is improved, the blood flow's velocity is increased, and the oxygen content in the brain is restored. Furthermore, as mentioned above, this combination can cross the blood/brain barrier and kill leukemic cells "hiding" in the brain.

Another blood-quickening medicinal which is used not in the treatment of meningeal leukemia but rather in the treatment of elevated blood urea nitrogen (BUN) in chronic kidney failure with accompanying anemia is Radix Et Rhizoma Rhei (*Da Huang*). *Da Huang* quickens the blood and frees the flow of the network vessels. Combined with other blood-quickening medicinals, it improves the microcirculation in the kidneys and thus helps to activate renewed erythropoietin production. Furthermore, the combination of *Da Huang* with Radix Lateralis Praeparatus Aconiti Carmichaeli (*Fu Zi*) is a specifically effective combination for lowering blood urea nitrogen.

• Medicinals that enhance the body's ability to cope with low tissue oxygen concentrations

Radix Panacis Ginseng (*Ren Shen*) and Tuber Ophiopogonis Japonici (*Mai Dong*) have the function of enhancing the body's ability to cope with low oxygen concentrations. In all anemias, reduced oxygen flow to the tissues is one of the main problems. *Ren Shen* and *Mai Dong* lower the body tissues' requirement of oxygen for functional activities.

• Anti-allergy medicinals

Some of the best anti-allergic medicinals (which are applicable in allergic purpura, for example) are Herba Ephedrae (*Ma Huang*), Herba Asari Cum Radice (*Xi Xin*), Periostracum Cicadae (*Chan Tui*), and Lumbricus (*Di Long*). *Di Long* further lowers capillary perfusion and, during allergy attacks, functions as a histamine inhibitor.

• Immune-regulating medicinals

Medicinals that regulate the immune system are important in all diseases where the immune system has gone astray from its normal and beneficial function. Examples include all autoimmuune diseases and allergies. One combination which regulates the immune system is Bombyx Batryticatus (*Jiang Can*) and Cordyceps Chinensis (*Dong Chong Xia Cao*). A second combination is Herba Oldenlandiae Diffusae Cum Radice (*Bai Hua She She Cao*), Sclerotium Polypori Umbellati (*Zhu Ling*), and Radix Glycyrrhizae (*Gan Cao*).

Bai Hua She She Cao, in addition to regulating the immune system, is also an anti-viral and anti-microbial medicinal and is thus even more applicable in allergic reactions in which a malfunctioning of the immune system is initiated by a viral infection (such as in certain types of allergic purpura).

• Iron absorption-enhancing medicinals

In the treatment of iron deficiency anemia, iron supplementation is a very important part of the treatment plan. However, rather than simply administering iron supplements, a better effect can be achieved when iron-containing medicinals and medicinals which enhance the digestive system's iron absorption are combined. Medicinals with a high iron content or medicinals that help in iron absorption are the following: Fructificatio Ganodermae Lucidi (*Ling Zhi*), Radix Panacis Ginseng (*Ren Shen*), Radix Astragali Membranacei (*Huang Qi*), Rhizoma Atractylodis Macrocephalae (*Bai Zhu*), Placenta Hominis (*Zi He Che*), Radix Angelicae Sinensis (*Dang Gui*), Gelatinum Corii Asini (*E Jiao*), Herba Cynomorii Songarici (*Suo Yang*), Cornu Parvum Cervi (*Lu Rong*), Fructus Ligustri Lucidi (*Nu Zhen Zi*), uncooked and cooked Radix Rehmanniae (*Sheng Shu Di*), Radix Polygoni Multiflori (*He Shou Wu*), Rhizoma Polygonati (*Huang Jing*), Herba Sargassii (*Hai Zao*), and Melanteritum (*Lu Fan*). Of course, these medicinals should never be prescribed just as they are listed above. Rather, after differentiating the pattern and selecting a treatment formula, a few appropriate medicinals from the above list should be selected and added to the formula.

Other medicinals which are very effective and important for enhancing intestinal absorption of iron are Fructus Crataegi (*Shan Zha*) and Endothelium Corneum Gigeriae Galli (*Ji Nei Jin*). Both these medicinals increase the secretion of gastric fluids and digestive enzymes and thus improve stomach acid concentration and digestive function.

3
Acupuncture in the Treatment of Blood Diseases

In China today, acupuncture is not considered the standard of care for the treatment of Western hematological diseases. Patients with blood diseases are treated in the *nei ke* (internal medicine) department. In other words, patients with Western hematological diseases are treated by Chinese medical doctors prescribing orally administered, polypharmacy Chinese medicinal formulas. It is telling that, in the preparation of this book, I could only find three articles on the treatment of hematological diseases with acupuncture in the modern Chinese medical literature.

In the West in general and North America in particular, the practice of acupuncture became established before Chinese herbal medicine did, and thus acupuncture still represents Chinese medicine to a lot of Western patients seeking Chinese medical treatment. Because of this, many, if not most, Western patients routinely expect acupuncture treatment from Chinese medical practitioners who are most commonly legally defined as "acupuncturists," and they are often not satisfied receiving orally administered Chinese medicines alone. It is partly for this reason and partly due to the fact that acupuncture can be beneficial to most Western patients regardless of disease, that I have included this short and albeit limited discussion of the ways in which acupuncture may benefit patients who are also taking Chinese medicinals or modern Western drugs for the treatment of hematological diseases. Because Book II, the treatment section of this book, is based entirely on Chinese sources, it does not include any acupuncture references. However, based on the functions of acupuncture points as described below, one can formulate acupuncture treatment plans for any patient with any hematological disease simply by following the treatment principles listed for the different patterns of the respective diseases discussed in Book II.

Acupuncture principles & protocols

As Bob Flaws is fond of pointing out, the liver becomes depressed and the qi becomes stagnant if either one does not get what one wants or, conversely, gets what one does not want.[1] Since sufferers of chronic diseases are limited as to what they can and cannot do, virtually all chronic diseases are complicated by liver depression qi stagnation. In addition, living in modern Western society and having to cope with its many socio-economic stressors, severe liver qi depression first transforming into heat and then giving rise to heart fire is not uncommon. When fire harasses the heart spirit, this spirit becomes disquieted, resulting in various psycho-emotional complaints. In addition, most blood diseases tend to be enduring, and many of them are also relatively severe. Thus patients with these kinds of diseases are often depressed, anxious, and fearful. Therefore, one can expect to find liver depression and disquietude of the spirit complicating most cases of blood disease. Based on my experience, one of the ways acupuncture can benefit patients suffering from blood diseases is to course the liver and resolve depression, clear heat and quiet the spirit.

Although Chinese medicinals may also effectively relieve symptoms of liver depression qi stagnation, when trying to deal with the sometimes very complicated pathological mechanisms underlying some of the blood diseases discussed in this book, acupuncture treatments for the psychological imbalances arising from depressed liver qi and consequent heart fire may be a very useful and immediately acting adjunct. It is my experience that acupuncture is a very effective and relatively quick way of dealing with such problems.

• Liver-coursing & spirit-quieting points
The four basic points for freeing the orderly reaching of the liver qi are the so-called four bars (si guan). The four bars are made up of the two points, He Gu (LI 4) and Tai Chong (Liv 3), which are needled bilaterally (thus totaling four insertions). Inserting needles at these four points typically quickly leads to very deep relaxation, with patients often falling asleep within minutes of obtaining the qi.

Another effective four needle combination which not only courses the liver and rectifies the qi but also nourishes yin and quiets the spirit is the contralateral insertion of Nei Guan (Per 6) and Zhu Bin (Ki 9) and Shen Men (Ht 7) and Tai Xi (Ki 3). I like to use this combination in patients suffering from liver depression qi stagnation complicated by kidney yin vacuity with upward flaming of internal heat. Such internal heat is usually transformative heat from liver depression as well as heat from yin vacuity.

Nei Guan is the meeting point of the yin linking vessel (yin wei mai). It nourishes the blood and enriches yin, and loosens the chest and calms the mind. It is located on the hand jue yin pericardium channel and is, therefore, connected to the foot jue yin liver

---

[1]   Flaws, Bob, Blue Poppy Seminars *Chinese Medical Pediatric Certification Program*, lecture notes

channel. Thus, *Nei Guan* also has a function of coursing the liver and moving the qi. This point is combined, contralaterally, with *Zhu Bin*. *Zhu Bin* is the beginning and cleft (*xi*) point of the yin linking vessel. As such, it is connected to *Nei Guan* and functions more strongly when combined with that point. *Zhu Bin* further has the function of enriching yin and quieting the spirit. When the yin linking vessel is accessed through this combination, it powerfully nourishes yin and quiets the spirit, loosens the chest and relieves anxiety.

Shen Men is a point on the hand *shao yin* heart channel. It is a main point for quieting the spirit and nourishing heart blood. *Tai Xi* enriches yin and clears vacuity heat. It also lies on the lesser yin channel - the foot *shao yin* kidney channel—and is thus connected to the heart channel. When these four points are used together, they course the liver and rectify the qi, enrich yin, clear vacuity heat, and quiet the spirit.

• Points for patterns

As far as the treatment of specific blood diseases with acupuncture is concerned and based on my own clinical experience with Western patients, I believe the following approach is a rational one. Once the patient's pattern(s) and, therefore, the treatment principles for these patterns are established, a point prescription can be composed in a similar fashion to composing a Chinese medicinal formula. This approach to the creation of acupuncture protocols is standard in the People's Republic of China today. One of the modern proponents of this approach was Wang Le-ting, past director of the Acupuncture Department of the Beijing Chinese Medical Hospital.[2]

For instance, if a particular patient's pattern is a liver-spleen disharmony with qi and blood dual vacuity and damp accumulation, then the treatment principles necessary to rebalance these patterns are to course the liver and fortify the spleen, supplement the qi and nourish the blood, and also to eliminate dampness. *Tai Chong* (Liv 3) courses the liver and rectifies the qi. Because it is the earth point on the wood channel, it also harmonizes liver wood and spleen earth. Because the spleen is the latter heaven root of qi and blood engenderment, supplementing the spleen and supplementing the qi and blood are largely synonymous. To supplement the qi, one can choose *Zu San Li* (St 36), the earth point on the yang earth channel. To supplement the blood, one can combine *Zu San Li* with *San Yin Jiao* (Sp 6). This is the spleen network point which connects the spleen, liver, and kidneys, all three of which are closely connected to the blood. In addition, *San Yin Jiao* helps harmonize the liver. Since the spleen is in charge of moving and transforming water within the body, another spleen channel point may be added -

[2] For examples of Wang's use of this approach, see *Golden Needle Wang Le-ting: A 20th Century Master's Approach to Acupuncture*, Yu Hui-chan & Han Fu-ru, trans. by Shaui Xue-zhong, Blue Poppy Press, Boulder, CO, 1997

Shang Qiu (Sp 5). Dampness is associated with the earth phase and *Shang Qiu* is the child or draining point on the yin earth channel. Or, depending on where the dampness is located and the nature of its pathological manifestations, one might choose the water point on the yin earth channel—*Yin Ling Quan* (Sp 9).

Thus it is easy to see that acupuncture can be chosen for each of the elements in a statement of treatment principles which, in turn, is based on the patient's pattern discrimination. Depending on the relative proportions of patterns, more than a single point might be selected to accomplish a single function, while sometimes a single point may accomplish two or more functions. In addition, it is also possible and typically standard practice to add one or more points depending on the patient's symptomatology or major complaints. Certain points are known to have pronounced empirical effects on certain symptoms or areas of the body. Therefore, one or more points may be added for their symptomatic actions.

Below is a selection of the most commonly used points for the most common Chinese patterns. Using this list, one should be able to craft the core of acupuncture prescriptions for all of the patterns of all of the hematological diseases discussed in Book II.

• Common points for common treatment principles:

Boosting the qi: *Zu San Li* (St 36), *Qi Hai* (CV 6), *San Yin Jiao* (Sp 6), *Pi Shu* (Bl 20)

Lifting & upbearing the qi: *Bai Hui* (GV 20), *Dan Zhong* (CV 17)

Nourishing the blood: *San Yin Jiao* (Sp 6), *Qi Hai* (CV 6), *Guan Yuan* (CV 4), *Nei Guan* (Per 6), *Qu Quan* (Liv 8), *Tai Chong* (Liv 3), *Ge Shu* (Bl 17)

Enriching yin: *Tai Xi* (Ki 3), *Zhao Hai* (Ki 6), *San Yin Jiao* (Sp 6), *Guan Yuan* (CV 4), *Shen Shu* (Bl 23), *Zhu Bin* (Ki 9)

Invigorating yang: *Ming Men* (GV 4), *Guan Yuan* (CV 4), *Shen Shu* (Bl 23), *Fu Liu* (Ki 7)

Fortifying the spleen: *Zhong Wan* (CV 12), *Zu San Li* (St 36), *San Yin Jiao* (Sp 6), *Tai Bai* (Sp 3)

Warming the center: Moxibustion at *Zu San Li* (St 36), moxibustion at *Zhong Wan* (CV 12)

Coursing the liver: *Tai Chong* (Liv 3), *He Gu* (LI 4), *Zhang Men* (Liv 13), *Yang Ling Quan* (GB 34), *Nei Guan* (Per 6), *Zhi Gou* (TB 6)

Quieting the spirit: *Shen Men* (Ht 7), *Nei Guan* (Per 6), *Da Ling* (Per 7), *Yin Tang* (M-HN-3), *Tai Xi* (Ki 3), *San Yin Jiao* (Sp 6), *Xin Shu* (Bl 15), *Shen Tang* (Bl 44)

Quickening the blood: *Xue Hai* (Sp 10), *Tai Chong* (Liv 3), *He Gu* (LI 4), *Ge Shu* (Bl 17)

Resolving the exterior: *Fei Shu* (Bl 13), *Lie Que* (Lu 7), *He Gu* (LI 4)

Clearing heat: *Chi Ze* (Lu 5), *Qu Chi* (LI 11), *Wei Zhong* (Bl 40), *Shao Hai* (Ht 3), *Yin Xi* (Ht 6), *Lao Gong* (Per 8), *Shao Fu* (Ht 8), *Qu Ze* (Per 3), *Jie Xi* (St 41), *Xing Jian* (Liv 2), *Da Zhui* (GV 14)

Although acupuncture is not commonly used in China for the treatment of hematological diseases *per se*, that does not mean that one cannot or should not seek to redress the patient's pathological imbalance through the use of acupuncture based on the patient's pattern discrimination. All that is required in order to use this kind of acupuncture is to do a pattern discrimination, state the logically necessary treatment principles, and compose an acupuncture protocol based on those principles. In addition, acupuncture points may also be selected on the basis of their known empirical efficacy in eliminating or mitigating the patient's major clinical symptoms or complaints.

However, one should not use too many needles in any given treatment. It is my experience as a teacher and clinical preceptor that many Western practitioners, when not able to decide between two similar points, use both of them. This often leads to the use of an excessive number of needles. The use of too many needles can disperse a patient's qi and, if their qi is already vacuous, produce very exhausting treatments. Therefore, attention should be paid to keeping the number of needles to a minimum. Correct point selection and effective point combination is of much greater importance than using every applicable point.

Having said all this, I believe it needs to be pointed out once again in an unequivocal fashion that Chinese herbal medicine should be the predominant method of treatment of hematological diseases. This is the standard of care for the diseases discussed in this book in the People's Republic of China where Chinese medicine originated and has been the most extensively documented. If one also chooses to do acupuncture as well as prescribe Chinese medicinals for the diseases discussed in this book, the practitioner should keep in mind that this is nonstandard, experimental treatment which is primarily being used as an adjunctive modality.

4
The Role of Chinese Medicine in the Treatment of Blood Diseases

Many of the hematologic diseases discussed in this book are severe or even life-threatening in nature. Aplastic anemia, leukemia, and Hodgkin's disease, to name only a few, are all disorders which require Western medical treatment for their management. Chinese medicine, in and of itself, is not sufficient to treat these diseases and keep such patients alive. Therefore, it is absolutely essential that patients suffering from such grave illnesses receive professional Western medical care. However, as we have seen above, many of the Western medical treatments for the hematological diseases described in this book have serious side effects, while other Western hematological diseases have no effective Western medical treatments. Therefore, there are several ways that Chinese medicine can be used in the treatment of hematological diseases.

First, Chinese medicine can be used in less severe hematological diseases as part of a graduated series of responses culminating in more powerful Western therapies. Since correctly prescribed Chinese medicine has such a low potential for iatrogenic side effects, diseases which respond to Chinese medical treatment should first be treated with it. If and when Chinese medicine proves ineffective for curing or controlling a blood disease in a specific patient, more powerful Western therapies, with their higher incidence of side effects, can be tried. In addition, because Chinese medicine treats the whole person, when it succeeds in treating disease, it brings the entire patient's organism back into a more harmonious state of balance, thus often also ameliorating other concomitant complaints and conditions.

Secondly, Chinese medicine can be used to increase the healing effects of Western medicines and treatments in those conditions where Western medicine alone is not entirely satisfactory. Numerous Chinese studies on various diseases have shown that often the combination of Chinese medicine plus Western medicine achieves a better therapeutic outcome than Western medicine alone.[1]

---

[1] *E.g.,* She You-zhi, "Observations on the Treatment of 60 Cases of Gouty Arthritis with Integrated Chinese-Western Medicine," *Zhe Jiang Zhong Yi Za Zhi (Zhejiang Journal of Chinese Medicine)*, #11, 1996, p. 497

Third, Chinese medicine can be used to attempt treatment in conditions where Western medicine has no effective treatments. Because Chinese medicine works by bringing the entire organism back into a more harmonious state of balance, its treatments are not disease specific but rather patient specific. Western physicians require specific treatments for specific diseases. This makes Western medical treatment very focused. However, sometimes it makes Western medicine too focused. There are literally thousands of documented cases in the Chinese medical literature of all sorts of diseases which were untreatable by Western medicine but responded to Chinese medical treatment. Therefore, Chinese medicine provides a possible alternative to all those conditions for which modern biomedical medicine has no treatment.[2]

And fourth, Chinese medicine can be used to treat the side effects of Western medical treatment. Again, there are hundreds of published studies and case histories within the Chinese medical literature documenting Chinese medicine's ability to treat the side effects of Western pharmaceuticals and heroic treatments, such as radiation and chemotherapy.[3] Many of these studies show not only Chinese medicine's ability to

---

Chen Yong-zhen *et al.*, "Clinical Observations on the Treatment of 30 Cases of Acute Leukemia with Integrated Chinese-Western Medicine," *Zhong Guo Zhong Xi Yi Jie He Za Zhi (Chinese Journal of Integrated Chinese-Western Medicine)*, #1, 1998, p. 752-754

[2]   *E.g.*, Yuan Hai-yan, "The Use of Ear Press Tacks in the Treatment of Chronic Constipation," *Zhong Guo Zhen Jiu (Chinese Acupuncture & Moxibustion)*, #1, 1999, p. 18

Yang Xiao-lin, "*Si Wei Shao Yao Tang* (Four Flavors Peony Decoction) in the Treatment of Trigeminal Neuralgia," *Xin Zhong Yi (New Chinese Medicine)*, #2, 1999, p. 14

Shi Zheng-fang & Wang Fan-hong, "The Chinese Medical Treatment of 28 Cases of Primary Gout," *Zhe Jiang Zhong Yi Za Zhi (Zhejiang Journal of Chinese Medicine)*, #5, 1994, p. 208

Sun Wei-bin, "The Treatment of 30 Cases of Genital Herpes with Chinese Medicinals," *Xin Zhong Yi (New Chinese Medicine)*, #10, 1999, p. 47

Wan Li-jian *et al.*, "Clinical Analysis of the Treatment of Difficult-to-Treat Idiopathic Thrombocytopenic Purpura by the Methods of Boosting the Qi & Replenishing Essence," *Zhong Yi Za Zhi (Journal of Chinese Medicine)*, #8, 1995, p. 478-480

[3]   *E.g.,* Jin Pu-fang, "The Treatment of 58 Cases of Post Liver Cancer Chemotherapy Vomiting with *Zhu Ye Shi Gao Tang* (Bamboo Leaf & Gypsum Decoction)," *Zhe Jiang Zhong Yi Za Zhi (Zhejiang Journal of Chinese Medicine)*, #5, 1995, p. 200

Gong Hao, "The Treatment of 17 Cases of Cancer Chemotherapy Reactions with *Bu Yang Huan Wu Tang* (Supplement Yang & Restore the Five [Viscera] Decoction)," *Zhe Jiang Zhong Yi Za Zhi (Zhejiang Journal of Chinese Medicine)*, #2, 1996, p. 67

Wei Chang-chun *et al.*, "The Treatment of 20 Cases of Anti-tubercular Medicine's Gastrointestinal Tract Reactions with Chinese Medicinals," *Ji Lin Zhong Yi Yao (Jilin Chinese Medicine & Medicinals)*, #4, 1999, p. 17

mitigate Western medical side effects, but, in that process, the Chinese medicine also often seems to potentize the Western medicine's therapeutic effects.

In China, there are three separate health care delivery systems: 1) Chinese medicine alone, 2) Western medicine alone, and 3) integrated Chinese-Western medicine. Patients with relatively benign blood diseases and those for which no effective Western biomedical treatments exist are typically treated within the Chinese medical health care delivery system alone, while patients with severe blood diseases typically are treated within the integrated Chinese-Western medicine delivery system. Patients suffering side effects due to Western treatments and medications may be treated with either the Chinese medicine alone or integrated Chinese-Western delivery systems.

Here in the West, there is, as yet, no integrated Chinese-Western medical delivery system. Therefore, most Western practitioners of Chinese medicine work on their own. However, when it comes to the treatment of hematological diseases, practitioners are often called on to treat patients who are concurrently under the care of Western physicians. In such cases, it is important to open a dialogue with the patient's Western medical care-giver. Both sets of care-givers presumably have the patient's best interests at heart. Therefore, they should try to work together as best as possible. When it comes to the treatment of some of the serious, potentially life-threatening diseases described in this book, it is important for Western practitioners of Chinese medicine to recognize that integrated Chinese-Western medicine is a medical necessity.

In terms of treating the side effects of Western medicinals, the basic prescriptive methodology is exactly the same as for any other complaint. One does a Chinese pattern discrimination, states one's treatment principles, and chooses medicinals or acupuncture points based on those principles and the main symptoms of those side effects. Therefore, drug-induced diarrhea, night-sweats, or thirst are treated exactly the same, with the same points and prescriptions, as any other diarrhea, night-sweats, or thirst.

Zhou Xiong-gen, "A Clinical Audit of the Preventive Treatment of Chemotherapy Gastrointestinal Tract Reactions with Chinese Medicinals," *Shang Hai Zhong Yi Yao Za Zhi (Shanghai Journal of Chinese Medicine & Medicinals)*, #6, 1999, p. 24-25

Lin Bei-hong *et al.*, "The Treatment of 30 Cases of Post-chemotherapy Gastrointestinal Tract Reactions with Acupuncture & Massage," *Si Chuan Zhong Yi (Sichuan Chinese Medicine)*, #9, 1999, p. 52-53

Li Zong-ju, "The Treatment of 59 Cases of Cancer Chemotherapy Toxic Reactions by the Methods of Regulating & Rectifying the Spleen & Stomach," *Si Chuan Zhong Yi (Sichuan Chinese Medicine)*, #10, 1999, p. 24-25

When patients have been first treated with Western medicine and then concurrently initiate treatment with Chinese medicine, it is common to see a decrease in or elimination of the patient's presenting symptoms. In that case, the patient should be referred back to the prescribing Western physician in order to adjust or suspend their Western medical prescription. On the other hand, practitioners of Chinese medicine also have the obligation to encourage those patients who are naïvely prejudiced against Western medicine to continue with their Western medications when those medications are truly necessary for the patient's life and well-being. If the patient's dislike of their Western medications is due to unacceptable side effects, then at least one of the Chinese medical practitioner's focuses should be on eliminating those side effects.

Book II:

The Treatment of Hematological Diseases With Chinese Medicine

Section I
Red Blood Cell Disorders

1 Anemias

Anemia refers to a decrease in the number of red blood cells (RBCs) or hemoglobin (Hgb) content. Because there are fewer RBCs or less Hgb in anemic patients to carry oxygen from the lungs to the tissues of the body, tissue hypoxia ensues. Symptoms are characteristic of a cardiovascular-pulmonary compensatory response to the hypoxia. Severe anemia can be associated with weakness, vertigo, headache, tinnitus, spots before the eyes, ease of fatigue, drowsiness, irritability, and even bizarre behavior. Amenorrhea, loss of libido, gastrointestinal complaints, and sometimes jaundice and splenomegaly can occur. Finally, shock and heart failure are a possibility.

It is important to understand that anemia *per se* is not a diagnosis but rather a complex of signs and symptoms, and it is critical to determine the cause of the decrease of RBCs or Hgb content. The three basic mechanisms giving rise to anemia are the following: blood loss, decreased RBC production, and increased RBC destruction.

Blood loss often follows trauma or childbirth, and anemias due to such acute blood loss are not further discussed in this work. Within Chinese medicine, such post-traumatic or postpartum anemias fall within the province of traumatology and gynecology respectively. However, chronic blood loss, such as due to gastrointestinal bleeding or excessive menstruation, is also a frequent cause of iron deficiency anemia. One should always first consider such low-grade blood loss in patients suffering from anemia. Once it is ruled out, the two other mechanisms remain.

Hemocytoblasts are the stem cells from which all formed elements of the blood are produced. A defect at this level not only gives rise to a decrease of RBCs but also to a decrease of white blood cells (WBCs) and platelets. Aplastic anemia (AA), myelodysplastic syndrome (MDS)[1], and paroxysmal nocturnal hematuria (PNH) are all anemias due to stem cell disorders.

Once the hemocytoblast commits to the erythrocyte pathway, it differentiates into a proerythroblast which is referred to as the progenitor cell. Since the progenitor cell has already committed to the erythrocyte pathway, a disorder at this level of blood cell production does not affect other blood elements. Anemias due to such progenitor cell disorders are pure red cell anemia and anemia due to chronic renal disease.

The proerythroblast, which is a committed cell, next differentiates into what is called an early erythroblast. The early erythroblast starts on the developmental pathway of the erythrocyte and, after having differentiated into the late erythroblast, normoblast, and reticulocyte, becomes the erythrocyte which circulates in the blood. A disorder anywhere in the developmental pathway of the erythrocyte production is called an erythrocyte precursor disorder. Anemias due to such erythrocyte precursor disorders are megaloblastic anemia, iron deficiency anemia, and thalassemia.

The second mechanism, increased destruction of RBCs, can further be differentiated into three different pathologies. In the first, hemoglobin may be abnormal, giving rise to deformed RBCs which occlude small vessels and are lysed in the process. Sickle cell anemia is the most common example of hemoglobinopathic hemolytic anemias. In the second, the membrane of the red blood cell may be abnormal, giving rise to abnormally shaped RBCs. Spherocytosis (round), acanthocytosis (deformed), and elliptocytosis (elliptical) are examples of such membrane defect hemolytic anemias. And in the third, RBCs can be lysed when the immune system malfunctions and attacks its own red blood cells. Two main types, warm-reacting and cold-reacting autoimmune hemolytic anemias, are differentiated, their names referring to the temperature of maximal activity (warm: 37°C; cold: 37°C). Furthermore, hemolytic anemia can also be induced by a number of Western drugs. The following table lists anemias according to their underlying pathology.

---

[1]   Classifying MDS as a type of anemia is somewhat controversial as other, well-respected textbooks sometimes add it to the category of white blood cell disorders on the basis that MDS can be considered a pre-leukemic disease. It is grouped with the anemias in this book following the example of *Essential Pathology*. The main clinical signs in all types of MDS are anemia signs with varying degrees of leukopenia and thrombocytopenia. Furthermore, four of the five FAB types of MDS (see section 1.2 below) are types of refractory anemias, *i.e.*, the anemia is not responsive to iron, folic acid, vitamin B$_{12}$, or any other hematinic therapy. The MDS disease type termed Chronic Myelomonocytic Leukemia (CMML), the type most obviously differing from anemias, is actually controversial in regard to its classification as an MDS. Only blood and bone marrow abnormalities resemble other types of MDS. Therefore, on clinical grounds, CMML is more closely related to chronic myeloproliferative disorders.

Decreased RBC production		Increased RBC destruction	
Stem cell disorders	Aplastic Anemia MDS PNH	Hemoglobinopathies	Sickle cell anemia
Progenitor cell disorders	Pure Red Cell Anemia Anemia due to chronic renal disease	Abnormally shaped RBCs	Spherocytosis, Acanthocytosis, Elliptocytosis
Erythrocyte precursor disorders	Megaloblastic anemia Iron deficiency anemia Thalassemia	Immunologically induced	Warm reacting autoimmuune anemia Cold reacting autoimmuune anemia

1.1 Aplastic Anemia

Aplastic anemia (AA) is a chronic disorder of the hemopoietic stem cells that results in the cellular depletion of the bone marrow and pancytopenia (a decrease in all circulating elements). Aplastic anemia is most common in adolescents and young adults. In most cases, no cause is found for the bone marrow aplasia. In a few cases, a variety of drugs, including chemotherapeutic agents, benzene, and even non-steroidal anti-inflammatory agents (NSAIDs), as well as ionizing radiation or certain viruses may precipitate the onset of disease. In such cases, a genetic component is believed to exist. Even though the cause for AA is not clear, since this condition can be cured by bone marrow transplantation, the defect must be intrinsic in the hemopoietic cells (the cells giving rise to the formed elements of the blood). Furthermore, the successful use of anti-T-lymphocyte antibodies in the treatment of AA suggests that there is an immunologic component to either the pathogenesis or the subsequent progression of this disease.

In terms of pathology, the bone marrow in AA is, to a large extent, replaced by fat. The anemia is usually macrocytic[2] with an increased erythrocyte content of fetal hemoglobin, and erythropoietin levels in the blood tend to be high. Because this disorder affects the stem cell in the marrow, all formed elements of the blood are depleted (pancytopenia). This means that patients suffering from AA are immuno-compromised (lack of WBCs) and have a tendency to bleed (decreased platelet count).

Signs vary with the severity of the pancytopenia, and general symptoms of anemia are usually severe. A waxy pallor of the skin and mucous membranes is characteristic. Splenomegaly is mostly absent. Thrombocytopenia leads to bleeding into the skin and mucous membranes, and hemorrhages into the ocular fundi are frequent. Life-threatening infections are common. Untreated patients with severe AA have a median survival of 3-6 months, and only 20% survive one year. Western medical treatment focuses on the

---

[2]   Macrocytic refers to abnormally large red blood cells (*i.e.*, more than 10 microns in diameter).

therapeutic use of blood components, immuno-suppressive agents, and eventual bone marrow transplantation.

Chinese medical disease explanation:

In Chinese medicine, aplastic anemia is divided into chronic and acute types, a distinction not frequently found in modern Western medicine. Chronic aplastic anemia manifests with a prolonged history and primarily symptoms of anemia. Bleeding is only slight and mainly limited to the external parts of the body, and infections are not severe and are easily controlled. This corresponds to the Chinese medical categories of vacuity taxation (*xu lao*), blood vacuity (*xue xu*), and bleeding conditions (*xue zheng*). The basic disease mechanism is an underlying kidney vacuity essence detriment. Because essence is one of the material components in the production of blood, if essence is depleted, blood cannot be engendered sufficiently. In addition, kidney yang is the foundation of all yang in the body, supporting and empowering all warm transformations. In particular, former heaven yang bolsters and supports latter heaven yang. Thus, kidney yang vacuity may reach the spleen, causing compromise to and weakness of the spleen's functions of engenderment and transformation. This then also contributes to blood vacuity. Furthermore, if both the former and latter heaven roots are vacuous and insufficient, then the heart and lung qi, *i.e.*, the ancestral qi, also becomes vacuous, leading to a loss of strength of blood movement. Therefore, not only is the blood vacuous and insufficient, but it also tends to become inhibited and static. To make matters worse, insufficiency of lung qi also leads to easy and recurrent contraction of external evils, since the lungs govern the defensive qi. If evils enter the body and transform into heat, they cause even further detriment and consumption of the qi and blood, yin and yang. Thus, three main patterns are differentiated in chronic aplastic anemia: 1) yin vacuity, 2) yang vacuity, and 3) yin and yang dual vacuity. Hence, treatment should focus on enriching and invigorating the kidneys and fortifying the spleen, assisted by quickening the blood and transforming stasis. If heat evils have assailed the body, it is also important to clear heat and resolve toxins.

Acute aplastic anemia, on the other hand, belongs to the Chinese medical categories of warm heat (*wen re*), acute taxation (*ji lao*), heat taxation (*re lao*), and bleeding conditions (*xue zheng*). It manifests with sudden onset of high fever, severe and life-threatening infections, severe bleeding diathesis (including bleeding of internal organs), and pronounced symptoms of anemia. Similar to chronic anemia, the main Chinese disease mechanism here is kidney depletion with essence vacuity. This leads to generalized qi and blood vacuity and consequent contraction of evil heat. Modern Chinese medical authors say that radiation and Western drugs as well as viruses may all be counted as disease evils. Once in the body, these evils transform into heat and deplete and cause detriment to essence and marrow. Bleeding is due to either qi vacuity not containing the blood or frenetic movement due to hot blood. Because the blood spills outside the vessels and the qi becomes too weak to move the blood, the blood becomes static. Thus, the most common pattern of acute aplastic anemia is yin vacuity marrow depletion with exuberance of toxic heat evils and blood stasis. The treatment principles in this case need to focus on enriching the kidneys and nourishing the essence, clearing heat and resolving toxins, and quickening the blood and transforming stasis.

Treatment based on pattern discrimination:

A. Chronic aplastic anemia

1. Kidney yang vacuity pattern

Main symptoms: A lusterless, sallow yellow facial complexion, bodily emaciation, dizziness, lack of strength, heart palpitations, shortness of breath, fear of cold, cold hands and feet, lumbar aching, profuse urination, loose stools, fat but vacuous body, puffy swellings of the lower limbs, subcutaneous purple patches dispersed on the four limbs, profuse menstruation in women, no or only low-grade fever, a pale, enlarged tongue with teeth-marks on its edges, and a deep, fine pulse

Treatment principles: Warm the kidneys and reinforce yang, replenish essence and supplement the marrow

Chinese medicinal formulas:

ZAI ZHANG BU YANG TANG (Aplastic Anemia Supplement Yang Formula)
Radix Pseudostellariae Heterophyllae (*Tai Zi Shen*), Radix Astragali Membranacei (*Huang Qi*), Fructus Psoraleae Corylifoliae (*Bu Gu Zhi*), Rhizoma Polygonati (*Huang Jing*), Herba Cistanchis Deserticolae (*Rou Cong Rong*), Herba Agrimoniae Pilosae (*Xian He Cao*), Caulis Milletiae Seu Spatholobi (*Ji Xue Teng*), Radix Angelicae Sinensis (*Dang Gui*), Herba Epimedii (*Yin Yang Huo*), Cortex Cinnamomi Cassiae (*Rou Gui*), Radix Lateralis Praeparatus Aconiti Carmichaeli (*Fu Zi*), cooked Radix Rehmanniae (*Shu Di*), Radix Glycyrrhizae (*Gan Cao*)

SHI QUAN DA BU TANG (Ten [Ingredients] Completely & Greatly Supplementing Decoction)
Radix Panacis Ginseng (*Ren Shen*), Rhizoma Atractylodis Macrocephalae (*Bai Zhu*), Sclerotium Poriae Cocos (*Fu Ling*), Radix Glycyrrhizae (*Gan Cao*), Radix Angelicae Sinensis (*Dang Gui*), cooked Radix Rehmanniae (*Shu Di*), Radix Ligustici Wallichii

(*Chuan Xiong*), Radix Albus Paeoniae Lactiflorae (*Bai Shao*), Cortex Cinnamomi Cassiae (*Rou Gui*), Radix Astragali Membranacei (*Huang Qi*)

LU RONG WAN (Deer Antler Pills)

Cornu Parvum Cervi (*Lu Rong*), Radix Lateralis Praeparatus Aconiti Carmichaeli (*Fu Zi*), Lignum Aquilariae Agallochae (*Chen Xiang*), Radix Angelicae Sinensis (*Dang Gui*), Fructus Foeniculi Vulgaris (*Xiao Hui Xiang*), Semen Cuscutae Chinensis (*Tu Si Zi*), Fructus Psoraleae Corylifoliae (*Bu Gu Zhi*), Semen Trigonellae Foenigraeci (*Hu Lu Ba*)

SHEN QI XIAN BU TANG (Ginseng, Astragalus, Epimedium & Psoralea Decoction)

Radix Panacis Ginseng (*Ren Shen*), Radix Astragali Membranacei (*Huang Qi*), Fructus Psoraleae Corylifoliae (*Bu Gu Zhi*), Herba Epimedii (*Yin Yang Huo*), Rhizoma Curculiginis Orchioidis (*Xian Mao*), Fructus Lycii Chinensis (*Gou Qi Zi*), Herba Cistanchis Deserticolae (*Rou Cong Rong*), Herba Agrimoniae Pilosae (*Xian He Cao*), Radix Angelicae Sinensis (*Quan Dang Gui*), Caulis Milletiae Seu Spatholobi (*Ji Xue Teng*), Radix Glycyrrhizae (*Gan Cao*)

HUO XUE YI SUI TANG # 1 (Quicken the Blood & Boost the Marrow Decoction # 1)

Radix Angelicae Sinensis (*Dang Gui*), Caulis Milletiae Seu Spatholobi (*Ji Xue Teng*), Herba Leonuri Heterophylli (*Yi Mu Cao*), Semen Cuscutae Chinensis (*Tu Si Zi*), Radix Astragali Membranacei (*Huang Qi*), Rhizoma Drynariae (*Gu Sui Bu*), Radix Salviae Miltiorrhizae (*Dan Shen*), Fructus Lycii Chinensis (*Gou Qi Zi*), Radix Ligustici Wallichii (*Chuan Xiong*), Rhizoma Curculiginis Orchioidis (*Xian Mao*), Herba Epimedii (*Yin Yang Huo*), Fructus Psoraleae Corylifoliae (*Bu Gu Zhi*), Cortex Cinnamomi Cassiae (*Rou Gui*)

Of all of the above formulas, this last one moves the blood the strongest and is indicated when signs of stasis, such as purple macules on the four limbs, are relatively pronounced.

2. Kidney yin vacuity pattern

Main symptoms: A lusterless, sallow yellow facial complexion, bodily emaciation, dizziness, lack of strength, heart palpitations, shortness of breath, thirst, a dry mouth and throat, low-grade fever, heat in the palms of the hands and feet, night sweats, marked bleeding, lumbar aching, limp knees, typically accompanying infections, a red tongue with scanty fur, and a rapid pulse

Treatment principles: Supplement the kidneys, enrich yin, and nourish the blood

Chinese medicinal formulas:

TU SI ZI JIAN **(Cuscuta Decoction)**
Semen Cuscutae Chinensis (*Tu Si Zi*), Fructus Schisandrae Chinensis (*Wu Wei Zi*), uncooked Radix Rehmanniae (*Sheng Di*)

JU HUA WAN **(Chrysanthemum Flower Pills)**
Flos Chrysanthemi Morifolii (*Ju Hua*), Fructus Lycii Chinensis (*Gou Qi Zi*), Herba Cistanchis Deserticolae (*Rou Cong Rong*), Radix Morindae Officinalis (*Ba Ji Tian*)

HUO XUE YI SUI TANG **#2 (Quicken the Blood & Boost the Marrow Decoction # 2)**
Radix Angelicae Sinensis (*Dang Gui*), Caulis Milletiae Seu Spatholobi (*Ji Xue Teng*), Herba Leonuri Heterophylli (*Yi Mu* Cao), Semen Cuscutae Chinensis (*Tu Si Zi*), Radix Astragali Membranacei (*Huang Qi*), Rhizoma Drynariae (*Gu Sui Bu*), Radix Salviae Miltiorrhizae (*Dan Shen*), Fructus Lycii Chinensis (*Gou Qi Zi*), Radix Ligustici Wallichii (*Chuan Xiong*), cooked Radix Rehmanniae (*Shu Di*), uncooked Radix Rehmanniae (*Sheng Di*), Fructus Ligustri Lucidi (*Nu Zhen Zi*), Herba Ecliptae Prostratae (*Han Lian Cao*), Cortex Radicis Moutan (*Dan Pi*)

Like the similarly named formula above, this is a relatively strong blood-moving formula and, therefore, is particularly indicated if blood stasis symptoms are present.

3. Yin & yang dual vacuity pattern

Main symptoms: A lusterless, sallow yellow facial complexion, bodily emaciation, dizziness, lack of strength, heart palpitations, shortness of breath, lumbar aching, long, clear urination, loose stools or constipation, subcutaneous purple macules dispersed on the four limbs, profuse menstruation in women, seminal emission in men, a dry mouth and throat, low-grade fever, possibly heat in the palms of the hands and feet, night sweats, low to medium-grade infections, a red tongue with scanty fur or a pale, enlarged tongue with teeth-marks on its edges, and a fine, forceless, possibly slightly rapid pulse

Treatment principles: Enrich yin and invigorate yang, boost the qi and nourish the blood

Chinese medicinal formulas:

WA NA BU TIAN WAN **(Seal Penis Heavenly Supplementing Pills)**
Testes Et Penis Otariae (*Wa Na Qi* [*Hai Gou Shen*]), Radix Panacis Ginseng (*Ren Shen*), Sclerotium Poriae Cocos (*Fu Ling*), Radix Angelicae Sinensis (*Dang Gui*), Radix Ligustici Wallichii (*Chuan Xiong*), Fructus Lycii Chinensis (*Gou Qi Zi*), Fructus Foeniculi Vulgaris (*Xiao Hui Xiang*), Rhizoma Atractylodis Macrocephalae

(*Bai Zhu*), mixed-fried Radix Glycyrrhizae (*Gan Cao*), Radix Auklandiae Lappae (*Mu Xiang*), Sclerotium Pararadicis Poriae Cocos (*Fu Shen*), Radix Albus Paeoniae Lactiflorae (*Bai Shao*), Radix Astragali Membranacei (*Huang Qi*), cooked Radix Rehmanniae (*Shu Di*), Cortex Eucommiae Ulmoidis (*Du Zhong*), Radix Achyranthis Bidentatae (*Niu Xi*), Fructus Psoraleae Corylifoliae (*Bu Gu Zhi*), Fructus Meliae Toosendan (*Chuan Lian Zi*), Radix Polygalae Tenuifoliae (*Yuan Zhi*), Semen Juglandis Regiae (*Hu Tao Ren*), Lignum Aquilariae Agallochae (*Chen Xiang*)

TU SI JIAN (Cuscuta Decoction)
Radix Panacis Ginseng (*Ren Shen*), Radix Dioscoreae Oppositae (*Shan Yao*), Radix Angelicae Sinensis (*Dang Gui*), Semen Cuscutae Chinensis (*Tu Si Zi*), Fructus Zizyphi Jujubae (*Da Zao*), Sclerotium Poriae Cocos (*Fu Ling*), mix-fried Radix Glycyrrhizae (*Gan Cao*), Radix Polygalae Tenuifoliae (*Yuan Zhi*), Cornu Deglatinatum Cervi (*Lu Jiao Shuang*)

This formula focuses strongly on supplementing the spleen and is, therefore, indicated if spleen vacuity signs are pronounced.

MU GUA SAN (Chaenomeles Powder)
Fructus Chaenomelis Lagenariae (*Mu Gua*), Os Suis (*Zhu Gu*), Cortex Radicis Acanthopanacis Gracilistylis (*Wu Jia Pi*), Radix Angelicae Sinensis (*Dang Gui*), Ramulus Loranthi Seu Visci (*Sang Ji Shen*), Semen Ziziphi Spinosae (*Suan Zao Ren*), Radix Panacis Ginseng (*Ren Shen*), Semen Biotae Orientalis (*Bai Zi Ren*), Radix Astragali Membranacei (*Huang Qi*), mix-fried Radix Glycyrrhizae (*Gan Cao*), uncooked Rhizoma Zingiberis (*Sheng Jiang*)

This formula strongly nourishes the blood and supplements the qi. It is indicated for severe qi and blood vacuity not nourishing the sinews and bones with manifestations such as hypertonicity of the hands and feet, pain of the ten fingernails, a shrunken and contracted tongue, and greenish blue lips.

BU TIAN DA ZAO WAN (Supplementing Heaven Great Construction Pills)
Radix Panacis Ginseng (*Ren Shen*), mix-fried Radix Astragali Membranacei (*Huang Qi*), Rhizoma Atractylodis Macrocephalae (*Bai Zhu*), Radix Angelicae Sinensis (*Dang Gui*), Semen Zizyphi Spinosae (*Suan Zao Ren*), Radix Polygalae Tenuifoliae (*Yuan Zhi*), Radix Albus Paeoniae Lactiflorae (*Bai Shao*), Sclerotium Poriae Cocos (*Fu Ling*), Fructus Lycii Chinensis (*Gou Qi Zi*), cooked Radix Rehmanniae (*Shu Di*), Placenta Hominis (*Zi He Che*), Cervi Cornu (*Lu Jiao*), Plastrum Testudinis (*Gui Ban*)

Because this formula contains ingredients to supplement and boost all five viscera, it is appropriate for use when there is severe vacuity involving all the viscera.

HUO XUE YI SUI TANG SAN HAO (Quicken the Blood & Boost the Marrow Decoction # 3)

Radix Angelicae Sinensis (*Dang Gui*), Caulis Milletiae Seu Spatholobi (*Ji Xue Teng*), Herba Leonuri Heterophylli (*Yi Mu Cao*), Semen Cuscutae Chinensis (*Tu Si Zi*), Radix Astragali Membranacei (*Huang Qi*), Rhizoma Drynariae (*Gu Sui Bu*), Radix Salviae Miltiorrhizae (*Dan Shen*), Fructus Lycii Chinensis (*Gou Qi Zi*), Radix Ligustici Wallichii (*Chuan Xiong*), uncooked Radix Rehmanniae (*Sheng Di*), cooked Radix Rehmanniae (*Shu Di*), Fructus Psoraleae Corylifoliae (*Bu Gu Zhi*), Radix Codonopsitis Pilosulae (*Dang Shen*), Radix Polygoni Multiflori (*He Shou Wu*)

TIAN GU SUI JIAN (Bone Marrow Replenishing Decoction)

Sclerotium Poriae Cocos (*Fu Ling*), Fructus Corni Officinalis (*Shan Zhu Yu*), Radix Angelicae Sinensis (*Dang Gui*), Radix Morindae Officinalis (*Ba Ji Tian*), Fructus Schisandrae Chinensis (*Wu Wei Zi*), Radix Panacis Ginseng (*Ren Shen*), Radix Polygalae Tenuifoliae (*Yuan Zhi*), Cortex Cinnamomi Cassiae (*Gui Xin*), Radix Lateralis Praparatus Aconiti Carmichaeli (*Fu Zi*), Semen Cuscutae Chinensis (*Tu Si Zi*), Tuber Asparagi Cochinensis (*Tian Men Dong*), Semen Germinatus Glycinis (*Da Dou Huang Juan*), Herba Cistanchis Deserticolae (*Rou Cong Rong*), Herba Dendrobii (*Shi Hu*), Folium Pyrrosiae (*Shi Wei*), uncooked Radix Rehmanniae (*Sheng Di*), bovine marrow (*Niu Sui*)

SHOU WU DI HUANG TANG (Polygonum Multiflorum & Rehmannia Decoction)

Radix Polygoni Multiflori (*He Shou Wu*), cooked Radix Rehmanniae (*Shu Di*), Fructus Ligustri Lucidi (*Nu Zhen Zi*), Radix Angelicae Sinensis (*Dang Gui*), Semen Cuscutae Chinensis (*Tu Si Zi*), Herba Epimedii (*Xian Ling Pi*), Fructus Psoraleae Corylifoliae (*Bu Gu Zhi*), Radix Codonopsitis Pilosulae (*Dang Shen*), Rhizoma Atractylodis Macrocephalae (*Bai Zhu*), Sclerotium Poriae Cocos (*Fu Ling*), Caulis Milletiae Seu Spatholobi (*Ji Xue Teng*), Radix Salviae Miltiorrhizae (*Dan Shen*), Radix Rubiae Cordifoliae (*Qian Cao*), Radix Glycyrrhizae (*Gan Cao*)

Additions & subtractions: For profuse sweating due to qi vacuity, add Radix Astragali Membranacei (*Huang Qi*) and Radix Albus Paeoniae Lactiflorae (*Bai Shao*). For upper respiratory tract infections, add Flos Lonicerae Japonicae (*Jin Yin Hua*), Fructus Forsythiae Suspensae (*Lian Qiao*), and Folium Daqingye (*Da Qing Ye*). For decreased food intake, add Endothelium Corneum Gigeriae Galli (*Ji Nei Jin*), Massa Medica Fermentata (*Shen Qu*), and Fructus Crataegi (*Shan Zha*).

All of the above patterns can be benefitted by administering the following short formula:

SHEN MA LU RONG SAN **(Ginseng, Strychnos & Deer Antler Powder)**

Radix Panacis Ginseng (*Hong Ren Shen*), processed Semen Strychnotis (*Ma Qian Zi*)[3], Cornu Parvum Cervi (*Lu Rong*)

B. Acute aplastic anemia

Yin vacuity marrow depletion, exuberance of toxic heat & blood stasis pattern

Main symptoms: Shortage of qi[4], laziness to speak, decreased activity, heart palpitations, shortness of breath upon activity, severe bleeding into the skin and membranes or, if very severe, bleeding of internal organs, vexation and agitation, a red face and cheeks, high fever, a dry mouth and throat, thirst with a desire for cool drinks, sores in the mouth and on the tongue, dry, bound stools, short, reddish urination, a pale or crimson tongue body with yellow fur, and a fine, rapid or vacuous, large, forceless pulse. If severe, there may be spirit clouding, deranged speech, and a crimson tongue with raised prickles and purple and black macules.

Treatment principles: Enrich yin and clear heat, transform stasis and engender the blood, clear heat and resolve toxins

---

[3] Processing Semen Strychnotis (*Ma Qian Zi*): *Ma Qian Zi* has the traditional functions of invigorating yang and securing the kidneys. Recent research has shown that it can also excite the spinal cord nerves, improve microcirculation of the bone marrow, and thus increase the marrow's production of blood cells and platelets. However, *Ma Qian Zi* is a very toxic medicinal, and the correct processing is of great importance to reduce its toxicity without damaging its therapeutic functions. Therefore, one should boil 500g of uncooked *Ma Qian Zi* and 50g of Semen Phaseoli Radiati (*Lu Dou*) in 3 liters of water. Cook until the beans have completely split (*i.e.*, opened). Remove the *Ma Qian Zi* and drop them in cold water. Dispose of the mung beans and water. With a knife, scrape off the fur from the *Ma Qian Zi* and let them air dry. Then, take sand, put it in a pot, and stir-fry until hot. Add in the *Ma Qian Zi* and stir-fry until the seeds become yellow-brown. Sift the sand in order to separate back out the *Ma Qian Zi*. This method of preparation reduces the toxicity of *Ma Qian Zi*. Nevertheless, one must still be very careful to use this medicinal in small amounts. Recommended dosages for the internal use of this medicinal is 0.3-0.6g per day. However, overdoses with such manifestations as crawling sensations in the cervical area, difficulty swallowing, and irritability have been recorded with as little as 50mg of this medicinal per day

[4] Shortage of qi refers to weak, short, hasty breathing, a weak voice, and a tendency to take deep breaths in order to continue speaking. It is a sign of visceral qi vacuity. When shortness of breath is due to a vacuity disease mechanism, it is usually accompanied by shortage of qi, although these are, strictly speaking, not one and the same thing.

Chinese medicinal formulas:

MAI DONG QIN DAN TANG (**Ophiopogon, Scutellaria & Salvia Decoction**)
Tuber Ophiopogonis Japonici (*Mai Dong*), Fructus Ligustri Lucidi (*Nu Zhen Zi*), Radix Polygoni Multiflori (*He Shou Wu*), Semen Cuscutae Chinensis (*Tu Si Zi*), Herba Epimedii (*Yin Yang Huo*), Radix Salviae Miltiorrhizae (*Dan Shen*), uncooked Radix Rehmanniae (*Sheng Di*), Caulis Milletiae Seu Spatholobi (*Ji Xue Teng*), Herba Agrimoniae Pilosae (*Xian He Cao*), Radix Pseudoginseng (*San Qi*), Flos Lonicerae Japonicae (*Jin Yin Hua*), Radix Scutellariae Baicalensis (*Huang Qin*), Radix Glycyrrhizae (*Gan Cao*)

Additions & subtractions: For severe bleeding, add uncooked Pollen Typhae (*Pu Huang*), Radix Rubiae Cordifoliae (*Qian Cao*), and Fructus Gardeniae Jasminoidis (*Zhi Zi*). For profuse sweating due to qi vacuity, add Radix Astragali Membranacei (*Huang Qi*). For accompanying manifestations of spleen vacuity, such as decreased appetite, add Rhizoma Atractylodis Macrocephalae (*Bai Zhu*), Sclerotium Poriae Cocos (*Fu Ling*), Endothelium Corneum Gigeriae Galli *(Ji Nei Jin)*, and Massa Medica Fermentata (*Shen Qu*).

HUANG QI TANG (**Astragalus Decoction**)
Radix Astragali Membranacei (*Huang Qi*), Cortex Radicis Lycii Chinensis (*Di Gu Pi*), Carapax Amydae Sinensis (*Bie Jia*), mix-fried Radix Glycyrrhizae (*Gan Cao*), Tuber Ophiopogonis Japonici (*Mai Men Dong*), Ramulus Cinnamomi Cassiae (*Gui Zhi*)

REN SHEN TANG (**Ginseng Decoction**)
Radix Panacis Ginseng (*Ren Shen*), Cortex Radicis Lycii Chinensis (*Di Gu Pi*), Herba Artemisiae Apiaceae (*Qing Hao*), Fructus Gardeniae Jasminoidis (*Zhi Zi*), mix-fried Radix Glycyrrhizae (*Gan Cao*)

LIANG XUE JIE DU TANG (**Cool the Blood & Resolve Toxins Decoction**)
Uncooked Radix Rehmanniae (*Sheng Di*), Gypsum Fibrosum (*Shi Gao*), Rhizoma Anemarrhenae Asphodeloidis (*Zhi Mu*), Radix Lithospermi Seu Arnebiae (*Zi Cao*), Herba Cephalanoploris Segeti *(Xiao Ji)*, Herba Taraxaci Mongolici Cum Radice (*Pu Gong Ying)*, Radix Glycyrrhizae (*Gan Cao*)

JIE DU LIANG XUE TANG (**Resolve Toxins & Cool the Blood Decoction**)
Uncooked Radix Rehmanniae (*Sheng Di*), Radix Isatidis Seu Baphicacanthi (*Ban Lan Gen*), Radix Achyranthis Bidentatae (*Niu Xi*), Radix Rubrus Paeoniae Lactiflorae (*Chi Shao*), Rhizoma Guanzhong (*Guan Zhong*), Herba Cephalanoploris Segeti (*Xiao Ji*), Herba Taraxaci Mongolici Cum Radice (*Pu Gong Ying*), Gypsum Fibrosum (*Shi Gao*), Radix Lithospermi Seu Arnebiae (*Zi Cao*), Radix Raphontici Seu Echinopsis (*Lou Lu*),

Radix Pseudostellariae Heterophyllae (*Tai Zi Shen*), Rhizoma Anemarrhenae Asphodeloidis (*Zhi Mu*), Radix Glycyrrhizae (*Gan Cao*)

Additions & subtractions: For severe bleeding, add Cortex Radicis Moutan (*Dan Pi*) and Herba Agrimoniae Pilosae (*Xian He Cao*). For constipation, add Radix Et Rhizoma Rhei (*Da Huang*) and Mirabilitum (*Mang Xiao*). For clouding of the spirit with delirium, add *An Gong Niu Huang Wan* (Spirit-quieting Bezoar Pills).

1.2 Myelodysplastic Syndrome (MDS)

Myelodysplastic syndrome (MDS) is a type of anemia resulting from clonal proliferation of abnormal stem cells. As such, it is very similar to aplastic anemia. All the symptoms of MDS result from pancytopenia of varying severity. The cause of this disease is obscure, but some patients have evidence of exposure to toxic chemicals. Benzene is the best defined of these agents. Furthermore, the use of alkylating chemotherapeutic drugs is also associated with a risk of subsequent MDS.

Pathologically, the bone marrow is normal or hypercellular, and, because of ineffective hemopoiesis, there are variable cytopenias (cell deficiencies), the most frequently seen being anemia. Extramedullary hemopoiesis can be seen with a subsequent enlargement of the spleen and liver. The WBC count may be normal, increased, or decreased.

Clinical manifestations are highly variable. Myelodysplastic syndrome may smolder for years and require only occasional transfusions or antibiotics for infections. However, this disorder transforms into acute myelogenic leukemia (AML) in 20-40% of patients. Western medical treatment so far is only experimental, and the use of chemotherapeutic agents has been largely ineffective. Therefore, Western medical therapy focuses on supportive care with RBC transfusions as indicated, platelet transfusions for bleeding, and antibiotic therapy for episodes of infection.

Myelodysplastic syndrome is commonly classified according to the FAB (French-American-British) system, and classification is strongly related to development of AML. The following table shows both this classification system and associated prognosis in different types of MDS.

Refractory anemia (RA)	Patients may survive for several years with expected median survivals of 2 to 3 years. Less likely to demonstrate progression to the more aggressive forms and patients may die from unrelated causes.
RA with sideroblasts (RA-S)	
RA with excess blasts (RAEB)	Median survival of one and a half years
Chronic myelomonocytic leukemia (CMML)	
RAEB in transformation (RAEB-T)	Median survival of half a year

Chinese medical disease explanation:

In Chinese medicine, MDS is related to an abnormality of the marrow. It is said that the kidneys govern the bones, engender the marrow, and store the essence. Marrow is engendered from kidney essence, and marrow itself is crucial in blood production. Furthermore, essence and blood have the same source. Kidney essence, besides being the material basis of marrow and thus blood, is also the material basis for former heaven source qi, while the spleen and stomach are the latter heaven root of qi and blood engenderment and transformation. Qi vacuity, due to either essence vacuity or spleen vacuity, leads to a lack of force of propelling the blood throughout the body, and hence the blood may become static. Such stasis may affect the bone marrow, obstructing it and thus interfering with its engenderment of essence and blood. This then creates a repetitive cycle or loop. In addition and over time, stasis and obstruction may also lead to transformative heat. The Chinese disease categories which correspond to MDS are vacuity taxation (*xu lao*), warm heat (*wen re*), and bleeding conditions (*xue zheng*).

Therefore, based on the above disease mechanisms, one pattern for MDS is qi and blood dual depletion with depressive heat. Because this is the milder one of the two patterns identified in the Chinese medical literature, it is often found in patients suffering from MDS-RA or MDS-RA-S. If the disease persists for a long time, the spleen and stomach suffer further damage. This can then lead to the engenderment of dampness which mutually binds with depressive heat, thus giving rise to the pattern of qi and blood dual depletion with internal exuberance of damp heat. This pattern is often seen in patients suffering from MDS-RAEB or RAEB-T and is usually very difficult to treat. Since it is a statement of fact that, "if there is stomach qi, there is flourishing; and if the stomach qi is lost, there is collapse," and since damp conditions are often very difficult to treat, this second pattern leads to a clinically poorer prognosis. It thus can be seen that early treatment of MDS is important and leads to much better treatment results.

According to the proceedings of the Fifth All China Scientific Conference on Integrated Chinese-Western Medicine Hematology held in 1998, Chinese doctors think that there are as yet no ideal treatments for MDS in Chinese medicine and that more research is needed to validate different theories, formulas, and medicinals. However, it is clear that the amelioration rate of treated patients is higher by combining Chinese and Western medical treatments. For example, a study by Guo Pei-jing *et al.* points out that:

> If MDS is treated with Western medicine alone, the amelioration rate is 41.2-76.9%. By using mainly Chinese medicine [assisted by Western drugs], considerably more satisfying results, with an [average] amelioration rate of 75%, can be achieved.[5]

For milder cases of MDS (*i.e.,* RA or RA-S types), good results can be achieved by using Chinese medicine alone. For the RAEB and RAEB-T types, Western drugs should certainly be added. In China, frequently used Western drugs for these stages of MDS are retinoic acid (acid of vitamin A) and stanozolol.

Treatment based on pattern discrimination:

1. Qi & blood dual depletion with depressive heat pattern

Main symptoms: A lusterless facial complexion, dizziness, lack of strength, flusteredness[6], shortness of breath which gets worse upon activity, occasional fevers, blood ejection, a pale tongue with white fur, and a deep, fine, rapid, and forceless pulse

Treatment principles: Boost the qi and nourish the blood, move the qi and clear heat

Chinese medicinal formulas:

YI SUI KANG (**Boost Marrow Health [Capsules]**)
Radix Astragali Membranacei (*Huang Qi*), Radix Angelicae Sinensis (*Dang Gui*), Rhizoma Polygonati (*Huang Jing*), Rhizoma Atractylodis Macrocephalae (*Bai Zhu*), Sclerotium Poriae Cocos (*Fu Ling*), Herba Leonuri Heterophylli (*Yi Mu Cao*), Rhizoma Dioscoreae Bulbiferae (*Huang Yao Zi*), Rhizoma Paridis Polyphyllae (*Zao*

---

[5]   Guo Pei-jing *et al.*, "Clinical Observation of the Treatment of Myelodysplastic Syndrome with *Yi Sui Kang* (Boost Marrow Health [Capsules])," *Zhong Guo Zhong Xi Yi Jie He Za Zhi (Chinese Journal of Integrated Chinese-Western Medicine)*, #2, 1995, p. 74-76

[6]   Flusteredness (*xin huang*) refers to a state of mental discomposure and confusion.

Xiu), Radix Sophorae Flavescentis (*Ku Shen*), Radix Lithospermi Seu Arnebiae (*Zi Cao*)

YI SUI CHU XIE PIAN (Boost the Marrow & Dispel Evils Tablets)

Radix Astragali Membranacei (*Huang Qi*), Fructus Ligustri Lucidi (*Nu Zhen Zi*), Radix Polygoni Multiflori (*He Shou Wu*), Spica Prunellae Vulgaris (*Xia Ku Cao*), Caulis Milletiae Seu Spatholobi (*Ji Xue Teng*), Rhizoma Curcumae Zedoariae (*E Zhu*), Radix Pinelliae Ternatae (*Ban Xia*), Semen Coicis Lachryma-jobi (*Yi Yi Ren*), Herba Solani Nigri (*Long Kui*)[7], Herba Solani Lyrati (*Bai Ying*)[8]

2. Qi & blood dual depletion pattern with internal exuberance of damp heat

Main symptoms: A lusterless facial complexion, pronounced dizziness, lack of strength, flusteredness, shortness of breath which gets worse upon activity, lingering fevers, a marked tendency to blood ejection, heavy-headedness, decreased appetite, nausea, vexation, susceptibility to oppression, a pale tongue body with slimy, yellow fur, and a slippery, rapid or floating, large pulse

Treatment principles: Boost the qi and nourish the blood, eliminate dampness, clear heat, and resolve toxins

Chinese medicinal formulas:

The same formulas as for the preceding pattern can be administered for this pattern as well. However, in this pattern, the amounts of the medicinals which clear heat, eliminate and percolate dampness, and resolve toxins should be increased. Such medicinals include Rhizoma Dioscoreae Bulbiferae (*Huang Yao Zi*), Rhizoma Paridis Polyphyllae (*Zao Xiu*), Radix Sophorae Flavescentis (*Ku Shen*), Radix Pinelliae Ternatae (*Ban Xia*), Semen Coicis Lachryma-jobi (*Yi Yi Ren*), Herba Solani Nigri (*Long Kui*), and Herba Solani Lyrati (*Bai Ying*).

---

[7] Herba Solani Nigri (*Long Kui*) is bitter and sweet, and cold in nature and enters the lungs and liver. It clears heat and resolves toxins, quickens the blood and disperses swellings.

[8] Herba Solani Lyrati (*Bai Ying*) is sweet and cold in nature and enters the heart and lungs. It clears heat and resolves toxins, disinhibits urination and dispels wind.

1.3 Paroxysmal Nocturnal Hemoglobinuria (PNH)

Paroxysmal nocturnal hemoglobinuria (PNH) is a rare disease most common in men in their 20s but possibly occurring at any age and in either sex. This disease is a type of hemolytic anemia. Red blood cells are lysed by normal complement in plasma because of a membrane defect. Its cause is unknown. Crises may be precipitated by infections, administration of iron, vaccines, or menstruation. As a clonal stem cell disease, all hemopoietic cells are affected, and thrombocytopenia and leukopenia are common.

Paroxysmal nocturnal hemoglobinuria is characterized by intermittent or sustained periods of hemolysis and hemoglobinuria, the latter being accentuated during sleep. This leads to the excretion of red urine in the morning. Other common symptoms are abdominal and lumbar pain with splenomegaly, hemoglobinuria, and hemoglobinemia. Loss of hemoglobin in the urine can lead to severe anemia, with hemoglobin levels below 5g/dL. Patients suffering from PNH are strongly predisposed to thrombotic complications, mostly affecting the deep abdominal veins. The thrombotic diathesis are poorly understood but are thought to be related to complement-mediated activation of platelets. Such arterial and venous thrombi together with complications of pancytopenia are the two most common causes of death.

Western medical treatment of PNH is purely symptomatic. The use of corticosteroids may result in controlling symptoms and stabilizing RBC values in more than 50% of patients. Transfusions containing plasma (which contains complement) should be avoided. Heparin, a drug that may accelerate hemolysis, should be used cautiously except in patients suffering from thrombosis where it may be warranted. Bone marrow transplantation has resulted in long-term remissions in some patients.

The course of PNH is variable. Some patients succumb within months of diagnosis, whereas others live for decades. Progression to bone marrow hypoplasia with all the symptoms of aplastic anemia is present in some patients. Others may develop myelodysplastic syndrome or acute leukemia.

Chinese medical disease explanation:

In Chinese medicine, PNH belongs to the disease categories of vacuity taxation (*xu lao*), bleeding conditions (*xue zheng*), and jaundice (*huang dan*). Chinese medicine divides PNH into acute and chronic (or remission) phases. The acute phase often manifests as jaundice due to excessive bilirubin in the blood (bilirubinemia) secondary to hemolysis. In Chinese medicine, jaundice is due to damp heat or damp cold smoldering internally and obstructing the free flow of bile. The jaundice of acute PNH corresponds to yang jaundice which is caused by damp heat and manifests as a vivid yellow, commonly described within the Chinese medical literature as being the color of tangerines. Such damp heat can be attributed to either contraction of external evils or internal accumulation because of problems with water metabolism.

Water metabolism within the human body relies on the proper functioning of the lungs, spleen, and kidneys. If the spleen is damaged due to eating too many uncooked, chilled, or dampening foods, then it cannot move and transform and dampness accumulates. Dampness, being a yin substance, blocks the free flow of yang qi. Over time, this transforms into heat and leads to mingling of dampness with heat, thus giving rise to damp heat. Heat may cause the blood to move frenetically and spill outside the vessels. Therefore, there is blood in the urine. Furthermore, if blood spills outside the vessels, it becomes malign and stagnates in the tissues. Thus, blood stasis often accompanies the damp heat pattern of PNH.

In chronic or remission stage PNH, anemia rather than acute jaundice is the main manifestation. This belongs to the category of vacuity taxation (*xu lao*) and mainly manifests as lack of strength, fatigue, and shortness of breath. Chronic PNH is divided into the two patterns of qi and yin dual vacuity and spleen-kidney dual vacuity. Recurrent bleeding during acute phases leads to damage of the qi and blood (or yin). Heat, on the other hand, scorches the fluids and consumes yin. Thus, after acute flare-ups, the body is left with a dual vacuity of qi and yin. Moreover, many long term chronic diseases or acute febrile diseases easily lead to a dual vacuity of qi and yin.

Dual vacuity of the spleen and kidneys can be caused by long-term disease, prolonged damage of the spleen affecting the kidneys, or congenital kidney vacuity leading to a weak spleen. A dual vacuity of the spleen and kidneys also leads to the accumulation of dampness since the kidneys are the source of the spleen yang which is necessary for the spleen's functions of movement and transformation. Furthermore, the kidneys are responsible for providing the bladder with the yang qi necessary to excrete fluids. Therefore, impairment of the spleen and kidneys can lead to accumulation of cold dampness and hence to yin jaundice. This, in contrast to yang jaundice discussed above under the acute patterns, manifests as a somber or sallow yellow, sometimes also referred to as dirty yellow complexion.

The patterns seen during the remission phase usually follow acute flare-ups of this disease, and there often is some remaining static blood. Furthermore, if qi and yin become vacuous, blood cannot be moved adequately. In the first instance, there may not be enough qi to move the blood, while in the second, the blood may be too dry. Hence both qi and yin vacuity may cause or aggravate blood stasis. In the pattern of spleen-kidney dual vacuity, dampness may obstruct the flow of blood, thus also leading to stasis.

The Chinese medical treatment of this disease is based upon the saying, "During the acute [phase], treat the tip (or branch); during the chronic [phase], treat the root." Thus, if there is acute PNH with damp heat smoldering internally, the treatment principles are to clear heat and disinhibit dampness, while during chronic PNH, treatment focuses on supplementation of either qi and yin or the spleen and kidneys. For both acute and chronic patterns, if there are symptoms of blood stasis, it is appropriate to also use blood-quickening medicinals.

Treatment based on pattern discrimination:

1. Damp heat smoldering internally pattern

Main symptoms: Tangerine-colored jaundice, soy sauce colored urine, slimy, yellow tongue fur, and a slippery, rapid pulse

Treatment principles: Clear heat and disinhibit dampness, possibly assisted by quickening the blood and transforming stasis

Chinese medicinal formulas:

YIN CHEN WU LING SAN (Artemesia Capillaris Five [Ingredients] Poria Powder)
Herba Artemesiae Capillaris (*Yin Chen Hao*), Rhizoma Atractylodis Macropcephalae (*Bai Zhu*), Sclerotium Poriae Cocos (*Fu Ling*), Sclerotium Polypori Umbellati (*Zhu Ling*), Ramulus Cinnamomi Cassiae (*Gui Zhi*), Rhizoma Alismatis (*Ze Xie*)

TAO HUA HUA ZHUO TANG (Persica & Carthamus Transform Turbidity Decoction)
Semen Pruni Persicae (*Tao Ren*), Flos Carthami Tinctorii (*Hong Hua*), Radix Achyranthis Bidentatae (*Niu Xi*), Rhizoma Corydalis Yanhusuo (*Yan Hu Suo*), Extremitas Radicis Angelicae Sinensis (*Dang Gui Wei*), Radix Rubrus Paeoniae Lactiflorae (*Chi Shao*), Radix Salviae Miltiorrhizae (*Dan Shen*), Herba Artemisiae Capillaris (*Yin Chen Hao*), Rhizoma Alismatis (*Ze Xie*), Semen Plantaginis (*Che Qian Zi*), Lignum Dalbergiae Odoriferae (*Jiang Xiang*), Crinis Carbonisatus (*Xue Yu Tan*)

This formula treats acute PNH with concurrent manifestations of blood stasis in the urinary bladder and lower abdomen, such as lower abdominal fullness, a black-colored forehead, heat in the lower legs, and black, loose stools.

YIN CHEN DI HUANG TANG (Artemisia Capillaris & Rehmannia Decoction)
Uncooked Radix Rehmanniae (*Sheng Di*), Radix Rubrus Paeoniae Lactiflorae (*Chi Shao*), Radix Ligustici Wallichii (*Chuan Xiong*), Radix Angelicae Sinensis (*Dang Gui*), Radix Trichosanthis Kirlowii (*Tian Hua Fen*), Sclerotium Rubrum Poriae Cocos (*Chi Fu Ling*), Sclerotium Polypori Umbellati (*Zhu Ling*), Herba Artemisiae Capillaris (*Yin Chen Hao*), Rhizoma Alismatis (*Ze Xie*)

This formula is particularly indicated if, in addition to the damp heat condition, there are symptoms of blood vacuity.

WEI LING XIAN FANG (Clematis Formula)
Radix Clematidis Chinensis (*Wei Ling Xian*), Ramulus Cinnamomi Cassiae (*Gui Zhi*), mix-fried Resina Myrrhae (*Mo Yao*), mix-fried Resina Olibani (*Ru Xiang*), Radix Et Rhizoma Rhei (*Da Huang*), Herba Artemisiae Capillaris (*Yin Chen Hao*), Rhizoma Alismatis (*Ze Xie*), Radix Codonopsitis Pilosulae (*Dang Shen*), Radix Astragali Membranacei (*Huang Qi*), Sclerotium Poriae Cocos (*Fu Ling*), stir-fried Rhizoma Atractylodis Macrocephalae (*Bai Zhu*), Fructus Corni Officinalis (*Shan Zhu Yu*)

2. Qi & yin dual vacuity pattern

Main symptoms: Short, reddish urination, a dark facial complexion, dizziness, tinnitus, heart palpitations, shortness of breath, torpid intake and scanty eating, vexatious heat in the five hearts, lumbar aching, knee limpness, sometimes spontaneous bleeding of the flesh with effusion of macules, a pale tongue with possibly static macules, and a fine, rapid pulse

Treatment principles: Boost the qi and enrich yin, clear heat and cool the blood, possibly assisted by quickening the blood and transforming stasis

Chinese medicinal formulas:

LIU WEI DI MAI YIN (Six Flavors Rehmannia & Ophiopogon Drink)
Cooked Radix Rehmanniae (*Shu Di*), Sclerotium Poriae Cocos (*Fu Ling*), Radix Dioscoreae Oppositae (*Shan Yao*), Fructus Corni Officinalis (*Shan Zhu Yu*), Cortex Radicis Moutan (*Dan Pi*), Rhizoma Alismatis (*Ze Xie*), Radix Panacis Ginseng (*Ren Shen*), Tuber Ophiopogonis Japonici (*Mai Men Dong*), Fructus Schisandrae Chinensis (*Wu Wei Zi*)

CHE QIAN YE TANG **(Plantain Leaf Decoction)**
Folium Plantaginis (*Che Qian Ye*)[9], Radix Rubiae Cordifoliae (*Qian Cao Gen*), Radix Scutellariae Baicalensis (*Huang Qin*), Gelatinum Corii Asini (*E Jiao*), Cortex Radicis Lycii Chinensis (*Di Gu Pi*), Flos Carthami Tinctorii (*Hong Hua*)

This formula quickens the blood and transforms turbidity. If this formula is used for cases not manifesting any signs of stasis, the blood-quickening medicinals should be eliminated or used in small quantity.

BU XUE YI QI TANG **(Supplement the Blood & Boost the Qi Decoction)**
Radix Panacis Ginseng (*Ren Shen*), mix-fried Radix Astragali Membranacei (*Huang Qi*), Sclerotium Poriae Cocos (*Fu Ling*), stir-fried Rhizoma Atractylodis Macrocephalae (*Bai Zhu*), Radix Angelicae Sinensis (*Dang Gui*), Radix Salviae Miltiorrhizae (*Dan Shen*), Radix Albus Paeoniae Lactiflorae (*Bai Shao*), Herba Artemisiae Capillaris (*Yin Chen Hao*), Rhizoma Alismatis (*Ze Xie*), Gelatinum Corii Asini (*E Jiao*), Rhizoma Polygonati (*Huang Jing*), Radix Polygoni Multiflori (*He Shou Wu*)

3. Spleen-kidney dual vacuity pattern

Main symptoms: A somber white facial complexion, dark colored, smoky looking jaundice, dizziness, essence spirit listlessness, shortage of qi, laziness to talk, decreased appetite, lumbar pain, knee limpness, impotence in men, long, clear urination, fear of cold, a pale, tender tongue with teeth-marks on its edges and slightly slimy, white fur, and a deep, fine pulse

Treatment principles: Fortify the spleen and boost the qi, invigorate the kidneys and warm yang

Chinese medicinal formulas:

YIN CHEN ZHU FU TANG **(Artemisia Capillaris, Atractylodes & Aconite Decoction)**
Herba Artemisiae Capillaris (*Yin Chen Hao*), Rhizoma Atractylodis Macrocephalae (*Bai Zhu*), Radix Lateralis Praeparatus Aconiti Carmichaeli (*Fu Zi*), dry Rhizoma Zingiberis (*Gan Jiang*), mix-fried Radix Glycyrrhizae (*Gan Cao*), Cortex Cinnamomi Cassiae (*Rou Gui*)

---

[9]   Folium Plantaginis (*Che Qian Ye*): this refers to the leaves of the plantago plant, and thus has similar properties to Herba Plantaginis (*Che Qian Cao*), which refers to the entire plantago plant

SHEN QI WAN (Kidney Qi Pills)

Uncooked Radix Rehmanniae (*Sheng Di*), Radix Dioscoreae Oppositae (*Shan Yao*), Fructus Corni Officinalis (*Shan Zhu Yu*), Cortex Radicis Moutan (*Dan Pi*), Rhizoma Alismatis (*Ze Xie*), Sclerotium Poriae Cocos (*Fu Ling*), Ramulus Cinnamomi Cassiae (*Gui Zhi*), Radix Lateralis Praeparatus Aconiti Carmichaeli (*Fu Zi*)

SHEN RONG GU BEN WAN (Ginseng & Antler Secure the Root Pills)

Radix Rubrus Panacis Ginseng (*Hong Shen*), Cornu Parvum Cervi (*Lu Rong*), cooked Radix Rehmanniae (*Shu Di*), Fructus Lycii Chinensis (*Gou Qi Zi*), Herba Epimedii (*Xian Ling Pi*), Radix Albus Paeoniae Lactiflorae (*Bai Shao*), Radix Astragali Membranacei (*Huang Qi*), Rhizoma Atractylodis Macrocephalae (*Bai Zhu*), Radix Angelicae Sinensis (*Dang Gui*), Radix Ligustici Wallichii (*Chuan Xiong*), Sclerotium Poriae Cocos (*Fu Ling*), Tuber Asparagi Cochinensis (*Tian Men Dong*), Pericarpium Citri Reticulatae (*Chen Pi*), mix-fried Radix Glycyrrhizae (*Gan Cao*)

LU RONG SAN (Deer Antler Powder)

Cornu Parvum Cervi (*Lu Rong*), cooked Radix Rehmanniae (*Shu Di*), Fructus Corni Officinalis (*Shan Zhu Yu*), Fructus Schisandrae Chinensis (*Wu Wei Zi*), Radix Astragali Membranacei (*Huang Qi*), Conchae Ostreae (*Mu Li*)

This last formula is indicated for PNH during periods of remission in children with decreased intelligence and slow development (*i.e.,* retardation). It is generally used for cases suffering from severe anemia.

HONG SHEN JIAN PI BU SHEN TANG (Red Ginseng Fortify the Spleen & Supplement the Kidneys Decoction)

Radix Rubrus Panacis Ginseng (*Hong Shen*), mix-fried Radix Astragali Membranacei (*Huang Qi*), Sclerotium Poriae Cocos (*Fu Ling*), stir-fried Rhizoma Atractylodis Macrocephalae (*Bai Zhu*), Radix Angelicae Sinensis (*Dang Gui*), Radix Salviae Miltiorrhizae (*Dan Shen*), Radix Albus Paeoniae Lactiflorae (*Bai Shao*), Herba Artemisiae Capillaris (*Yin Chen Hao*), Rhizoma Alismatis (*Ze Xie*), Semen Cuscutae Chinensis (*Tu Si Zi*), Herba Epimedii (*Xian Ling Pi*), Gelatinum Cornu Cervi (*Lu Jiao Jiao*)

1.4 Pure Red Cell Aplasia

Pure red cell aplasia (PRCA) is believed to be an autoimmune disease in which erythroid progenitor and precursor cells are suppressed. This leads to the absence of the formation of red blood cells and thus to anemia. However, in contrast to aplastic anemia, in pure red cell aplasia, because only the erythroid progenitor cells are involved, white blood cells and thrombocytes are not affected. This means that there are no debilitating and life-threatening infections or bleeding diathesis as is the case in aplastic anemia.

Acute PRCA often follows a viral infection and is most commonly seen in children. Infection with the human parvovirus appears to be the most common cause leading to the destruction of erythroid precursors. Acute PRCA may also be drug-induced. In these cases, the drug stimulates the formation of antibodies which then attack the erythroid precursors. Clinical signs are often not apparent in acute PRCA, except that the recovery from an infection may be prolonged. In patients suffering from underlying disorders characterized by a shortened life-span of circulating erythrocytes (such as sickle cell anemia or hereditary spherocytosis), the temporary decrease in the production of erythrocytes may cause a rapidly developing but brief anemia, referred to as an aplastic crisis.

Chronic PRCA can be divided into two types: a rare constitutional PRCA called Diamond-Blackfan anemia, and an acquired PRCA. Diamond-Blackfan anemia is usually detected in the first year of life. However, cases are known in which the characteristic changes develop in adulthood. The pathologic lesions are defective erythroid progenitor cells which are believed to be inherited. The fact that patients suffering from this type of PRCA respond so dramatically to corticosteroids suggests an immunologic component, but no firm evidence for this concept has been obtained.

Chronic acquired PRCA usually presents in middle-aged patients. Concurrent thymomas are present in 5% of all cases. In most patients, immunologic rejection of the erythroid progenitor cells can be demonstrated. The marrow of patients with acquired PRCA is usually depleted of erythroblasts, but some cases are marked by a maturation arrest with the presence of large abnormal proerythroblasts. As in the other form of chronic PRCA, corticosteroids and immuno-suppressive agents are therapeutically beneficial, inducing shorter or longer remissions. However, because the thymus seems to be so closely associated with this disease, a test (CT or MRI) for an enlargement of the thymus is often undertaken, and, if the thymus is enlarged, its removal may result in clinical remission. The medium survival in acquired PRCA is now more than 10 years.

Clinical manifestations for both types of chronic PRCA are anemia, lack of strength, somnolence, and reduced appetite.

Chinese medical disease explanation:

In Chinese medicine, this disease belongs to the category of vacuity taxation (*xu lao*) and is attributed to a relatively severe blood vacuity. However, because blood is the mother of qi, blood vacuity typically leads to qi vacuity. Thus, its manifestations usually reflect both a qi and blood dual vacuity. The reason for this dual vacuity is attributed to either former heaven kidney essence depletion and detriment if the disease arises in children or to a dual vacuity of spleen and kidneys if the disease comes on later in life. Within Chinese medicine, there are the related sayings that, "When essence is exuberant, blood is full," and, "When essence is depleted, blood is scanty." It is qi's transformative function which converts the finest essence of the bone marrow into blood. If either essence or qi are depleted, this conversion cannot take place, and, therefore, the blood is not engendered in sufficient quantities.

Furthermore, the spleen is the root of transformation and engenderment of qi and blood, but the spleen relies on kidney essence for its fortification. If the essence is depleted due to either former heaven insufficiency or kidney vacuity arising later in life, or if the spleen is weak due to faulty diet or excessive thinking, the transformation and engenderment of qi and blood loses its harmony and thus contributes to both blood detriment and qi vacuity. In addition, because essence is supplemented by surplus qi at the end of the day and since the blood and essence have the same source and transform into one another, a weak spleen also aggravates essence depletion.

Based on the above disease mechanisms, the treatment principles for dealing with this disease are to fortify the spleen and supplement the kidneys, nourish the blood and replenish the essence.

Treatment based on pattern discrimination:

Kidney vacuity-essence detriment, spleen vacuity-blood depletion pattern

Main symptoms: Progressively worsening withered, white nails, membranes, and facial complexion, fatigue, lack of strength, heart palpitations, shortness of breath, possible lymph node swelling but no swelling of the liver and spleen, a pale tongue with white fur, and a fine, forceless pulse

Treatment principles: Supplement the kidneys and replenish essence, fortify the spleen and nourish the blood

Chinese medicinal formulas:

ZI YIN GOU QI TANG (Yin-enriching Lycium Decoction)
Radix Polygoni Multiflori (*He Shou Wu*), cooked Radix Rehmanniae (*Shu Di*), Fructus Lycii Chinensis (*Gou Qi Zi*), Radix Angelicae Sinensis (*Dang Gui*), Semen Cuscutae Chinensis (*Tu Si Zi*), Herba Epimedii (*Yin Yang Huo*), Endothelium Corneum Gigeriae

Galli (*Ji Nei Jin*), Bombyx Batryticatus (*Bai Jiang Can*), Cordyceps Sinensis (*Dong Chong Xia Cao*), Radix Glycyrrhizae (*Gan Cao*)

Additions & subtractions: For severe anemia with frequent heart palpitations, hasty breathing, and a fine, rapid pulse, add Radix Panacis Ginseng (*Ren Shen*), Radix Astragali Membranacei (*Huang Qi*), Tuber Ophiopogonis Japonici (*Mai Dong*), and uncooked Radix Rehmanniae (*Sheng Di*). For reduced appetite with torpid intake, abdominal distention, and unhealthy dispersal and transformation (*i.e.*, indigestion), add Rhizoma Atractylodis Macrocephalae (*Bai Zhu*), Sclerotium Poriae Cocos (*Fu Ling*), Massa Medica Fermentata (*Shen Qu*), and Radix Auklandiae Lappae (*Mu Xiang*). For vexation and agitation, add Ramulus Uncariae Cum Uncis (*Gou Teng*), Periostracum Cicadae (*Chan Tui*), Concretio Silicea Bambusae (*Tian Zhu Huang*), and Lumbricus (*Di Long*).

SHENG XUE WAN (Engender the Blood Pills)

Uncooked Radix Rehmanniae (*Sheng Di*), cooked Radix Rehmanniae (*Shu Di*), Fructus Corni Officinalis (*Shan Zhu Yu*), Herba Ecliptae Prostratae (*Han Lian Cao*), Cortex Radicis Lycii Chinensis (*Di Gu Pi*), Cortex Radicis Moutan (*Dan Pi*), Radix Dioscoreae Oppositae (*Shan Yao*), Fructus Lycii Chinensis (*Gou Qi Zi*), Radix Polygoni Multiflori (*He Shou Wu*), Radix Albus Paeoniae Lactiflorae (*Bai Shao*), Radix Achyranthis Bidentatae (*Niu Xi*), Gelatinum Corii Asini (*E Jiao*), Radix Angelicae Sinensis (*Dang Gui*), Rhizoma Anemarrhenae Asphodeloidis (*Zhi Mu*), Fructus Psoraleae Corylifoliae (*Bu Gu Zhi*), Radix Salviae Miltiorrhizae (*Dan Shen*), Fructus Ligustri Lucidi (*Nu Zhen Zi*), Radix Astragali Membranacei (*Huang Qi*), Radix Panacis Ginseng (*Hong Shen*), Radix Pseudoginseng (*San Qi*), Cortex Phellodendri (*Huang Bai*)

ZAI ZHANG JIAN (Aplasia Decoction)

Radix Astragali Membranacei (*Huang Qi*), Radix Codonopsitis Pilosulae (*Dang Shen*), Radix Angelicae Sinensis (*Dang Gui*), Gelatinum Cornu Cervi (*Lu Jiao Jiao*), Plastrum Testudinis (*Gui Ban*), Gelatinum Corii Asini (*E Jiao*), Radix Rubrus Paeoniae Lactiflorae (*Chi Shao*), Radix Albus Paeoniae Lactiflorae (*Bai Shao*), Pericarpium Citri Reticulatae (*Chen Pi*), Radix Polygoni Multiflori (*He Shou Wu*), Fructus Lycii Chinensis (*Gou Qi Zi*), uncooked Radix Rehmanniae (*Sheng Di*), Herba Epimedii (*Yin Yang Huo*), Placenta Hominis (*Zi He Che*), Fructus Zizyphi Jujubae (*Hong Zao*)

1.5 Megaloblastic Anemia

When differentiating anemias according to stem cell disorders (aplastic anemia), erythroid progenitor cell disorders (pure red cell anemia), and erythroid precursor disorders, megaloblastic anemia belongs to the last category. The name megaloblastic, which literally means "big cell," accurately describes the red blood cells of megaloblastic anemia. Thus, this disease, according to anemic cell size differentiation, falls into the category of macrocytic anemias. The reason why the red blood cells are so abnormally large and contain segmented nuclei lies in a deficiency of either vitamin B_{12} or folic acid. Both these substances are important in DNA synthesis, and a deficiency of either one leads to defective DNA synthesis which, in turn, causes the megaloblastic transformation of hemopoietic cells. The consequences of impaired DNA synthesis, although occurring in a variety of cells in the body, are mainly expressed in rapidly dividing cells, such as those in the bone marrow (blood cells) and the gastrointestinal epithelium.

Megaloblastic anemia due to vitamin B_{12} deficiency is referred to as pernicious anemia. Vitamin B_{12} deficiency is caused by an intestinal malabsorption owing to a lack of intrinsic factor. The reason for the lack of intrinsic factor is often attributed to an autoimmune attack on the gastric mucosa and, in particular, on the gastric parietal cells (which secrete intrinsic factor). However, vitamin B_{12} deficiency can also be due to veganism, gastrectomy, overgrowth of vitamin B_{12}-consuming microorganisms (mostly happening in a surgically constructed intestinal blind loop), inflammatory and neoplastic disorders involving the ileum, and intestinal infestation of a fish tapeworm (*Diphyllobothrium latum*) that consumes vitamin $B_{12.}$

Vitamin B_{12} is stored in large quantities in the liver and a deficiency comes on gradually. However, attention needs to be paid to breast-fed babies of vegan mothers. Because the stores of vitamin B_{12} of such babies are inherently low, they may show hematologic and neurologic changes relatively quickly.

Folic acid is an essential nutrient which is present in leafy vegetables and in meat and egg products. Folic acid deficiency manifests mainly in alcoholics or in people with very poor nutrition. However, celiac and tropical sprue as well as anticonvulsive drugs, such as phenytoin, can also lead to intestinal malabsorption of folic acid.

It is important to note that, since all cellular proliferation, from the stem cell on, is defective (the impairment lies at the DNA level), patients with this condition suffer from anemia, neutropenia, and thrombocytopenia. Besides anemic signs, such as dizziness, lack of strength, heart palpitations, and shortness of breath, various gastrointestinal manifestations may be present, including anorexia, intermittent constipation and diarrhea, and poorly localized abdominal pain. Glossitis, manifesting as burning of the tongue, may be an early symptom of a deficiency of B vitamins. Marked weight loss is common. Splenomegaly and hepatomegaly may also occasionally be seen. Furthermore, some patients suffering from pernicious anemia experience degeneration of the posterior and lateral columns of the spinal cord which leads to irreversible ataxia and other neurologic abnormalities, such as a loss of vibratory sense and loss of proprioception.[10]

Western medical treatment focuses on providing the body with the deficient nutrients, either vitamin B_{12} or folic acid.

Chinese medical disease explanation:

Chinese medicine does not recognize the disease megaloblastic anemia as such. However, the symptoms of this disease closely match those discussed in the *Sheng Ji Zong Lu* (*Record of Sagely Aid*) under the rubric "cold taxation" (*han lao*), namely, a sallow yellow facial complexion, non-transformation of food and drink with heart and abdominal glomus and fullness, nausea and vomiting, and diarrhea. The neurologic symptoms present in this disease belong, according to Chinese medicine, to the categories of insensitivity (*bu ren*) and impediment (*bi*). In addition, some Chinese texts also categorize megaloblastic anemia as a species of vacuity taxation (*xu lao*).

The main disease mechanisms initially involve the spleen and, in later stages, the spleen and kidneys. Insufficient eating and drinking or one-sided eating and drinking (*i.e.*, not eating a wide variety of foods) leads to spleen and stomach vacuity weakness. The *Za Bing Guang Yao* (*Important Expansions on Miscellaneous Diseases*) points out that:

> If the spleen is not harmonious, then food is not transformed. If the stomach is not harmonious, then there is no thought of food. If the spleen and stomach are both not harmonious, then there is no thought of food and food is not transformed. [Then] there is vomiting and diarrhea, distention and fullness, acid regurgitation and belching,...

Weakness of the spleen and stomach leads to debilitation of the source of qi and blood engenderment and transformation, and this then gives rise to qi and blood dual vacuity.

The kidneys store essence, govern the bones, and engender marrow. Because essence and blood have the same source and mutually transform into each other and because marrow aids in blood engenderment, blood production, besides relying on the spleen's

---

[10] Proprioception is the awareness of posture, movement, and changes in equilibrium and the knowledge of position, weight, and the resistance of objects in relation to the body.

transformation of the finest essence of food and drink, also depends on sufficient kidney essence and marrow.

Based on the above disease mechanisms, megaloblastic anemia is thus differentiated into the three patterns of spleen-stomach disharmony with qi and blood dual depletion, spleen-kidney dual vacuity, and liver-kidney dual vacuity.

Treatment based on pattern discrimination:

1. Spleen-stomach disharmony with qi & blood dual depletion pattern

Main symptoms: A relatively lusterless facial complexion, devitalized essence spirit, lack of strength in the four limbs, no pleasure in eating, aversion to food, torpid intake, abdominal fullness after eating, diarrhea or loose stools, pale lips, a pale tongue, and a fine, forceless pulse

Treatment principles: Fortify the spleen and open the stomach, boost the qi and nourish the blood

Chinese medicinal formulas:

BU XUE TANG JIANG (Supplement the Blood Syrup)
Radix Angelicae Sinensis (*Dang Gui*), Radix Astragali Membranacei (*Huang Qi*), Fructus Crataegi (*Shan Zha*), Massa Medica Fermentata (*Shen Qu*), Fructus Germinatus Hordei Vulgaris (*Mai Ya*), Pericarpium Citri Reticulatae (*Chen Pi*), Caulis Milletiae Seu Spatholobi (*Ji Xue Teng*), Flos Carthami Tinctorii (*Hong Hua*), Endothelium Corneum Gigeriae Galli (*Ji Nei Jin*), uncooked Radix Rehmanniae (*Sheng Di*), Fructus Lycii Chinensis (*Gou Qi Zi*), Radix Polygoni Multiflori (*He Shou Wu*), Radix Panacis Ginseng (*Ren Shen*), Rhizoma Atractylodis Macrocephalae (*Bai Zhu*), Rhizoma Dioscoreae Oppositae (*Shan Yao*), Fructus Zizyphi Jujubae (*Da Zao*), honey (*Feng Mi*)

YI GONG BU XUE TANG (Special Achievement Supplement the Blood Decoction)
Radix Codonopsitis Pilosulae (*Dang Shen*), Rhizoma Atractylodis Macrocephalae (*Bai Zhu*), Sclerotium Poriae Cocos (*Fu Ling*), mix-fried Radix Glycyrrhizae (*Gan Cao*), Pericarpium Citri Reticulatae (*Chen Pi*), Radix Astragali Membranacei (*Huang Qi*), Radix Angelicae Sinensis (*Dang Gui*)

JIAN PI BU QI FANG (**Fortify the Spleen & Boost the Qi Formula**)

Radix Panacis Ginseng (*Ren Shen*), Radix Astragali Membranacei (*Huang Qi*), mix-fried Radix Glycyrrhizae (*Gan Cao*), Rhizoma Atractylodis Macrocephalae (*Bai Zhu*), Radix Dioscoreae Oppositae (*Shan Yao*), Fructus Zizyphi Jujubae (*Da Zao*), uncooked Rhizoma Zingiberis (*Sheng Jiang*), Ramulus Cinnamomi Cassiae (*Gui Zhi*), Fructus Schisandrae Chinensis (*Wu Wei Zi*), Fructus Amomi (*Sha Ren*)

Additions & subtractions: For simultaneous phlegm and dampness, add Sclerotium Poriae Cocos (*Fu Ling*), Rhizoma Pinelliae Ternatae (*Ban Xia*), and Semen Coicis Lachrymae-jobi (*Yi Yi Ren*). For accompanying blood stasis and qi stagnation, add Radix Salviae Miltiorrhizae (*Dan Shen*), Radix Rubrus Paeoniae Lactiflorae (*Chi Shao*), Rhizoma Curcumae (*Jiang Huang*), and Sanguis Draconis (*Xue Jie*). If there is accompanying seeping of blood outside the network vessels, add Nodus Nelumbinis Nuciferae (*Ou Jie*), Cacumen Biotae Orientalis (*Ce Bai Ye*), and powdered Radix Pseudoginseng (*San Qi*). If cold is severe, add Rhizoma Alpiniae Officinari (*Gao Liang Jiang*) and Fructus Evodiae Rutacarpae (*Wu Zhu Yu*).

2. Spleen-kidney dual vacuity pattern

Main symptoms: Dizziness, tinnitus, heart palpitations, shortness of breath, fear of cold, cold limbs, lumbar aching and knee pain, abdominal distention, loose stools, numbness and tingling or insensitivity of the lower limbs, a pale tongue with thin or no fur, and a deep, fine pulse

Treatment principles: Fortify the spleen and boost the kidneys

Chinese medicinal formulas:

BAI ZHU SAN (**Atractylodes Powder**)

Rhizoma Atractylodis Macrocephalae (*Bai Zhu*), Radix Angelicae Dahuricae (*Bai Zhi*), Plastrum Testudinis (*Gui Ban*), Rhizoma Atractylodis (*Cang Zhu*), Radix Ledebouriellae Divaricatae (*Fang Feng*), Cortex Magnoliae Officinalis (*Hou Po*), Ramulus Cinnamomi Cassiae (*Gui Zhi*), Radix Panacis Ginseng (*Ren Shen*), Pericarpium Citri Reticulatae (*Chen Pi*), dry Rhizoma Zingiberis (*Gan Jiang*), Rhizoma Alpiniae Officinari (*Gao Liang Jiang*), Fructus Evodiae Rutaecarpae (*Wu Zhu Yu*), Radix Bupleuri (*Chai Hu*), Fructus Zanthoxyli Bungeani (*Shu Jiao*), Radix Ligusticii Wallichii (*Chuan Xiong*), Sclerotium Poriae Cocos (*Bai Fu Ling*), Pasta Ulmi Macrocarpi (*Bai Wu Yi*)[11], Fructus Amomi (*Sha Ren*), Radix Lateralis

---

[11] Pasta Ulmi Macrocarpi (*Bai Wu Yi*) is sweet, astringent, and neutral in nature and enters the stomach and large intestine channel. It kills worms, stops diarrhea, and guides out accumulations.

Praeparatus Aconiti Carmichaeli (*Fu Zi*), Lignum Aquilariae Agallochae (*Chen Xiang*), Flos Caryophylli (*Ding Xiang*), Radix Angelicae Sinensis (*Dang Gui*), Radix Auklandiae Lappae (*Mu Xiang*), pig liver (*Zhu Gan*)

HUANG QI GUI ZHI WU WU TANG (Astragalus & Cinnamon Twig Five Materials Decoction)
Radix Astragali Membranacei (*Huang Qi*), Radix Albus Paeoniae Lactiflorae (*Bai Shao*), Ramulus Cinnamomi Cassiae (*Gui Zhi*), uncooked Rhizoma Zingiberis (*Sheng Jiang*), Fructus Zizyphi Jujubae (*Da Zao*)

3. Liver-kidney dual vacuity pattern

Main symptoms: Dizziness, heart palpitations, a thin face with a pale complexion, pale lips and nails, insomnia with profuse dreams, dry skin, hypertonicity of the sinews and vessels, tingling in the limbs, night sweats, vexation and agitation, a pale tongue, and a fine, weak pulse

Treatment principles: Enrich and supplement the liver and kidneys, nourish the blood and boost the essence

Chinese medicinal formulas:

SI WU E JIAO TANG (Four Materials Donkey Skin Glue Decoction)
Radix Angelicae Sinensis (*Dang Gui*), Radix Ligustici Wallichii (*Chuan Xiong*), cooked Radix Rehmanniae (*Shu Di*), Radix Albus Paeoniae Lactiflorae (*Bai Shao*), Gelatinum Corii Asini (*E Jiao*), Semen Plantaginis (*Che Qian Zi*), Radix Glycyrrhizae (*Gan Cao*)

DI HUANG GOU QI TANG (Rehmannia & Lycium Decoction)
Cooked Radix Rehmanniae (*Shu Di*), Fructus Lycii Chinensis (*Gou Qi Zi*), Rhizoma Polygonati (*Huang Jing*), Radix Angelicae Sinensis (*Dang Gui*), Radix Albus Paeoniae Lactiflorae (*Bai Shao*), Rhizoma Atractylodis (*Cang Zhu*), Excrementum Bombicis Mori (*Can Sha*)

BU SHEN LU RONG SAN (Supplement the Kidneys Deer Antler Powder)
Cornu Parvum Cervi (*Lu Rong*), Magnetitum (*Ci Shi*), Fructus Immaturus Citri Aurantii (*Zhi Shi*), blast-fried Radix Lateralis Praeparatus Aconiti Carmichaeli (*Fu Zi*), Fructus Corni Officinalis (*Shan Zhu Yu*), Conchae Ostreae (*Mu Li*), Herba Cistanchis

Deserticolae (*Rou Cong Rong*), Fructus Schisandrae Chinensis (*Wu Wei Zi*), Radix Morindae Officinalis (*Ba Ji Tian*), Fructus Broussonetiae (*Chu Shi*)[12]

YI JING JIAN (Essence-boosting Decoction)

Herba Cistanchis Deserticolae (*Rou Cong Rong*), Semen Cuscutae Chinensis (*Tu Si Zi*), Fructus Lycii Chinensis (*Gou Qi Zi*), Fructus Tribuli Terrestris (*Bai Ji Li*), Radix Achyranthis Bidentate (*Niu Xi*), Cortex Cinnamomi Cassiae (*Rou Gui*), Fructus Chaenomelis Lagenariae (*Mu Gua*), Radix Dioscoreae Oppositae (*Shan Yao*), Rhizoma Atractylodis Macrocephalae (*Bai Zhu*)

Additions & subtractions: For pronounced lumbar aching, add Radix Dipsaci (*Xu Duan*) and Fructus Psoraleae Corylifoliae (*Bu Gu Zhi*).

Addendum: In the early stages of pernicious anemia, the tongue is often tender, burning, and swollen. This is attributed to heart fire, and medicinals such as Radix Scutellariae Baicalensis (*Huang Qin*), Rhizoma Coptidis Chinensis (*Huang Lian*), Cortex Moutan Radicis (*Mu Dan Pi*), and Radix Rubrus Paeoniae Lactiflorae (*Chi Shao*) should be added accordingly.

1.6 Iron deficiency anemia

Iron is the most abundant mineral in the world. Iron deficiency anemia, however, is the most common of all the anemias. The two principal causes of iron deficiency are 1) a poor diet with inadequate dietary iron intake and 2) blood loss of any type. In men, the most frequent cause is chronic occult bleeding, most commonly from the gastrointestinal tract. In women, menstrual blood loss is the most common mechanism. In pregnant women, although they are not menstruating and thus not losing any blood, because of the net iron loss in the developing fetus, supplementary iron is needed and, if not administered, can lead to iron deficiency anemia. Iron deficiency in young children is mostly due to an iron poor diet. In adolescent females, it is commonly observed as a result of inadequate iron intake for growth requirements and added loss due to menstruation. The growth spurt in adolescent boys may also lead to iron deficiency anemia.

Iron deficiency anemia is characteristically a hypochromic, microcytic anemia. Signs and symptoms, besides the usual anemia manifestations of somber white facial complexion, shortness of breath, fatigue, heart palpitations, and dizziness, are pica (a craving for dirt or paint) or pagophagia (a craving for ice), glossitis (inflammation of the tongue), cheilosis (red lips with fissures at the angles), and koilonychia (thin and concave

---

[12] Fructus Broussonetiae (*Chu Shi*) is sweet and cold in nature and enters the liver, spleen, and kidney channels. It supplements the kidneys, clears the liver, brightens the eyes, and disinhibits urination.

fingernails with raised edges). All these manifestations, however, are characteristic of advanced iron deficiency anemia. Severe cases may even manifest with an esophageal web (Plummer-Vinson syndrome).

Iron supplementation for iron deficiency anemia without addressing the cause of this anemia if it is other than dietary is poor practice. Even in mild anemias, any site of bleeding should be located. Western medical treatment focuses on iron supplementation if no underlying cause of blood or iron loss can be located or once such has been corrected. As a rule, anemia should be corrected within two months. Treatment should then be continued for another six months so as to replenish tissue stores of iron. If anemia cannot be corrected, other bleeding sites may need to be sought. Furthermore, underlying infections, malignancy, or malabsorption of oral iron may lie at the center of the lack of response to treatment with iron supplements.

As shown below, certain Chinese medicinals contain iron or can help facilitate the iron absorption process. This has been shown to be much more efficacious than simple iron supplementation which is often the least effective way to correct iron deficiency anemia after the cause has been sought and corrected.

Chinese medical disease explanation:

In Chinese medicine, iron deficiency anemia corresponds to the disease categories of vacuity taxation (*xu lao*), vacuity jaundice (*xu huang*), yellow fat (*huang pang*)[13], and yellow swelling (*huang zhong*). The two viscera most closely involved in the pathology of this disease are the spleen and kidneys. It is a statement of fact in Chinese medicine that, "Blood is the essence of food and drink and is transformed and engendered in the spleen." It is also a statement of fact that, "When the middle burner receives qi and obtains fluids, what is transformed is called blood." Furthermore, Li Dong-yuan points out in his masterwork, the *Pei Wei Lun (Treatise on the Spleen & Stomach),* that, "If the spleen and stomach function lose their regulation, then this affects the production of blood." Thus it is easy to understand that if the spleen and stomach are not functioning properly, due to a spleen-damaging diet or excessive thinking or worry, qi and blood cannot be engendered. If the blood becomes vacuous, it cannot nourish and moisten the

---

[13] Yellow fat (*huang pang*) is another name for yellow swelling (*huang zhong*). Both refer to swelling of the face and ankles with a sallow yellow facial complexion, together with fatigued spirit and lack of strength. In some cases, these symptoms are also associated with nausea and vomiting of yellow water and a desire to eat uncooked rice, tea leaves, and coal. In Western medicine, this refers generally, but not exclusively, to hookworm infestation.

head and body, leading to such manifestations such as dizziness and flowery vision[14], fatigue, and tinnitus. If the blood cannot nourish the heart, palpitations arise.

The spleen and kidneys are closely related. Debilitation of one can, over time, affect the other. If there is former heaven kidney vacuity, this can lead to non-fortification of the spleen. On the other hand, a weak and debilitated spleen may lack the strength to supplement kidney yang. In both cases, one precipitates the severity of detriment of the other. Therefore, in spleen-kidney yang vacuity, there are signs of bodily cold as well as of non-transformation of food, *e.g.*, diarrhea with undigested food or simply loose stools.

A weak spleen and stomach not only leads to non-engenderment of blood but also to a lack of qi. Thus, the pattern of qi and blood dual vacuity is very similar to spleen-stomach vacuity weakness. The only difference is that there are pronounced digestive problems in the spleen-stomach vacuity weakness pattern, while digestive problems, other than possibly reduced appetite, are absent in the qi and blood dual vacuity pattern. This is because the main disease mechanisms involved in spleen-stomach vacuity weakness center on this viscus and bowel's non-transformation of food and liquids which then accumulate and obstruct the middle burner.

The liver is the sea of blood and stores the blood. Thus, any blood vacuity must affect the liver. This can manifest in either of two ways. One, there may simply present the signs and symptoms of liver blood vacuity. Two, when the liver is not nourished properly, it cannot satisfactorily fulfill its function of free coursing. Thus liver blood vacuity can also give rise, secondarily, to liver depression qi stagnation. Because qi is inherently warm in nature, this can then transform into heat, giving rise to the pattern of blood vacuity with fire and dryness.

Both the liver and kidneys and the blood and essence are said to have the same source. Thus, if liver blood is vacuous, kidney essence also typically becomes insufficient. Vice versa, because essence is the source of marrow engenderment and because the marrow plays an important role in blood production, insufficient essence not engendering adequate marrow further contributes to blood vacuity.

One last pattern of this disease which frequently appears in the Chinese medical literature is accumulation and lodging of intestinal worms. Worms accumulating in the intestines may cause detriment to the spleen and stomach by absorbing the finest essence of food and drink. The correct treatment principles for dealing with this last pattern is to kill the worms. However, because this can be damaging to the spleen and stomach, once

---

[14] Flowery vision refers to various kinds of visual disturbances, such as blurring, distortion, floaters, nearsightedness, etc. In the present instance, it refers to blurred vision and floaters due to blood vacuity.

the worms are killed, a spleen-supplementing formula usually needs to follow so as to fortify the spleen and strengthen the stomach.

Hence, there are six commonly encountered patterns of iron deficiency anemia, and Chinese medical treatment is based on these six patterns' discrimination. However, because this disease often arises due to either bleeding (be that hemoptysis, hematemesis, hemafecia, hematuria, or profuse menstruation) or due to insufficient intake/mal-absorption, it is also very important to focus treatment on the origin of this disease and address this cause accordingly by appropriately modifying the prescription selected for the pattern.

Treatment based on pattern discrimination:

1. Spleen-stomach vacuity weakness pattern

Main symptoms: Reduced appetite, loose stools, lack of strength in the four limbs, bodily emaciation, chest and duct glomus and blockage, abdominal distention, borborygmus, a sallow yellow facial complexion, pale lips, lusterless nails, a pale tongue with thin, white fur, and a deep, fine, weak pulse

Treatment principles: Fortify the spleen, boost the qi, and nourish the blood

Chinese medicinal formulas:

XIANG SHA LIU JUN ZI TANG (Auklandia & Amomum Six Gentlemen Decoction)
Radix Auklandiae Lappae (*Mu Xiang*), Fructus Amomi (*Sha Ren*), Radix Panacis Ginseng (*Ren Shen*), Rhizoma Atractylodis Macrocephalae (*Bai Zhu*), Sclerotium Poriae Cocos (*Fu Ling*), mix-fried Radix Glycyrrhizae (*Gan Cao*)

SHEN LING BAI ZHU SAN (Ginseng, Poria & Atractylodis Powder)
Radix Panacis Ginseng (*Ren Shen*), Fructus Amomi (*Sha Ren*), Rhizoma Atractylodis Macrocephalae (*Bai Zhu*), Sclerotium Poriae Cocos (*Fu Ling*), mix-fried Radix Glycyrrhizae (*Gan Cao*), Semen Nelumbinis Nuciferae (*Lian Zi*), Radix Platycodi Grandiflori (*Jie Geng*), Radix Dioscoreae Oppositae (*Shan Yao*), Semen Coicis Lachryma-jobi (*Yi Yi Ren*), Semen Dolichoris Lablab (*Bai Bian Dou*)

Besides fortifying the spleen, this formula also has the function of percolating dampness. Thus, it is indicated particularly when spleen vacuity has led to the accumulation of dampness, hence giving rise to such manifestations as generalized heaviness and slimy, white tongue fur.

LI PI YI YING TANG (**Rectify the Spleen & Boost the Constructive Decoction**)
Processed Radix Polygoni Multiflori (*He Shou Wu*), Stichopus Japonicus (*Hai Shen*), Semen Nelumbinis Nuciferae (*Lian Rou*), Semen Glycinis Sojae (*Hei Dou*)[15], Semen Phaseoli Radiati (*Lu Dou*), Radix Angelicae Sinensis (*Dang Gui*), uncooked Radix Rehmanniae (*Sheng Di*)

YONG SHOU DAN (**Longevity Pills**)
Rhizoma Atractylodis (*Cang Zhu*), cooked Radix Rehmanniae (*Shu Di*), uncooked Radix Rehmanniae (*Sheng Di*), Tuber Asparagi Cochinensis (*Tian Men Dong*), Sclerotium Poriae Cocos (*Fu Ling*), Radix Polygoni Multiflori (*He Shou Wu*), Cortex Radicis Lycii Chinensis (*Di Gu Pi*)

Besides fortifying the spleen, this formula also contains medicinals which enrich the kidneys. Thus it is suitable in the treatment of iron deficiency anemia in which the main pattern is spleen vacuity with damp encumbrance complicated by kidney yin vacuity.

ZHEN SHA WAN (**Needle Filings Pills**)
Acus Pulvis (*Zhen Sha*)[16], Cortex Magnoliae Officinalis (*Hou Po*), Rhizoma Atractylodis (*Cang Zhu*), Pericarpium Citri Reticulatae (*Chen Pi*), uncooked Rhizoma Zingiberis (*Sheng Jiang*), Fructus Zizyphi Jujubae (*Da Zao*), Radix Glycyrrhizae (*Gan Cao*), Fructus Amomi (*Sha Ren*), Rhizoma Cyperi Rotundi (*Xiang Fu*), Pericarpium Citri Reticulatae Viride (*Qing Pi*)

This formula treats iron-deficiency anemia due to spleen vacuity with damp encumbrance giving rise to yellow swelling.

JIAN PI SHENG XUE WAN (**Fortify the Spleen & Engender the Blood Pills**)
Radix Codonopsitis Pilosulae (*Dang Shen*), Rhizoma Atractylodis Macrocephalae (*Bai Zhu*), Sclerotium Poriae Cocos (*Fu Ling*), Pericarpim Citri Reticulatae (*Chen Pi*), calcined Melanteritum Rubrum (*Lu Fan*)

JIANG FAN WAN (**Melanterite Fortification Pills**)
Melanteritum Rubrum (*Lu Fan*), Rhizoma Atractylodis (*Cang Zhu*), Cortex Magnoliae Officinalis (*Hou Po*), Pericarpium Citri Reticulatae (*Chen Pi*)

This formula again focuses on dampness secondary to spleen vacuity and is better than the previous one if there are manifestations of damp accumulation.

---

[15] Semen Glycinis Sojae (*Hei Dou*) is sweet and neutral in nature. It supplements both the liver and kidneys.

[16] *I.e.*, powdered or pulverized iron needles

2. Qi & blood dual vacuity pattern

Main symptoms: A somber white facial complexion, fatigue, lack of strength, dizziness, shortage of qi, laziness to speak, heart palpitations, insomnia, essence spirit abstraction, reduced food intake, a pale tongue with thin fur, and a soggy, fine pulse

Treatment principles: Supplement and boost the qi and blood, fortify and move the spleen and stomach

Chinese medicinal formulas:

DANG GUI BU XUE TANG (**Dang Gui Supplement the Blood Decoction**)
Radix Angelicae Sinensis (*Dang Gui*), Radix Astragali Membranacei (*Huang Qi*)

REN SHEN SHAO YAO TANG (**Ginseng & Peony Decoction**)
Tuber Ophiopogonis Japonici (*Mai Men Dong*), Radix Angelicae Sinensis (*Dang Gui*), Radix Panacis Ginseng (*Ren Shen*), mix-fried Radix Glycyrrhizae (*Gan Cao*), Radix Albus Paeoniae Lactiflorae (*Bai Shao*), Radix Astragali Membranacei (*Huang Qi*), Fructus Schisandrae Chinensis (*Wu Wei Zi*)

HUANG QI SHI BU TANG (**Astragalus Ten [Ingredients] Supplementing Decoction**)
Mix-fried Radix Astragali Membranacei (*Huang Qi*), Radix Angelicae Sinensis (*Dang Gui*), cooked Radix Rehmanniae (*Shu Di*), Sclerotium Pararadicis Poriae Cocos (*Fu Shen*), Radix Albus Paeoniae Lactiflorae (*Bai Shao*), Radix Panacis Ginseng (*Ren Shen*), Rhizoma Atractylodis Macrocephalae (*Bai Zhu*), Semen Zizyphi Spinosae (*Suan Zao Ren*), Rhizoma Pinelliae Ternatae (*Ban Xia*), Pericarpium Citri Reticulatae (*Chen Pi*), Fructus Schisandrae Chinensis (*Wu Wei Zi*), Cortex Cinnamomi Cassiae (*Rou Gui*), Radix Linderae Strychnifoliae (*Wu Yao*), mix-fried Radix Glycyrrhizae (*Gan Cao*), Tuber Ophiopogonis Japonici (*Mai Men Dong*), Radix Auklandiae Lappae (*Mu Xiang*), Lignum Aquilariae Agallochae (*Chen Xiang*), uncooked Rhizoma Zingiberis (*Sheng Jiang*), Fructus Zizyphi Jujubae (*Da Zao*)

LE QIN HUANG QI TANG (**Qin's Astragalus Decoction**)
Radix Astragali Membranacei (*Huang Qi*), Radix Panacis Ginseng (*Ren Shen*), Pericarpium Citri Reticulatae (*Chen Pi*), Radix Angelicae Sinensis (*Dang Gui*), Herba Asari Cum Radice (*Xi Xin*), Radix Peucedani (*Qian Hu*), Radix Albus Paeoniae Lactiflorae (*Bai Shao*), Radix Glycyrrhizae (*Gan Cao*), Sclerotium Poriae Cocos (*Fu Ling*), Tuber Ophiopogonis Japonici (*Mai Dong*), uncooked Rhizoma Zingiberis (*Sheng Jiang*), Rhizoma Pinelliae Ternatae (*Ban Xia*), Fructus Zizyphi Jujubae (*Da Zao*)

SAN HUANG BU XUE TANG **(Three Yellows Supplement the Blood Decoction)**
Cortex Radicis Moutan (*Dan Pi*), Radix Astragali Membranacei (*Huang Qi*), uncooked Radix Rehmanniae (*Sheng Di*), cooked Radix Rehmanniae (*Shu Di*), Radix Ligustici Wallichi (*Chuan Xiong*), Rhizoma Cimicifugae (*Sheng Ma*), Radix Bupleuri (*Chai Hu*), Radix Albus Paeoniae Lactiflorae (*Bai Shao*)

This formula is indicated if iron deficiency anemia is due to excessive blood loss leading to blood vacuity with qi fall and fire harassing above. Because of fire harassing above, there are heat symptoms, such as a red facial complexion and a liking for coolness. In addition, the pulse is large but empty and vacuous upon pressure.

HUANG QI WU MEI TANG **(Astragalus & Mume Decoction)**
Radix Astragali Membranacei (*Huang Qi*), Fructus Pruni Mume (*Wu Mei*), Radix Glycyrrhizae (*Gan Cao*), Fructus Schisandrae Chinensis (*Wu Wei Zi*), Radix Codonopsitis Pilosulae (*Dang Shen*), Radix Angelicae Chinensis (*Dang Gui*), Radix Polygoni Multiflori (*He Shou Wu*), Pericarpium Citri Reticulatae (*Chen Pi*)

3. Liver blood insufficiency pattern

Main symptoms: Bodily rigidity, clouded and dark eyes, headache, dizziness, tinnitus, dry eyes, photophobia, clouded and flowery vision, rashness, impatience, irascibility, numbness and tingling of the limbs, jerking sinews and twitching flesh[17], a dry, red tongue, and a bowstring, fine, rapid pulse

Treatment principles: Nourish the blood and enrich yin, emolliate the liver and soothe the sinews

Chinese medicinal formulas:

BU GAN TANG **(Supplement the Liver Decoction)**
Uncooked Radix Rehmanniae (*Sheng Di*), Radix Angelicae Sinensis (*Dang Gui*), Radix Albus Paeoniae Lactiflorae (*Bai Shao*), Fructus Zizyphi Jujubae (*Da Zao*), Radix Ligustici Wallichii (*Chuan Xiong*), Fructus Chaenomelis Lagenariae (*Mu Gua*), mix-fried Radix Glycyrrhizae (*Gan Cao*)

---

[17] The term "jerking sinews and twitching flesh" first appears in Zhang Zhong-jing's *Shang Han Lun (Treatise [Due to] Cold Damage)*. It refers to spasmodic jerking of the sinews and flesh. This arises from insufficient blood and liquids not nourishing the sinews. Less commonly, it may also be due to cold and dampness damaging yang and thus preventing water qi transformation.

TIAO YING SAN GAN YIN (**Regulate the Constructive & Scatter the Liver Drink**)
Radix Angelicae Sinensis (*Dang Gui*), wine-processed Radix Albus Paeoniae Lactiflorae (*Bai Shao*), Gelatinum Corii Asini (*E Jiao*), Fructus Lycii Chinensis (*Gou Qi Zi*), Fructus Schisandrae Chinensis (*Wu Wei Zi*), Radix Ligustici Wallichii (*Chuan Xiong*), Semen Zizyphi Spinosae (*Suan Zao Ren*), Sclerotium Poriae Cocos (*Fu Ling*), Pericarpium Citri Reticulatae (*Chen Pi*), Radix Auklandiae Lappae (*Mu Xiang*), uncooked Rhizoma Zingiberis (*Sheng Jiang*), Fructus Zizyphi Jujubae (*Da Zao*)

Besides addressing liver blood insufficiency, this formula also contains medicinals for transverse counterflow of liver qi with chest and rib-side distention and pain which is more severe when fatigued, cumbersome essence spirit, and disquieted sleep.

4. Spleen-kidney yang vacuity pattern

Main symptoms: A lusterless, sallow yellow or somber white facial complexion, cold body and limbs, loose stools with undigested foods, fifth watch diarrhea, lumbar aching, knee limpness, torpid intake, a pale tongue with teeth-marks on its edges, and a deep, fine pulse

Treatment principles: Warm and supplement the spleen and kidneys

Chinese medicinal formula:

BU GU ZHI SAN (**Psoralea Powder**)
Cortex Cinnamomi Cassiae (*Rou Gui*), Fructus Psoraleae Corylifoliae (*Bu Gu Zhi*), Gelatinum Cornu Cervi (*Lu Jiao Jiao*), stir-fried Radix Dioscoreae Oppositae (*Shan Yao*), Radix Astragali Membranacei (*Huang Qi*), Radix Codonopsitis Pilosulae (*Dang Shen*), Rhizoma Nardostachytis (*Gan Song*), Radix Auklandiae Lappae (*Mu Xiang*), Pericarpium Citri Reticulatae (*Chen Pi*)

5. Blood vacuity with fire & dryness pattern

Main symptoms: Marked emaciation of the body and limbs, lack of strength, bone-steaming fever, afternoon tidal fever, menstrual irregularities, dream emissions, seminal emissions without dreams, a dry mouth and throat, disquieted sleep, insomnia, heart palpitations, vexation and agitation, a red tongue, and a bowstring, fine pulse

Treatment principles: Nourish yin and supplement the liver, clear heat and drain fire

Chinese medicinal formulas:

JI YIN ZHI BAO TANG (Yin's Treasure-saving Decoction)
Radix Angelicae Sinensis (*Dang Gui*), Radix Albus Paeoniae Lactiflorae (*Bai Shao*), Sclerotium Poriae Cocos (*Bai Fu Ling*), Rhizoma Atractylodis Macrocephalae (*Bai Zhu*), Pericarpium Citri Reticulatae (*Chen Pi*), Rhizoma Anemarrhenae Asphodeloidis (*Zhi Mu*), Bulbus Fritillariae Cirrhosae (*Chuan Bei Mu*), Rhizoma Cyperi Rotundi (*Xiang Fu*), Radix Bupleuri (*Chai Hu*), Herba Menthae Haplocalycis (*Bo He*), Cortex Radicis Lycii Chinensis (*Di Gu Pi*), Radix Glycyrrhizae (*Gan Cao*), Tuber Ophiopogonis Japonici (*Mai Dong*), uncooked Rhizoma Zingiberis (*Sheng Jiang*)

ZI YIN BAI BU WAN (Yin-enriching One Hundred Supplementations Pills)
Rhizoma Cyperi Rotundi (*Xiang Fu*), Herba Leonuri Heterophylli (*Yi Mu Cao*), Radix Angelicae Sinensis (*Dang Gui*), Radix Ligustici Wallichii (*Chuan Xiong*), cooked Radix Rehmanniae (*Shu Di*), Radix Albus Paeoniae Lactiflorae (*Bai Shao*), Rhizoma Atractylodis Macrocephalae (*Bai Zhu*), Radix Panacis Ginseng (*Ren Shen*), Sclerotium Poriae Cocos (*Fu Ling*), Rhizoma Corydalis Yanhusuo (*Yan Hu Suo*), Radix Glycyrrhizae (*Gan Cao*)

LIU WU TANG (Six Materials Decoction)
Radix Angelicae Sinensis (*Dang Gui*), Radix Ligustici Wallichii (*Chuan Xiong*), cooked Radix Rehmanniae (*Shu Di*), Radix Albus Paeoniae Lactiflorae (*Bai Shao*), Cortex Phellodendri (*Huang Bai*), Rhizoma Anemarrhenae Asphodeloidis (*Zhi Mu*)

6. Liver-kidney depletion & detriment with non-transformation of blood by essence pattern

Main symptoms: Dizziness, tinnitus, dry eyes, baking fever of the face, scorching pain of the ribs and rib-side, vexatious heat in the five hearts, tidal fever, bone-steaming, heat in the palms of the hands and feet, night sweats, a dry mouth and throat, lumbar aching, knee limpness, possible wriggling of hands and feet, a red tongue with scanty fur, and a bowstring, fine, rapid pulse

Treatment principles: Nourish yin and supplement the liver, replenish essence and boost the kidneys

Chinese medicinal formulas:

SI WU TANG JIA WEI **(Four Materials Decoction with Added Flavors)**
Radix Angelicae Sinensis (*Dang Gui*), Fructus Lycii Chinensis (*Gou Qi Zi*), Radix Ligustici Wallichii (*Chuan Xiong*), Radix Albus Paeoniae Lactiflorae (*Bai Shao*), Fructus Ligustri Lucidi (*Nu Zhen Zi*), cooked Radix Rehmanniae (*Shu Di*)

GUI SHAO DI HUANG TANG **(Dang Gui, Peony & Rehmannia Decoction)**
Radix Angelicae Sinensis (*Dang Gui*), Radix Albus Paeoniae Lactiflorae (*Bai Shao*), uncooked Radix Rehmanniae (*Sheng Di*), Cortex Radicis Moutan (*Dan Pi*), Sclerotium Poriae Cocos (*Fu Ling*), Radix Dioscoreae Oppositae (*Shan Yao*), Fructus Corni Officinalis (*Shan Zhu Yu*), Rhizoma Alismatis (*Ze Xie*)

BU XUE RONG JIN WAN **(Supplement the Blood & Construct the Sinews Pills)**
Herba Cistanchis Deserticolae (*Rou Cong Rong*), Radix Achyranthis Bidentatae (*Niu Xi*), Rhizoma Gastrodiae Elatae (*Tian Ma*), Fructus Chaenomelis Lagenariae (*Mu Gua*), Cornu Parvum Cervi (*Lu Rong*), cooked Radix Rehmanniae (*Shu Di*), Semen Cuscutae Chinensis (*Tu Si Zi*), Fructus Schisandrae Chinensis (*Wu Wei Zi*)

7. Accumulation & lodging of intestinal worms pattern

Main symptoms: Worm eggs or even entire worms can be found in the stools, a sallow yellow facial complexion, desiccated hair, abdominal distention, loose stools, a liking to eat and quick hungering, nausea and vomiting, abnormal liking for uncooked rice, soil, or tea leaves, lack of strength in the limbs, shortness of breath, dizziness, a pale tongue with white fur, and a vacuous, weak pulse

Treatment principles: Fortify the spleen and boost the qi, transform dampness and kill worms

Chinese medicinal formulas:

FEI ZI SHA CHONG WAN **(Torreya Seed Kill Worms Pills)**
Semen Torreyae Grandis (*Fei Zi*), Semen Arecae Catechu (*Bing Lang*), Cortex Radicis Meliae Azerdachis (*Ku Lian Gen Pi*), Caulis Sargentodoxae (*Hong Teng*), Radix Stemonae (*Bai Bu*), Realgar (*Xiong Huang*), Bulbus Allii Sativi (*Da Suan*)

GAN ZHI SAN **(Gan Accumulation Powder)**
Sclerotium Poriae Cocos (*Fu Ling*), Fructificatio Omphaliae Seu Lapidiscentis (*Lei Wan*), Os Sepiae Seu Sepiellae (*Wu Zei Gu*), Fructus Carpesii Abrotanoidis (*He Shi*), Semen Arecae Catechu (*Bing Lang*), Rhizoma Curcumae Zedoariae (*E Zhu*), Rhizoma

Sparganii (*San Leng*), Endothelium Corneum Gigeriae Galli (*Ji Nei Jin*), Flos Carthami Tinctorii (*Hong Hua*), Fructus Quisqualis Indicae (*Shui Jun Zi*)

After undergoing a course of treatment with either of the above two formulas, it is important to fortify the spleen and nourish the blood with such formulas as *Ba Zhen Tang* (Eight Pearls Decoction).

Chinese dietary therapy

Supplementation of body iron should not be sought through simple iron supplementation but can more effectively be achieved by taking in foods or medicinals which are particularly rich in iron. One method is to add iron-containing medicinals, such as Radix Panacis Ginseng (*Ren Shen*), Radix Astragali Membranacei (*Huang Qi*), Rhizoma Atractylodis Macrocephalae (*Bai Zhu*), Radix Angelicae Sinensis (*Dang Gui*), Gelatinum Corii Asini (*E Jiao*), Rhizoma Polygoni Multiflori (*He Shou Wu*), cooked Radix Rehmanniae (*Shu Di*), Rhizoma Polygonati (*Huang Jing*), Cornu Parvum Cervi (*Lu Rong*), and Stichopus Japonicus (*Hai Shen*), to commonly consumed, iron-rich foods and prepare delicious meals. The consumption of such dishes several times per week can have very beneficial effects on the iron supplementation treatment phase of iron deficiency anemia.

Chinese medical doctors in China generally hold the opinion that it is far better to consume iron rich foods and Chinese medicinals than to simply take iron supplements. Further, attention needs to be paid to eating easily digestible foods or to combine foods which contain more *wei*[18] with Chinese medicinals which promote gastrointestinal absorption (*i.e.,* move qi in the middle burner and keep the spleen and stomach from being obstructed). Below are four dishes which are especially suitable for patients suffering from iron deficiency anemia. All of these dishes contain meat. This underscores the fact that Chinese medicine does not advocate a purely vegetarian diet and that meats can have a very beneficial and important function in health and well-being.

ANGELICA, GINGER & LAMB SOUP
Cook Radix Angelicae Sinensis (*Dang Gui*), 15g, lamb meat, 75g, fresh ginger, 3 slices, and Fructus Zizyphi Jujubae (*Da Zao*), 3 pieces, in 200 mL of water and eat. Add salt as needed.

---

[18] *Wei* literally means flavor. However, in Chinese dietary therapy, it is a technical term which refers to foods that are very nutritious, typically are derived from animal sources, and are, therefore, more suitable for iron supplementation. However, foods rich in *wei* are also harder to digest.

GINSENG & CHICKEN STEW

Cook Radix Panacis Ginseng (*Ren Shen*), 10g, chicken meat, 75g, fresh ginger, 3 slices, and honey mix-fried Fructus Zizyphi Jujubae (*Da Zao*), 1 piece, in 200 mL of water and eat. Add salt as needed.

SHIITAKE MUSHROOM, TREE EARS & PORK LIVER STIR FRY

Stir-fry Shiitake mushrooms (soaked in water), 25g, Tree Ear fungus (soaked in water), 15g, and pork liver (cut into small pieces), 75g, in oil, adding salt as needed. Add a little water and cook until done.

PORK CONGEE

Cook 75g of rice in a suitable amount of water into porridge. Add pork blood and 50g of lean pork meat, a little fresh ginger, and some green onions. Cook until done. Add salt as needed.

Chinese ready-made medicines

Besides the list of iron rich medicinals given above, the following Chinese ready-made or so-called patent medicines are all high in iron content and can be used in the treatment of iron deficiency anemia based on pattern discrimination.

XUE BAO WAN (Protect the Blood Pills)

Cornu Parvum Cervi (*Lu Rong*), Placenta Hominis (*Zi He Che*), Radix Panacis Ginseng (*Ren Shen*), Radix Acanthopanacis Senticosi (*Ci Wu Jia*)[19], Cornu Bubali (*Shui Niu Jiao*), Radix Achyranthis Bidentatae (*Niu Xi*), Radix Polygoni Multiflori (*He Shou Wu*)

YANG XUE DANG GUI JING (Nourish the Blood Dang Gui Essence)

Radix Ligustici Wallichii (*Chuan Xiong*), Radix Codonopsitis Pilosulae (*Dang Shen*), cooked Radix Rehmanniae (*Shu Di*), Sclerotium Poriae Cocos (*Fu Ling*), Radix Albus Paeoniae Lactiflorae (*Bai Shao*), Gelatinum Corii Asini (*E Jiao*), Radix Astragali Membranacei (*Huang Qi*), Radix Glycyrrhizae (*Gan Cao*)

YI XUE SHENG WAN (Blood-boosting & Engendering Pills)

Gelatinum Corii Asini (*E Jiao*), Gelatinum Plastri Testudinis (*Gui Ban Jiao*), Gelatinum Cornu Cervi (*Lu Jiao Jiao*), Radix Astragali Membranacei (*Huang Qi*), Radix Codonopsitis Pilosulae (*Dang Shen*), cooked Radix Rehmanniae (*Shu Di*), Rhizoma Polygoni Multiflori (*He Shou Wu*)

---

[19] Radix Acanthopanacis Senticosi (*Ci Wu Jia*), also called *Wu Jia Shen* and known in the West under its common name, Siberian Ginseng, is acrid and warm in nature and enters the liver and kidney channels. It supplements the qi, dispels wind dampness, and levels the liver.

1.7 Thalassemia

Hemoglobin consists of four chains–two alpha chains and two beta chains. Thalassemia is an inherited disease in which the synthesis of either the alpha or beta chains is defective. It is characterized by a hypochromic, microcytic anemia owing to reduced or absent synthesis of the complete hemoglobin molecule. The various types of thalassemias are one of the most common inherited disorders in humans.

Thalassemia was originally believed to occur exclusively in the Mediterranean basin (thus it is often referred to as Mediterranean anemia), but it is now realized that it is also commonly seen in a belt extending across the Middle East, through parts of Pakistan and India, to Southeast Asia. Furthermore, sporadic mutations may produce beta thalassemia in populations where it ordinarily does not occur.

Signs and symptoms are similar in all thalassemias but vary in severity. Patients are usually jaundiced due to hemolysis of the abnormal red blood cells. The spleen is often markedly enlarged. Compensatory bone marrow hyperactivity leads to thickening of the cranial bones and malar eminences, producing characteristic facies. Long-bone involvement makes pathological fractures common. Growth rates are often impaired, and puberty may be delayed or entirely absent. The iron released upon the breakdown of the RBCs is deposited in the heart muscle, ultimately leading to heart failure, and in the liver, leading to hepatic siderosis with functional impairment and eventual cirrhosis.

The outlook for patients suffering from thalassemia varies according to the type. If the gene is homozygous, the outlook is worse. If it is heterozygous, it is better. Involvement of the beta-chain in homozygotes, giving rise to beta-thalassemia major, is the most severe type of this disease, and patients typically only live till puberty or slightly beyond. Heterozygotes, or carriers which are referred to as "minors," have a normal life expectancy.

Thalassemia minor requires no treatment. Thalassemia major is mainly treated through blood transfusions. However, because the transfused RBCs are quickly sequestered by an enlarged spleen, transfusions add to iron overload, and iron-chelation is often necessary. Splenectomy may also be of benefit if the enlarged spleen causes concurrent hemolysis of RBCs. Because of their side effects, it is important to keep the number of transfusions to a minimum.

Chinese medical disease explanation:

Little information is found in the Chinese literature on thalassemia. This is probably partly due to the fact that, as mentioned above, only a small area of southern China lies within the belt stretching from the Middle East to Southeast Asia. Thus, this disease is relatively uncommon in the People's Republic of China. Furthermore, since the symptoms of this disease resemble the symptoms of hemolytic anemia[20], Chinese doctors typically treat this disease the same as hemolytic anemia based on the saying, "Different diseases, same treatment."

In terms of Chinese disease categorization, thalassemia corresponds to the categories of vacuity taxation (*xu lao*) and jaundice (*huang dan*). Because it occurs primarily in infants and young children (it is an inherited disorder), it is thought to be due to an insufficiency in qi engenderment and blood transformation in the middle burner with an underlying constitutional weakness. Yang cannot engender yin and, therefore, there is a lack of essence and blood. Water and grains cannot be dispersed, and the finest essence which normally is transformed into qi and blood contrarily turns into water dampness, obstructing the gallbladder fluids (*i.e.,* the bile). The bile then is forced outward and spills over into the skin and flesh, leading to jaundice. Furthermore, since qi, blood, yin, and yang are all insufficient, external evils can settle in the exterior, giving rise to mixed vacuity-repletion patterns.

Chinese medical treatment of this condition focuses on boosting the qi and engendering the blood, supplementing the kidneys and fortifying the spleen, reinforcing yang and enriching yin, as well as eliminating and dispersing externally contracted or internally engendered evils.

Treatment based on pattern discrimination:

1. Qi & blood dual vacuity pattern

Main symptoms: A somber white facial complexion, fatigue, lack of strength, shortness of breath, heart palpitations, dizziness, dull yellowing of the skin and membranes, an enlarged spleen, enlarged facial and cranial bones, a pale tongue with white fur, and a fine, forceless pulse

Treatment principles: Supplement and nourish the qi and blood

Chinese medicinal formula:

---

[20] This resemblance is only true for the main symptoms of thalassemia which is not considered a hemolytic anemia. The pathologic lesion is a defect in hemoglobin production, and thus this anemia, as pointed out in the introduction to anemias, belongs to the category of decreased erythrocyte production due to a disorder in erythroid precursors.

QI XUE SHUANG BU TANG (Qi & Blood Doubly Supplementing Decoction)
Radix Astragali Membranacei (*Huang Qi*), Radix Angelicae Sinensis (*Dang Gui*), Radix Codonopsitis Pilosulae (*Dang Shen*), red Radix Pseudostellariae Heterophyllae (*Hong Hai Shen*), processed Radix Polygoni Multiflori (*He Shou Wu*), mix-fried Radix Glycyrrhizae (*Gan Cao*)

2. Yin & yang dual vacuity pattern

Main symptoms: A somber white facial complexion, lack of strength, emaciation, heart palpitations, shortness of breath, lumbar aching, dizziness, long, clear urination, seminal emission with or without dreams, yellow skin and membranes, an enlarged spleen, enlarged facial and cranial bones, possible fever, possible night sweats, a red tongue with scanty fur or a pale, enlarged tongue with teeth-marks on its edges, and a fine, forceless, possibly slightly rapid pulse

Treatment principles: Supplement the spleen and kidneys, enrich yin and invigorate yang

Chinese medicinal formulas:

SHEN FU QIANG FANG TANG (Codonopsis, Aconite, Notopterygium & Ledebouriella Decoction)
Radix Codonopsitis Pilosulae (*Dang Shen*), Radix Astragali Membranacci (*Huang Qi*), Cortex Cinnamomi Cassiae (*Rou Gui*), Radix Angelicae Sinensis (*Dang Gui*), Radix Lateralis Praeparatus Aconiti Carmichaeli (*Fu Zi*), uncooked Radix Rehmanniae (*Sheng Di*), Radix Albus Paeoniae Lactiflorae (*Bai Shao*), Radix Ligustici Wallichii (*Chuan Xiong*), Radix Et Rhizoma Notopterygii (*Qiang Huo*), Radix Ledebouriellae Divaricatae (*Fang Feng*), mix-fried Radix Glycyrrhizae (*Gan Cao*), Tuber Ophiopogonis Japonici (*Mai Men Dong*), Fructus Zizyphi Jujubae (*Da Zao*), uncooked Rhizoma Zingiberis (*Sheng Jiang*)

Additions & subtractions: For insomnia with profuse dreams and night sweats, add Radix Salviae Miltiorrhizae (*Dan Shen*), Os Draconis (*Long Gu*), Conchae Ostreae (*Mu Li*), and Radix Panacis Quinquefolii (*Xi Yang Shen*).

SHU TU XIAN LU TANG (Rehmannia, Cuscuta, Epimedium & Deer [Antler] Decoction)
Cooked Radix Rehmanniae (*Shu Di*), Semen Cuscutae Chinensis (*Tu Si Zi*), Fructus Lycii Chinensis (*Gou Qi Zi*), Radix Dioscoreae Oppositae (*Shan Yao*), Radix Codonopsitis Pilosulae (*Dang Shen*), Radix Angelicae Sinensis (*Dang Gui*), Semen Nelumbinis Nuciferae (*Lian Zi*), Herba Epimedii (*Xian Ling Pi*), Tuber Asparagi

Cochinensis (*Tian Dong*), Radix Albus Paeoniae Lactiflorae (*Bai Shao*), Fructus Schisandrae Chinensis (*Wu Wei Zi*), Cornu Cervi (*Lu Jiao*), Radix Astragali Membranacei (*Huang Qi*), Fructus Alpiniae Oxyphyllae (*Yi Zhi Ren*), Herba Artemesiae Capillaris (*Yin Chen Hao*)

This formula supplements the kidneys and fortifies the spleen, reinforces yang and engenders yin at the same time as it also courses the liver and rectifies the qi, clears heat and resolves dampness, thus receding jaundice.

Additions & subtractions: For swollen and painful lymph nodes, ductal (*i.e.*, epigastric) oppression, a fine and rapid pulse, and a red tongue tip, remove *Gou Qi Zi, Shu Di,* and *Bai Shao*, and add Radix Isatidis Seu Baphicacanthi (*Ban Lan Gen*), Fructus Crataegi (*Shan Zha*), Rhizoma Atractylodis Macrocephalae (*Bai Zhu*), Semen Coicis Lachryma-jobi (*Yi Yi Ren*), Sclerotium Poriae Cocos (*Fu Ling*), and Pericarpium Citri Reticulatae (*Chen Pi*). For coughing with scanty phlegm and a dry throat, add Radix Glehniae Littoralis (*Sha Shen*), Radix Platycodi Grandiflori (*Jie Geng*), Arillus Euphoriae Longanae (*Long Yan Rou*), and stir-fried Gelatinum Mantidis (*Piao Jiao*, ground into powder and taken as granules). For accompanying night sweats and/or afternoon low-grade fever, remove *Xian Ling Pi, Lu Jiao, Wu Wei Zi,* and *Dang Shen*, and add Radix Pseudostellariae Heterophyllae (*Tai Zi Shen*), Fructus Rosae Laevigatae (*Jin Ying Zi*), and Fructus Psoraleae Corylifoliae (*Bu Gu Zhi*). For accompanying purple-colored skin macules, a bitter taste in the mouth, and dizziness due to heart-liver fire effulgence, remove *Yi Zhi Ren* and add stir-fried Carapax Erethmochelyos (*Dai Mao*).[21]

1.8 Anemia Due to Chronic Renal Failure

Physiologically, a small amount of erythropoietin, which is secreted mainly by the kidneys, circulates in the blood at all times. When the renal cells become hypoxic due to either a lack of red blood cells, reduced oxygen availability to the blood, or increased oxygen demand by tissues, the kidneys step up their release of erythropoietin. This glycoprotein hormone then stimulates red marrow cells which have already been committed to becoming erythrocytes. Thus, the production of red blood cells is increased and the oxygen demands can be met. Conversely, kidney damage due to a wide variety of reasons leads to a decrease in erythropoietin secretion which then leads to a decrease in red bone marrow stimulation and RBC production. The resulting anemia is normocytic

---

[21] Carapax Erethmochelyos (*Dai Mao*) is sweet and cold in nature and enters the heart and liver channel. It subdues yang and downbears counterflow, settles the liver and extinguishes wind, and resolves toxins.

and normochromic[22] and is proportional to the amount of renal failure exhibited by the patient.

Two different types of hemolytic anemia may contribute to the anemia of chronic renal failure. Uremia[23] is associated with increased hemolysis. (It is believed that the retained metabolic debris of uremia injures RBCs.) Red blood cell fragmentation, called microangiopathic hemolytic anemia, occurs when the renal vascular endothelium is injured, thus damaging the red blood cells when they circulate through the renal vasculature. However, only the hypoproliferative hypoerythropoietinemic type anemia refers to anemia of renal failure.

The symptoms of this disorder are characteristic of the underlying renal disease and of moderate to severe anemia. Similarly, Western medical treatment is directed at the underlying renal disease. Administration of recombinant erythropoietin has led to the near-elimination of anemia accompanying renal failure.

Chinese medical disease explanation:

In Chinese medicine, it is recognized that this disease is a complication of an obviously prolonged and uncured primary disease. The prolonged and uncured disease damages the qi and yang and thus sets up the disease mechanism for this illness. Like so many of the anemias, the two main viscera involved are the spleen and kidneys. Kidney yang is the source yang of the body and serves as the foundation for spleen yang. Thus, if kidney yang becomes vacuous, spleen yang will become debilitated and weak. On the other hand, the spleen nourishes the kidneys via the surplus of qi and blood engendered and transformed from the finest essence of food and drink. Therefore, if spleen qi or spleen yang is weak and debilitated for a prolonged period of time, the kidneys will eventually be affected. Thus the mutual warming and nourishing of the former and latter heavens loses its harmony and disease is engendered.

In terms of pattern discrimination, two main patterns of this disease are differentiated, with the second pattern being a progression of the first with the exact same disease mechanisms. The only difference is that the second pattern is much more severe. If spleen and kidney yang become vacuous and weak, the form (*i.e.,* the body) is not

---

[22] Normocytic refers to blood of normal size; normochromic refers to blood of normal color and hemoglobin content. This means that the red blood cells are normal in this particular type of anemia; however, they are insufficient in quantity.

[23] Uremia refers to a toxic condition associated with renal insufficiency produced by the retention in the blood of nitrogenous substances normally excreted by the kidneys. Symptoms are nausea, vomiting, headache, dizziness, dimness of vision, coma or convulsions, and urinous odor of breath and perspiration.

warmed and nourished properly, the engenderment and transformation of qi and blood is decreased, and movement and transformation cannot perform their duties, thus causing water and dampness to accumulate. Dampness then spills over into the tissues, and water evils gather internally. Furthermore, when yang is vacuous, there is cold inside. Cold's nature is congealing and contracting and thus internal cold can lead to blood stasis and stagnation of turbid qi.

In the second and more severe pattern, static and turbid evils smolder internally and damage the network vessels, thus causing blood to seep into the flesh and skin. If such obstruction occurs within the viscera and bowels, bleeding from these organs may arise and death will ensue.

In general, the treatment principles for dealing with both patterns is to warm yang and supplement the spleen, transform stasis and engender blood. In the second pattern, it is further important to focus on moving water and downbearing turbidity.

Treatment based on pattern discrimination:

1. Spleen-kidney dual vacuity with blood stasis pattern

Main symptoms: A somber white facial complexion with yellow-brown spots, puffy swelling[24], cold and painful lumbus and knees, lower abdominal cold and pain, reduced food intake, constipation and/or loose stools, a pale, enlarged, tender tongue with teeth-marks on its edges and slimy, white fur, and a floating, vacuous or deep, fine pulse

Treatment principles: Warm and supplement the spleen and kidneys, transform stasis and engender blood

Chinese medicinal formula:

DANG SHEN ZI ZHU TANG (**Codonopsis, Salvia, Lycium & Atractylodes Decoction**)
Radix Codonopsitis Pilosulae (*Dang Shen*), Rhizoma Atractylodis Macrocephalae (*Bai Zhu*), Sclerotium Poriae Cocos (*Fu Ling*), Herba Epimedii (*Xian Ling Pi*), Fructus Lycii Chinensis (*Gou Qi Zi*), Rhizoma Drynariae (*Gu Sui Bu*), Semen Cuscutae Chinensis (*Tu Si Zi*), Rhizoma Alismatis (*Ze Xie*), Radix Et Rhizoma Rhei (*Da Huang*), Semen Plantaginis (*Che Qian Zi*), Radix Salviae Miltiorrhizae (*Dan Shen*), Caulis Milletiae Seu Spatholobi (*Ji Xue Teng*), Lumbricus (*Di Long*), Cordyceps Chinensis (*Dong Chong Xia Cao*), Radix Glycyrrhizae (*Gan Cao*)

---

[24] Puffy swelling (*fu zhong*) refers to swelling due to a vacuity of the lungs, spleen, or kidneys. Puffy swelling is sometimes distinguished from water swelling, with the former being due to vacuity and the latter due to repletion.

Additions & subtractions: For congenital renal cysts leading to renal failure, add stir-fried Squama Manitis Pentadactylis (*Chuan Shan Jia*) and Endothelium Corneum Gigeriae Galli (*Ji Nei Jin*). For accompanying exterior vacuity with profuse sweating, vexation, and agitation, add Radix Astragali Membranacei (*Huang Qi*), Os Draconis (*Long Gu*), and Conchae Ostreae (*Mu Li*). For accompanying infection of the urinary tract system, add Herba Lysimachiae Seu Desmodii Styracifolii (*Jin Qian Cao*) and Flos Lonicerae Japonicae (*Jin Yin Hua*).

2. Spleen-kidney vacuity detriment with blood stasis pattern

Main symptoms: A somber white facial complexion with yellow-brown spots, listless and devitalized essence spirit[25], fatigued and exhausted body and limbs, inactivity, heart palpitations, qi panting, purple lips, a pale, enlarged, tender tongue with teeth-marks on its edges and thick, slimy, white fur, and a deep, fine pulse

Treatment principles: Warm yang and move water, transform stasis and downbear turbidity

Chinese medicinal formula:

FU ZI DI HUANG ZE XIE TANG (**Aconite, Rehmannia & Alisma Decoction**)
Radix Lateralis Praeparatus Aconiti Carmichaeli (*Fu Zi*), Radix Et Rhizoma Rhei (*Da Huang*), Radix Panacis Ginseng (*Ren Shen*), Herba Epimedii (*Xian Ling Pi*), Rhizoma Atractylodis Macrocephalae (*Bai Zhu*), Sclerotium Poriae Cocos (*Fu Ling*), Rhizoma Alismatis (*Ze Xie*), Caulis Akebiae (*Mu Tong*), Flos Carthami Tinctorii (*Hong Hua*), Semen Pruni Persicae (*Tao Ren*), Radix Salviae Miltiorrhizae (*Dan Shen*), Radix Pseudoginseng (*San Qi*), Bombyx Batryticatus (*Bai Jiang Can*), Radix Glycyrrhizae (*Gan Cao*)

Additions & subtractions: For pronounced bleeding, increase *San Qi* and add Pollen Typhae (*Pu Huang*), Herba Agrimoniae Pilosae (*Xian He Cao*), Herba Cephalanoplori Segeti (*Xiao Ji*), and Herba Cirsii Japonici (*Da Ji*). For very high BUN (blood urea nitrogen), administer an enema consisting of Radix Et Rhizoma Rhei (*Da Huang*) and Mirabilitum (*Mang Xiao*). For accompanying nausea and abdominal distention, add Pericarpium Citri Reticulatae (*Chen Pi*), Rhizoma Pinelliae Ternatae (*Ban Xia*), and Radix Auklandiae Lappae (*Mu Xiang*).

---

[25] Essence spirit (*jing shen*) refers to the outward manifestation of a person's life force or vitality. In modern terms, this is sometimes referred to as the mind.

1.9 Hemolytic Anemia

Red blood cells have a normal life span of about 120 days. At that point in their life cycle, RBCs are trapped in the smaller circulatory channels of particularly the spleen but also of the liver. Dying erythrocytes are engulfed and destroyed by macrophages. The heme of their hemoglobin is degraded to bilirubin, and the globin part is metabolized into amino acids which are then released into the circulation. In hemolytic anemia, the RBC life span is shortened and bone marrow production of RBCs cannot keep up with the rate of destruction. Although there are various types of hemolytic anemias, they most commonly are due to an extravascular hemolysis of the red blood cells in the phagocytic cells of the spleen, liver, and bone marrow. It is this phagocytosis of the dying RBCs in the spleen and liver which leads to splenomegaly and, in some cases, hepatomegaly. Intravascular hemolysis is uncommon.

The signs and symptoms of hemolytic anemias resemble those of other anemias. If hemolysis is acute (hemolytic crisis), fever, chills, pains in the back and abdomen, prostration, and even shock may be seen. Hemolytic crisis, however, is relatively uncommon. In chronic and episodic hemolysis, the symptoms are less severe. Anemia symptoms are exacerbated if there is a temporary failure of RBC production, usually due to infections by the parvovirus.

As explained above, during the breakdown of RBCs, the heme part of hemoglobin is transformed into bilirubin. During acute hemolytic attacks, the amount of bilirubin released exceeds the excretory function of the liver. This then leads to jaundice.

Hemolytic anemias can be divided into three different categories: hemoglobinopathies, membrane defects, and autoimmuune disorders. These categories have been discussed above in the introduction to anemias at the beginning of this chapter. The Western medical treatment of hemolytic anemia is individualized and follows the specific mechanisms of hemolysis. Splenectomy is beneficial when the RBC defect is associated with selective spleen sequestration.

Chinese medical disease explanation:

All hemolytic anemias are characterized by very similar symptoms: anemia, jaundice, and possibly splenomegaly or hepato-splenomegaly. Therefore, the main traditional Chinese disease categories corresponding to hemolytic anemia are vacuity taxation (*xu lao*), jaundice (*huang dan*), and concretions and conglomerations (*zheng jia*). Furthermore, in Chinese medicine, the underlying biomedical abnormality is not usually of great importance because Chinese medicine focuses on patterns rather than diseases, and because pattern discrimination does not rely on or take into account Western medical pathologies. Therefore, in this work, all the different types of hemolytic anemias are grouped into one disease: hemolytic anemia.

If the spleen and stomach function is not fortified and qi and blood cannot be engendered and transformed, qi and blood become vacuous. Over time, a weak middle burner, the latter heaven source, leaves the kidneys, the former heaven source, depleted. If kidney yang, which depends on spleen yang for fortification, is not roused, and yang consequently does not engender yin, an insufficiency in the production of both yin and blood arises.

Vice versa, a weak spleen, dependant on kidney yang for fortification and warming, cannot move and transform if the kidneys become vacuous and weak. Thus water dampness collects. Damp depression leads to obstruction of the free flow of qi. Because qi is inherently warm by nature, if qi depression is severe, it may transform into depressive heat. If this heat mixes with the dampness, it may give rise to damp heat. If damp heat steams the gallbladder and obstructs the discharge of bile, bile is forced outward and spills over into the skin and flesh, resulting in jaundice. Further, prolonged internal brewing and gathering of damp heat leads to a disharmony of qi and blood, resulting in qi stagnation and blood stasis with attendant swelling of the spleen and liver.

Because jaundice is its own disease category within Chinese medicine, jaundice associated with hemolytic anemia is treated by Chinese medicine similar to all other types of jaundice. This is despite the fact that, from a Western medical perspective, jaundice due to hemolytic anemia has, apart from the bile overload, no connection to the biomedical pathologies of jaundice due to either liver failure or cholecystitis. Therefore, in Chinese medicine, the standard "jaundice" medicinals and formulas are used to treat most types of hemolytic anemias. This again underscores the Chinese medical prescriptive methodology of basing treatment on patterns and not diseases. In this case, the underlying biomedical disease causing the jaundice is not important. What is important is that the main symptoms match the defining pattern.

Commonly, patients suffering from jaundice due to hemolytic anemia will also display symptoms of qi and blood vacuity besides those of damp heat. Formula modifications are then made to address this qi and blood vacuity. Whereas, in most cases of jaundice due to cholecystitis, there are few if any vacuity signs, and the formulas addressing that type of jaundice are consequently typically modified differently.

The Chinese patterns differentiating hemolytic anemia likewise differentiate the acute form from the more low-grade, chronic form of this disease. If jaundice is pronounced (due to an acute breakdown of red blood cells with bilirubin overload), this is usually categorized as liver-gallbladder damp heat with spleen accumulation and blood stasis. For less severe hemolytic anemia, the most commonly presenting pattern is yin and yang dual vacuity with spleen accumulation and blood stasis. In both of the above two patterns, spleen accumulation and blood stasis reflects the enlargement of the spleen and liver and may be relatively severe (in the former pattern) or less severe (in the latter pattern). According to the severity of the enlargement of the liver and spleen, the dosages of the medicinals in the formula addressing this condition (*i.e.,* the blood-quickening, stasis-transforming medicinals) must be modified.

Hereditary spherocytosis is yet another type of hemolytic anemia. It too falls into the Chinese medical categories and is caused by the Chinese disease mechanisms explained above. Hereditary spherocytosis is due to a former heaven natural endowment insufficiency which leads to a loss of regulation of yin and yang. Thus the treatment principles for spherocytosis are to enrich yin and invigorate yang, move blood and transform stasis.

Treatment based on pattern discrimination:

1. Yin-yang dual vacuity with spleen accumulation & blood stasis pattern

Main symptoms: A somber white facial complexion, reduced food intake, emaciated and fatigued limbs and body, enlargement of the spleen but not of the liver, a relatively pale tongue with a normal body and white fur, and a floating, rapid or floating, vacuous pulse. As discussed above, the symptoms of anemia, jaundice, and hepato-splenomegaly are mild in this pattern of hemolytic anemia.

Treatment principles: Enrich yin and supplement the blood, quicken the blood and transform stasis

Chinese medicinal formula:

SHENG YIN HUA YU TANG (**Engender Yin & Transform Stasis Decoction**)
Radix Polygoni Multiflori (*He Shou Wu*), Fructus Ligustri Lucidi (*Nu Zhen Zi*), Herba Epimedii (*Yin Yang Huo*), Semen Cuscutae Chinensis (*Tu Si Zi*), Rhizoma Curcumae Zedoariae (*E Zhu*), Radix Salviae Miltiorrhizae (*Dan Shen*), Flos Carthami Tinctorii (*Hong Hua*), Carapax Amydae Sinensis (*Bie Jia*), blast-fried Squama Manitis Pentadactylis (*Chuan Shan Jia*), Endothelium Corneum Gigeriae Galli (*Ji Nei Jin*), Caulis Milletiae Seu Spatholobi (*Ji Xue Teng*), Radix Glycyrrhizae (*Gan Cao*)

Additions & subtractions: For reduced food intake with abdominal distention, add Rhizoma Atractylodis Macrocephalae (*Bai Zhu*), Sclerotium Poriae Cocos (*Fu Ling*), *San Xian* (*i.e.,* Fructus Germinatus Hordei Vulgaris, *Mai Ya*, Massa Medica Fermentata, *Shen Qu*, and Fructus Crataegi, *Shan Zha*), and Radix Auklandiae Lappae (*Mu Xiang*). For accompanying nausea, add Rhizoma Pinelliae Ternatae (*Ban Xia*) and Pericarpium Citri Reticulatae (*Chen Pi*). For pronounced qi vacuity with weakness of the body and limbs, add Radix Astragali Membranacei (*Huang Qi*) and Radix Codonopsitis Pilosulae (*Dang Shen*). In case of contraction of external evils during the course of treatment, add heat-clearing, toxin-resolving medicinals.

2. Liver-gallbladder damp heat with spleen accumulation & blood stasis pattern

Main symptoms: Pronounced manifestations of anemia, such as dizziness, heart palpitations, shortness of breath, and fatigue, jaundiced skin and membranes, an obviously enlarged spleen as well as an enlarged liver, a pale tongue, and a floating, vacuous pulse

Treatment principles: Disinhibit the gallbladder and recede jaundice, transform stasis and soften hardness

Chinese medicinal formula:

JIN CHEN SAN **(Lysimachia & Artemisia Capillaris Powder)**
  Herba Lysimachiae Seu Desmodii Styracifolii (*Jin Qian Cao*), Herba Artemisiae Capillaris (*Yin Chen Hao*), Tuber Curcumae (*Yu Jin*), Rhizoma Curcumae Zedoariae (*E Zhu*), Plastrum Testudinis (*Gui Ban*), Carapax Amydae Sinensis (*Bie Jia*), Radix Salviae Miltiorrhizae (*Dan Shen*), Rhizoma Corydalis Yanhusuo (*Yan Hu Suo*), Flos Carthami Tinctorii (*Hong Hua*), Radix Achyranthis Bidentatae (*Niu Xi*), Radix Glycyrrhizae (*Gan Cao*)

If the above formula does not yield satisfactory results, the following powder can be used: *Hua Yu Ruan Jian San* (Stasis-transforming, Hardness-softening Powder)

Blast-fried Squama Manitis Pentadactylis (*Chuan Shan Jia*), Hirudo Seu Whitmania (*Shui Zhi*), Radix Et Rhizoma Rhei (*Da Huang*), Rhizoma Curcumae Zedoariae (*E Zhu*), Endothelium Corneum Gigeriae Galli (*Ji Nei Jin*), Rhizoma Corydalis Yanhusuo (*Yan Hu Suo*), Rhizoma Polygoni Multiflori (*He Shou Wu*), Radix Angelicae Sinensis (*Dang Gui*), Radix Glycyrrhizae (*Gan Cao*)

Addendum: Sickle cell anemia

Sickle cell anemia is predominantly a disease of blacks of African descent. This disease is extremely rare among Asians. Therefore, there is almost nothing that I have been able to find in the Chinese medical literature about this disease. However, sickle cell anemia is the most common type of severe hemoglobinopathy in North America and has a prevalence in the United States of one in 375 African-American live births. This translates to approximately 50,000 Americans as of this writing. Thus North American practitioners of Chinese medicine need to know something about this disease and its Chinese treatment.

Sickle cell anemia is a congenital disease in which a one-point mutation in the beta-globin chain leads to hemoglobin S (HbS). Hemoglobin S tends to aggregate and polymerize at low oxygen tension to form a rigid filamentous gel, thus rendering the erythrocyte rigid and less deformable. Because of membrane contraction around the aggregated polymers of the HbS, the erythrocyte takes on a characteristic appearance, resembling sickles or holly leaves. This sickling of cells is reversible up to a point. However, repeated sickling eventually damages the red blood cell membrane permanently, and the formation of rigid sickle cells is likely to plug small blood vessels, thus leading to tissue damage secondary to obstruction of blood flow and hypoxia.

Clinical manifestations in patients suffering from sickle cell anemia are many and varied but reflect the consequences of chronic hemolytic anemia and vaso-occlusion resulting in repeated ischemic tissue damage. All tissues and organs within the body are at risk, but the organs at greatest risk are the spleen, kidneys, and bone marrow.[26] In addition, due to the limited terminal arterial blood supply, the eyes and head of the femur are also targets for ischemic injury. Skin ulcers on the legs, osteomyelitis, avascular necrosis of the femoral head, renal complications such as renal papillary necrosis, an atrophic spleen secondary to repeated infarction and splenic fibrosis, pigment gallstones, iron overload in the heart and liver, retinopathy and blindness, infarcts of the lungs or pneumonia, and even stroke are the more common symptoms. Many afflicted persons are asymptomatic most of the time, only suffering sudden episodes of sickle crisis, which are sometimes fatal. Common causes of death are infections, multiple pulmonary emboli, occlusion of a vessel supplying a vital area, and renal failure.

Western medical treatment for sickle cell anemia is symptomatic since no effective *in vivo* anti-sickling agent has yet been found. Crises are managed with vigorous oral and IV hydration and analgesics, including narcotics for pain. Prophylactic antibiotics and early identification and treatment of serious bacterial infection have reduced mortality,

---

[26] This is because the blood flow is slow in the venous sinuses of these organs and there is reduced oxygen tension and a low pH, both factors which increase RBC sickling.

particularly during childhood. Life span has increased to more than 40 years of age over the years.

Chinese medical disease explanation & treatment:

I have only been able to find a single published piece on sickle cell anemia within the Chinese medical literature. This article, published in the *Zhong Yi Za Zhi (Journal of Chinese Medicine)* in 1994, discusses the treatment of sickle cell anemia with acupuncture and Chinese ready-made medicines.[27] According to its author, 32 cases of sickle cell anemia were thus treated and all 32 cases experienced definite treatment results. Interestingly, this is one of three Chinese articles reviewed for the preparation of this book which also specified acupuncture as part of the treatment protocol.

According to the author of this article, Dr. Li Qing-jiang from the Third Affiliated Hospital of the Beijing Medical University, sickle cell anemia in Chinese medicine should be categorized as basically a vacuity pattern (*xu zheng*) possibly complicated by elements of qi stagnation and blood stasis. He further holds that acupuncture is very good for stopping limb or abdominal pain in sickle cell anemia patients and seems to even prevent subsequent pain flare-ups. The Chinese medicinals Dr. Li used and advocates for this disease are mainly liver and kidney supplements to bank and boost former heaven insufficiency combined with spleen and stomach regulating medicinals to strengthen the latter heaven root. According to Dr. Li, such a combination of acupuncture and Chinese medicinals achieves a relatively good effect in treating sickle cell anemia patients by raising the body's resistance and improving patients' bodily condition, thereby prolonging their life span.

Similar to other congenital hematological diseases, it is apparent from the above comments that sickle cell anemia should also be considered as a form of former heaven vacuity. Sickle cell patients typically have a very vacuous, thin, and emaciated body, a pale facial complexion, and often suffer from multiple chronic illnesses (all related to their sickle cell condition). Symptoms of body pain experienced during sickle cell anemia crises should then be regarded as acute branch repletion conditions caused by the underlying vacuity. Therefore, Chinese medical treatment for this type of anemia should be a combination of supporting the righteous with dispelling evils as necessary. Formulas and medicinals under pattern #1 of hemolytic anemia above might be considered as models for experimental treatment.

---

[27]   Li Qing-jiang, "Experiences in the Clinical Treatment of Sickle Cell Anemia," *Zhong Yi Za Zhi (Journal of Chinese Medicine)*, #3, 1994, p. 161

2 Polycythemia Vera (PV)

Polycythemia vera is a rare disease with an incidence of about 5/1,000,000 and is more common in Jews and males. It often occurs in old age with only 5% of patients younger than 40 years at onset. Hyperplasia of all elements of the marrow is evident and replaces marrow fat. This leads to increased production and turnover not only of RBCs but also of neutrophils and platelets. The main manifestations of PV are related to expanded blood volume and hyperviscosity, such as weakness, headaches, light-headedness, visual disturbances, and fatigue or dyspnea. Bleeding due to abnormalities of platelet function is common, and pruritus is frequent, particularly after a hot bath. The face is often red, and the retinal veins are engorged. More than 75% of patients manifest with splenomegaly due to extramedullary hematopoiesis. As erythroid activity in the marrow decreases, immature white blood cells and RBC precursors can be found in the peripheral blood, developing into anemia and thrombocytopenia.

A healthy male has a red blood cell count of 5.1-5.8 million cells per ml and a healthy female, 4.3-5.3 million cells per ml. Expressed in different numbers, this equals a hematocrit of 42-52% (0.42-0.52 volume fraction) in males and 37-47% (0.37-0.47 volume fraction) in females. Red blood cell mass in normal males ranges from 25.5-31.1 ml/kg and in normal females from 22.8-28.0ml/kg. In polycythemia vera, the number of RBCs is increased (erythrocytosis), leading to thickening of the blood.

Erythrocytosis has several causes. If blood oxygen is at a low level for prolonged periods of time, the kidneys stimulate the production of erythrocytes through their secretion of erythropoietin, thus leading to an increased RBC count. On the other hand, when plasma volume decreases, the erythrocyte count may be elevated in relation to the decreased plasma volume. Since hematocrit is the ratio between the number of circulating RBCs per unit volume of whole blood, it is not a reliable test to diagnose PV. Such relative erythrocytosis is termed Gaisbock's syndrome. Therefore, the three major criteria for making the diagnosis of PV are 1) an increased RBC mass (>36ml/kg in men and >32ml/kg in women), 2) arterial oxygen saturation of more than 92%, and 3) splenomegaly.

Prognosis of PV is relatively poor, with 50% of untreated symptomatic patients dying within 18 months. With Western medical treatment, median survival ranges from 7-15 years. Thrombosis is the most common cause of death. Development of leukemia, myeloid metaplasia, and hemorrhage are other causes of death.

Western medical treatment for this condition focuses on reducing the RBC numbers through phlebotomy (surgical opening of a vein to withdraw blood) or myelosuppressive drugs. However, some myelosuppressive drugs may increase the risk of acute leukemic transformations and thus need to be administered carefully.

Chinese medical disease explanation:

In Chinese medicine, the main clinical symptoms of this disease correspond to the categories of bleeding conditions (*xue zheng*) and blood stasis (*xue yu*) patterns and are sometimes referred to as profuse blood of viscera, bowels, vessels, and network vessels disease (*zang fu mai luo duo xue bing*). Its onset is precipitated by a contraction of toxic evils due to righteous qi vacuity or due to a disharmony of either qi and blood or yin and yang.

If yin and yang are disharmonious and yang is exuberant, then, following the statement of fact that, "if yang is engendered, yin grows," exuberant yang may engender too much yin or blood. In that case, blood exuberance can lead to blood congestion and accumulation with inhibition of free movement of the blood. This may further progress into stasis obstruction of the vessels and network vessels and viscera and bowels. If there is stasis in the viscera and bowels, their blood nourishment is compromised and qi production suffers detriment. Thus, the viscera and bowel qi and, therefore, the whole body's qi becomes vacuous and debilitated. In such cases, qi supplementation is accomplished by merely quickening the blood and freeing the flow of the network vessels.

Because static blood may also obstruct the free flow of qi, the resulting qi stagnation and blood stasis easily transform into heat, giving rise to exuberant heat signs. Such heat can lead to frenetic movement of the blood manifesting as bleeding of the nose and gums as well as hematuria and hemafecia. Furthermore, debilitation of the viscera may give rise to kidney and liver yin vacuity with upward flaming of internal (albeit vacuous) heat.

The source spirit or spirit brilliance, the brain, and the heart vessels are all very sensitive to stagnation and stasis. If stasis progresses to obstruct the spirit brilliance's house (*i.e.*, the heart), the network vessels of the sea of marrow (*i.e.*, the brain), and the heart vessels, then symptoms corresponding to each of these entities may arise. Technically, these are not diseases due to polycythemia vera but rather complications of polycythemia vera.

Furthermore, if static blood obstructs the vessels and network vessels and transform into heat by inhibiting the free flow of qi, vessel impediment may arise. This is yet another complication of polycythemia vera. In addition, concretions and accumulations, masses of definite form and fixed location, may also appear as the result of long-term blood stasis.

Thus, this disease is differentiated into three primary patterns and five complicating patterns. The three primary patterns are 1) toxins and stasis transforming heat and assailing the liver, 2) qi stagnation and blood stasis, and 3) mutual binding of stasis and heat stirring blood. The five complication patterns, all due to obstruction by static blood, are 1) static blood in the spirit brilliance's house, 2) wind stroke, 3) chest impediment, 4) vessel impediment, and 5) concretions and accumulations. Common treatment principles used to deal with this disease are breaking the blood, quickening the blood, transforming stasis, rectifying the qi, boosting the qi, clearing heat, and cooling the blood.

In Chinese medicine, swellings and tumors typically correspond to congelation and stagnation of static blood, and many types of swellings and tumors fall under the category of blood stasis. According to Western medical theory, polycythemia vera is a malignancy of the blood. Therefore, nowadays within Chinese medicine, anti-cancerous medicinals are often combined with blood-quickening and stasis-transforming medicinals to yield better results.

Treatment based on pattern discrimination:

1. Toxins & stasis transforming heat & assailing the liver pattern

Main symptoms: Dizziness, headache, tinnitus, red eyes, vexation and agitation, easy anger, rib-side distention and pain, insomnia, reddish purple face and limbs, a dry mouth and tongue, reddish urine, dry stools, a dark red or dark purple tongue with possible static macules or spots and yellowish fur, and a bowstring, rapid pulse

Note: This pattern is characterized by predominant replete heat signs and symptoms, sometimes also referred to as upward flaming of liver fire, and signs and symptoms of stasis are not yet very pronounced since the blood is still moving through the vessels, if at a slower speed. If manifestations of stasis are more pronounced, refer to pattern #2 listed below.

Treatment principles: Break the blood, clear the liver, and resolve toxins

Chinese medicinal formulas:

QING GAN HUA ZHI TANG **(Clear the Liver & Transform Stagnation Decoction)**
Radix Gentianae Scabrae (*Long Dan Cao*), Radix Scutellariae Baicalensis (*Huang Qin*), Rhizoma Alismatis (*Ze Xie*), Radix Ligustici Wallichii (*Chuan Xiong*), Nodus Nelumbinis Nuciferae (*Ou Jie*), Rhizoma Imperatae Cylindricae (*Bai Mao Gen*), Caulis Milletiae Seu Spatholobi (*Ji Xue Teng*), Fructus Gardeniae Jasminoidis (*Zhi Zi*), Semen Pruni Persicae (*Tao Ren*), Flos Carthami Tinctorii (*Hong Hua*), Rhizoma Sparganii (*San Leng*), Rhizoma Curcumae Zedoariae (*E Zhu*), Radix Stellariae Dichotomae (*Yin Chai Hu*), Cortex Radicis Moutan (*Dan Pi*), Herba Aloes (*Lu Hui*), Pulvis Indigonis (*Qing Dai*, added later)

This formula's functions are mainly to clear the liver and cool the blood, transform stasis and disperse stagnation. Therefore, it is appropriate if liver heat manifestations are pronounced.

LONG DAN XIE GAN TANG JIA JIAN **(Gentiana Drain the Liver Decoction with Additions & Subtractions)**
Hirudo Seu Whitmania (*Shui Zhi*), Rhizoma Curcumae Zedoariae (*E Zhu*), Semen Pruni Persicae (*Tao Ren*), Radix Ligustici Wallichii (*Chuan Xiong*), Radix Gentianae Scabrae (*Long Dan Cao*), Fructus Gardeniae Jasminoidis (*Zhi Zi*), Radix Scutellariae Baicalensis (*Huang Qin*), Radix Bupleuri (*Chai Hu*), uncooked Radix Rehmanniae (*Sheng Di*), Rhizoma Alismatis (*Ze Xie*), Caulis Akebiae (*Mu Tong*), Rhizoma Corydalis Yanhusuo (*Yan Hu Suo*), Radix Et Rhizoma Rhei (*Da Huang*), Radix Lithospermi Seu Arnebiae (*Zi Cao*)

GUI BAN TANG **(Tortoise Shell Decoction)**
Plastrum Testudinis (*Gui Ban*), Rhizoma Anemarrhenae Asphodeloidis (*Zhi Mu*), Cortex Phellodendri (*Huang Bai*), Radix Salviae Miltiorrhizae (*Dan Shen*), Flos Carthami Tinctorii (*Hong Hua*), Semen Pruni Persicae (*Tao Ren*), Radix Achyranthis Bidentatae (*Niu Xi*), Radix Ligustici Wallichii (*Chuan Xiong*), Flos Chrysanthemi Morifolii (*Ju Hua*), Lumbricus (*Di Long*), Radix Glycyrrhizae (*Gan Cao*)

Additions & subtractions: For reduced appetite with constipation, add Endothelium Corneum Gigeriae Galli (*Ji Nei Jin*) and Radix Et Rhizoma Rhei (*Da Huang*). For vexation and agitation with insomnia, add Ramulus Uncariae Cum Uncis (*Gou Teng*), Periostracum Cicadae (*Chan Tui*), and Sclerotium Pararadicis Poria Cocos (*Fu Shen*). For abdominal pain, add Radix Auklandiae Lappae (*Mu Xiang*) and Rhizoma Corydalis Yanhusuo (*Yan Hu Suo*).

2. Qi stagnation & blood stasis pattern

Main symptoms: A dark red facial complexion and skin, purple and/or dark lips, all worsening in the winter, fixed location rib-side distention and pain, tinnitus, decreased hearing, decreased eyesight, heart palpitations, insomnia, accumulations and gatherings below the rib-sides (*i.e.,* enlargement of the liver and spleen), a purplish and/or dark tongue with static macules and spots with thin, pale yellow fur, and a bowstring or tight pulse

Treatment principles: Break the blood and disperse thrombi, free the flow of the network vessels and rectify the qi

Chinese medicinal formulas:

ZHENG HONG HUAN JIE TANG JIA WEI (**Moderating & Resolving True Red Decoction with Added Flavors**)
Herba Selaginellae (*Juan Bai*)[1], Radix Lithospermi Seu Arnebiae (*Zi Cao*), Rhizoma Curcumae Zedoariae (*E Zhu*), Flos Carthami Tinctorii (*Hong Hua*), Semen Pruni Persicae (*Tao Ren*), Radix Ligustici Wallichii (*Chuan Xiong*), Radix Rubrus Paeoniae Lactiflorae (*Chi Shao*)

XUE FU ZHU YU TANG JIA JIAN (**Blood Mansion Dispel Stasis Decoction with Additions & Subtractions**)
Hirudo Seu Whitmania (*Shui Zhi*), Rhizoma Curcumae Zedoariae (*E Zhu*), Semen Pruni Persicae (*Tao Ren*), Radix Ligustici Wallichii (*Chuan Xiong*), uncooked Radix Rehmanniae (*Sheng Di*), Radix Bupleuri (*Chai Hu*), Rhizoma Cyperi Rotundi (*Xiang Fu*), Fructus Citri Aurantii (*Zhi Ke*), Radix Achyranthis Bidentatae (*Niu Xi*), Herba Selaginellae (*Juan Bai*), Radix Lithospermi Seu Arnebiae (*Zi Cao*)

DAN SHEN HUO XUE FANG (**Salvia Quicken the Blood Formula**)
Radix Salviae Miltiorrhizae (*Dan Shen*), Rhizoma Curcumae Zedoariae (*E Zhu*), Hirudo Seu Whitmania (*Shui Zhi*), Flos Carthami Tinctorii (*Hong Hua*), Semen Pruni Persicae (*Tao Ren*), Radix Et Rhizoma Rhei (*Da Huang*), Lumbricus (*Di Long*), Radix Auklandiae Lappae (*Mu Xiang*), Rhizoma Corydalis Yanhusuo (*Yan Hu Suo*), Radix Glycyrrhizae (*Gan Cao*)

Additions & subtractions: For marked swelling of the liver and spleen with local tenderness and pain, add Plastrum Testudinis (*Gui Ban*), Eupolyphaga Seu Opisthoplatia

---

[1] Herba Selaginellae (*Juan Bai*) is acrid and neutral in nature and enters the liver and kidney channels. It boosts the essence, supplements and quickens the blood, quiets the spirit and disinhibits urination.

(*Zhe Chong*), and Tuber Curcumae (*Yu Jin*). For marked vacuity of heart qi, add Radix Astragali Membranacei (*Huang Qi*), uncooked Radix Rehmanniae (*Sheng Di*), Rhizoma Polygonati Odorati (*Yu Zhu*), and Buthus Martensis tail (*Xie Wei*). For hasty panting with expectoration of blood, add uncooked Pollen Typhae (*Pu Huang*), Rhizoma Bletillae Striatae (*Bai Ji*), and Radix Pseudoginseng (*San Qi*). For thrombotic angitis or thrombotic phlebitis, add Squama Manitis Pentadactylis (*Chuan Shan Jia*), Resina Olibani (*Ru Xiang*), Resina Myrrhae (*Mo Yao*), Radix Scrophulariae Ningpoensis (*Xuan Shen*), and Radix Achyranthis Bidentatae (*Niu Xi*). For fevers from infections, add Flos Lonicerae Japonicae *(Jin Yin Hua),* Herba Taraxaci Mongolici Cum Radice (*Pu Gong Ying*), and Herba Violae Yedoensitis Cum Radice (*Di Ding*). For elevated WBC counts without fever, add Pulvis Indigonis (*Qing Dai*). For dizziness with brain (*i.e.,* head) distention, add Rhizoma Gastrodiae Elatae (*Tian Ma*) and Ramulus Uncariae Cum Uncis (*Gou Teng*).

HUA YU JIANG HONG TANG YI HAO (Stasis-transforming Red [Blood Cell]-downbearing Decoction #1)

Radix Angelicae Sinensis (*Dang Gui*), uncooked Radix Rehmanniae (*Sheng Di*), Semen Pruni Persicae (*Tao Ren*), Flos Carthami Tinctorii (*Hong Hua*), Fructus Citri Aurantii (*Zhi Ke*), Radix Rubrus Paeoniae Lactiflorae (*Chi Shao*), Tuber Curcumae (*Yu Jin*), Radix Bupleuri (*Chai Hu*), Radix Glycyrrhizae (*Gan Cao*), Radix Ligustici Wallichii (*Chuan Xiong*), Radix Achyranthis Bidentatae (*Niu Xi*), Rhizoma Sparganii (*San Leng*), Rhizoma Curcumae Zedoariae (*E Zhu*)

JUAN BAI BIE JIA FANG (Selaginella & Carapax Amydae Formula)

Carapax Amydae Sinensis (*Bie Jia*), Squama Manitis Pentadactylis (*Jia Zhu*), Eupolyphaga Seu Opisthoplatia (*Zhe Chong*), Radix Rubrus Paeoniae Lactiflorae (*Chi Shao*), Cortex Radicis Moutan (*Dan Pi*), Flos Carthami Tinctori (*Hong Hua*), Radix Bupleuri (*Chai Hu*), Radix Angelicae Sinenesis (*Dang Gui*), Ramulus Cinnamomi Cassiae (*Gui Zhi*), Cortex Magnoliae Officinalis (*Hou Po*), Fructus Citri Aurantii (*Zhi Ke*), Herba Selaginellae (*Juan Bai*), Pulvis Indigonis (*Qing Dai*), Radix Glycyrrhizae (*Gan Cao*)

HUO XUE JIANG HONG FANG (Blood-quickening Red [Blood Cell]-downbearing Decoction)

Radix Salviae Miltiorrhizae (*Dan Shen*), Radix Angelicae Sinensis (*Dang Gui*), Radix Albus Paeoniae Lactiflorae (*Bai Shao*), Radix Rubrus Paeoniae Lactiflorae (*Chi Shao*), Pollen Typhae (*Pu Huang*), Excrementum Trogopterori Seu Pteromi (*Wu Ling Zhi*), carbonized Radix Et Rhizoma Rhei (*Da Huang*), Fructus Amomi (*Sha Ren*), Cortex Magnoliae Officinalis (*Hou Po*), Fructus Citri Sacrodactylis (*Fo Shou*),

Rhizoma Pinelliae Ternatae (*Ban Xia*), Sclerotium Poriae Cocos (*Fu Ling*), Radix Glycyrrhizae (*Gan Cao*)

Besides quickening the blood and transforming stasis, this formula also rectifies the qi and harmonizes the stomach and can thus be used in cases where either long-standing stasis or other causes have damaged the stomach, giving rise to such symptoms as torpid intake and abdominal fullness.

3. Mutual binding of stasis & heat stirring blood pattern

Main symptoms: Heart vexation, bodily heat, dizziness, abdominal distention, insomnia, profuse dreams, dry mouth, thirst, constipation, bloody stools, bloody urination, gum and nose bleeding, a dark red tongue with static macules and spots and yellow fur, and a slippery, rapid pulse

Treatment principles: Cool the blood, quicken the blood, and stop bleeding

Chinese medicinal formulas:

HUA YU JIANG HONG TANG ER HAO (Stasis-transforming Red [Blood Cell]-downbearing Decoction #2)
Cornu Bubali (*Shui Niu Jiao*), uncooked Radix Rehmanniae (*Sheng Di*), Radix Albus Paeoniae Lactiflorae (*Bai Shao*), Cortex Radicis Moutan (*Dan Pi*), Rhizoma Anemarrhenae Asphodeloidis (*Zhi Mu*), Tuber Ophiopogonis Japonici (*Mai Men Dong*), Radix Rubiae Cordifoliae (*Qian Cao Gen*), Gelatinum Corii Asini (*E Jiao*), Conchae Ostreae (*Mu Li*), Herba Ecliptae Prostratae (*Han Lian Cao*), Herba Cephalanoploris Segeti (*Xiao Ji*), Radix Codonopsitis Pilosulae (*Dang Shen*), Radix Astragali Membranacei (*Huang Qi*), Radix Glycyrrhizae (*Gan Cao*)

This formula addresses not only blood heat but also yin damage and stasis.

XI JIAO DI HUANG TANG JIA JIAN (Rhinoceros Horn & Rehmannia Decoction with Additions & Subtractions)
Cornu Bubali (*Shui Niu Jiao*), Radix Rubrus Paeoniae Lactiflorae (*Chi Shao*), Radix Albus Paeoniae Lactiflorae (*Bai Shao*), Cortex Radicis Moutan (*Dan Pi*), Radix Scutellariae Baicalensis (*Huang Qin*), Rhizoma Coptidis Chinensis (*Huang Lian*), uncooked Radix Rehmanniae (*Sheng Di*), Radix Scrophulariae Ningpoensis (*Xuan Shen*), Herba Agrimoniae Pilosae (*Xian He Cao*), Radix Pseudoginseng (*San Qi*), Rhizoma Imperatae Cylindricae (*Bai Mao Gen*), Radix Lithospermi Seu Arnebiae (*Zi Cao*)

QING FEI YANG WEI TANG (**Lung-clearing, Stomach-nourishing Decoction**)

Radix Adenophorae Strictae (*Nan Sha Shen*), Nodus Nelumbinis Nuciferae (*Ou Jie*), Cortex Radicis Mori Albi (*Sang Bai Pi*), Rhizoma Polygonati Odorati (*Yu Zhu*), Folium Eryobotryae Japonicae (*Pi Pa Ye*), Rhizoma Imperatae Cylindricae (*Bai Mao Gen*), Radix Glycyrrhizae (*Gan Cao*), Cortex Radicis Moutan (*Dan Pi*), Radix Isatidis Seu Baphicacanthi (*Ban Lan Gen*), Ramulus Mori Albi (*Sang Zhi*), Herba Oldenlandiae Diffusae Cum Radice (*Bai Hua She She Cao*)

This formula is indicated if heat has consumed the fluids. It not only moistens dryness but also nourishes the lungs and stomach.

Additions & subtractions: For pronounced kidney vacuity, add Semen Cuscutae Chinensis (*Tu Si Zi*) and Radix Dipsaci (*Xu Duan*). For an increased desire to eat, add uncooked Radix Rehmanniae (*Sheng Di*) and Gypsum Fibrosum (*Shi Gao*).

ZHENG HONG HUAN JIE TANG JIA WEI (**Moderating & Resolving True Red Decoction with Added Flavors**)

Herba Selaginellae (*Juan Bai*), Radix Lithospermi Seu Arnebiae (*Zi Cao*), Cortex Radicis Moutan (*Mu Dan Pi*), Rhizoma Anemarrhenae Asphodeloidis (*Zhi Mu*), Tuber Ophiopogonis Japonici (*Mai Men Dong*), Radix Rubiae Cordifoliae (*Qian Cao Gen*), Gypsum Fibrosum (*Shi Gao*)

Additions & subtractions: For an elevated WBC count without fever, add Pulvis Indigonis (*Qing Dai*). For qi vacuity and bodily weakness, add Radix Astragali Membranacei (*Huang Qi*) and Radix Codonopsitis Pilosulae (*Dang Shen*). For dizziness with brain (*i.e.,* head) distention, add Rhizoma Gastrodiae Elatae (*Tian Ma*) and Ramulus Uncariae Cum Uncis (*Gou Teng*).

4. Static blood in the mansion of the clear spirit pattern

Main symptoms: Initially, there is violent pain in the head and blurred vision followed by delirious ravings, delusion, talking nonsense, not recognizing one's relatives, a red facial complexion and purple lips, red eyes, and green-blue nails.

Treatment principles: Break the blood, transform phlegm, and open the orifices

Chinese medicinal formula:

SHUI ZHI HUANG PU TANG (Leech & Cat-tail Pollen Decoction)
Hirudo Seu Whitmania (*Shui Zhi*), Radix Angelicae Sinensis (*Dang Gui*), Radix Rubrus Paeoniae Lactiflorae (*Chi Shao*), Radix Albus Paeoniae Lactiflorae (*Bai Shao*), Pericarpium Citri Reticulatae (*Chen Pi*), Radix Pinelliae Ternatae (*Ban Xia*), Sclerotium Poriae Cocos (*Fu Ling*), Rhizoma Acori Graminei (*Shi Chang Pu*), bile-processed Rhizoma Arisaematis (*Dan Nan Xing*), Rhizoma Coptidis Chinensis (*Huang Lian*), Fructus Citri Aurantii (*Zhi Ke*)

Take a decoction of the above medicinals with one pill of *Ju Fang Zhi Bao Dan* (*Imperial Grace* Supreme Jewel Elixir).

5. Wind stroke (static blood obstructing the network vessels of the brain) pattern

Main symptoms: Numbness of the limbs, no strength in the muscles, a heavy head, limp legs, and decreased sensation possibly accompanied by non-freely flowing speech and deviation of the mouth and eyes, dark red cheeks and lips, and purple and dark nails

Treatment principles: Break the blood, quicken the blood, and free the flow of the network vessels accompanied by supplementing the qi

Chinese medicinal formulas:

ZHENG HONG HUAN JIE TANG JIA WEI (Moderating & Resolving True Red Decoction with Added Flavors)
Herba Selaginellae (*Juan Bai*), Radix Lithospermi Seu Arnebiae (*Zi Cao*), Spica Prunellae Vulgaris (*Xia Ku Cao*), Radix Gentianae Scabrae (*Long Dan Cao*), Fructus Gardeniae Jasminoidis (*Zhi Zi*), Flos Carthami Tinctorii (*Hong Hua*), Hirudo Seu Whitmania (*Shui Zhi*)

Additions & subtractions: For an elevated WBC count without fever, add Pulvis Indigonis (*Qing Dai*). For qi vacuity and bodily weakness, add Radix Astragali Membranacei (*Huang Qi*) and Radix Codonopsitis Pilosulae (*Dang Shen*). For dizziness with brain (*i.e.,* head) distention, add Rhizoma Gastrodiae Elatae (*Tian Ma*) and Ramulus Uncariae Cum Uncis (*Gou Teng*).

BU YANG HUAN WU TANG JIA JIAN (Supplement Yang & Restore Five [Tenths] Decoction with Additions & Subtractions)
Radix Astragali Membranacei (*Huang Qi*), Radix Rubrus Paeoniae Lactiflorae (*Chi Shao*), Radix Ligustici Wallichii (*Chuan Xiong*), Radix Angelicae Sinensis (*Dang Gui*), Lumbricus (*Di Long*), Semen Pruni Persicae (*Tao Ren*), Flos Carthami Tinctorii

(*Hong Hua*), Hirudo Seu Whitmania (*Shui Zhi*), Radix Achyranthis Bidentatae (*Niu Xi*), Rhizoma Acori Graminei (*Shi Chang Pu*), Radix Polygalae Tenuifoliae (*Yuan Zhi*), Bombyx Batryticatus (*Jiang Can*), Ramulus Mori Albi (*Sang Zhi*), Herba Selaginellae (*Juan Bai*)

6. Chest impediment (stasis obstruction of the heart vessels) pattern

Main symptoms: Stabbing pain in the chest which is fixed or chest oppression as if suffocating, pain radiating to the back, accompanying heart palpitations, shortness of breath, and hasty panting all of which symptoms are worse at night, a green-blue facial complexion, and dark lips

Treatment principles: Rectify the qi and quicken the blood assisted by boosting the qi

Chinese medicinal formula:

XUE FU ZHU YU TANG JIA JIAN (**Blood Mansion Dispel Stasis Decoction with Additions & Subtractions**)
   Semen Pruni Persicae (*Tao Ren*), Flos Carthami Tinctorii (*Hong Hua*), Radix Angelicae Sinensis (*Dang Gui*), Radix Ligustici Wallichii (*Chuan Xiong*), uncooked Radix Rehmanniae (*Sheng Di*), Fructus Citri Aurantii (*Zhi Ke*), Radix Rubrus Paeoniae Lactiflorae (*Chi Shao*), Radix Bupleuri (*Chai Hu*), Rhizoma Corydalis Yanhusuo (*Yan Hu Suo*), Tuber Curcumae (*Yu Jin*), Hirudo Seu Whitmania (*Shui Zhi*), Radix Panacis Quinquefolii (*Xi Yang Sheng*)

7. Vessel impediment (static blood transformative heat with obstruction of the vessels & network vessels) pattern

Main symptoms: Aching and pain of the body and limbs, swelling and distention, pressure pain or throbbing pain, dark red skin, increased skin temperature, symptoms possibly recurrent in nature

Treatment principles: Quicken the blood, clear heat, and free the flow of the network vessels

Chinese medicinal formula:

REN DONG TENG SAN (**Lonicera Stem Powder**)
   Caulis Lonicerae Japonicae (*Ren Dong Teng*), Radix Scrophulariae Ningpoensis (*Xuan Shen*), Radix Angelicae Sinensis (*Dang Gui*), Radix Rubrus Paeoniae

Lactiflorae (*Chi Shao*), Radix Albus Paeoniae Lactiflorae (*Bai Shao*), Radix Glycyrrhizae (*Gan Cao*), Cortex Radicis Moutan (*Dan Pi*), Radix Achyranthis Bidentatae (*Niu Xi*), Hirudo Seu Whitmania (*Shui Zhi*), Cornu Bubali (*Shui Niu Jiao*), Cortex Phellodendri (*Huang Bai*), Rhizoma Anemarrhenae Asphodeloidis (*Zhi Mu*), Rhizoma Corydalis Yanhusuo (*Yan Hu Suo*), Flos Lonicerae Japonicae (*Jin Yin Hua*), Fructus Forsythiae Suspensae (*Lian Qiao*)

8. Abdominal concretions & accumulations (static blood in the liver & gallbladder and the channels & network vessels) pattern

Main symptoms: An obvious accumulation lump either below both rib-sides or simply on one rib-side. The lump is hard, painful, and does not move. Associated pain is more severe at night and may penetrate to the lumbar area. Swelling signs increase progressively in severity, and there are possible static macules and spots subcutaneously.

Treatment principles: Rectify the qi and disperse concretions

Chinese medicinal formula:

GE XIA ZHU YU TANG JIA JIAN **(Below the Diaphragm Dispel Stasis Decoction with Additions & Subtractions)**

Radix Angelicae Sinensis (*Dang Gui*), Radix Ligustici Wallichii (*Chuan Xiong*), Semen Pruni Persicae (*Tao Ren*), Flos Carthami Tinctorii (*Hong Hua*), Cortex Radicis Moutan (*Dan Pi*), Radix Linderae Strychnifoliae (*Wu Yao*), Rhizoma Cyperi Rotundi (*Xiang Fu*), Fructus Citri Aurantii (*Zhi Ke*), Radix Bupleuri (*Chai Hu*), Rhizoma Corydalis Yanhusuo (*Yan Hu Suo*), Radix Auklandiae Lappae (*Mu Xiang*), Hirudo Seu Whitmania (*Shui Zhi*), Tuber Curcumae (*Yu Jin*), Radix Codonopsitis Pilosulae (*Dang Shen*)

Addendum: The formula below can be used for PV patients with symptoms of pronounced spleen vacuity with accumulation of phlegm and dampness. Its functions are to fortify the spleen and dispel dampness, transform phlegm and extinguish wind, and clear heat. This formula can also be modified so as to treat a wide variety of patterns in which phlegm and dampness occur simultaneously.

QU SHI HUA TAN XI FENG TANG **(Dispel Dampness, Transform Phlegm & Extinguish Wind Decoction)**

Rhizoma Pinelliae Ternatae (*Ban Xia*), Sclerotium Poriae Cocos (*Fu Ling*), Rhizoma Atractylodis Macrocephalae (*Bai Zhu*), Rhizoma Gastrodia Elatae (*Tian Ma*), Pericarpium Citri Reticulatae (*Chen Pi*), Rhizoma Acori Graminei (*Shi Chang Pu*), Flos Chrysanthemi Morifolii (*Ju Hua*), Radix Scutellariae Baicalensis (*Huang Qin*),

Bombyx Batryticatus (*Jiang Can*), bile-processed Rhizoma Arisaematis (*Dan Nan Xing*), Radix Glycyrrhizae (*Gan Cao*)

Additions & subtractions: For only mild symptoms of phlegm fire, remove *Shi Chang Pu* and *Ju Hua* and add Semen Coicis Lachryma-jobi (*Yi Yi Ren*) and Rhizoma Alismatis (*Ze Xie*). For static macules and spots on the skin which do not disperse, subtract *Jiang Can, Dan Xing,* and *Huang Qin*, and add Radix Salviae Miltiorrhizae (*Dan Shen*), Radix Rubrus Paeoniae Lactiflorae (*Chi Shao*), and Flos Carthami Tinctorii (*Hong Hua*).

Remarks: Research reported in the *Zhong Guo Zhong Xi Yi Jie He Za Zhi (Chinese Journal of the Integrated Chinese-Western Medicine)* on the treatment of 11 cases of polycythemia vera with a variation of *Zheng Hong Huan Jie Tang Jia Wei* depending on the pattern indicated that, in order to successfully treat polycythemia vera, it is good to take Chinese medicinals until remission has been initiated and the blood picture has become normal.[2] Then, the blood should be checked every one to two months. As soon as an increase of RBCs is detected, the herbal formula should be taken again. According to the above research report, this leads to the most prolonged benefits.

Furthermore, the same report points out that emphasis should not be put on seeking a complete cure but rather on improving life expectancy and prolonging periods of remission. It is further notable that, within three to six months of treatment, all 11 cases in this study improved, some of them going into long-term remission.

---

[2]   Han Jia-chang *et al.*, "The Treatment of 11 Cases of Polycythemia Vera with *Zheng Hong Huan Jie Tang* (Moderating & Resolving True Red Decoction)," *Zhong Guo Zhong Xi Yi Jie He Za Zhi (Chinese Journal of Integrated Chinese-Western Medicine)*, #9, 1995, p. 555-556

Section II
White Blood Cell Disorders

1 Infectious Mononucleosis

Infectious mononucleosis is an acute disease due to infection by the Epstein-Barr virus (EBV) and characterized by the tetrad of fever, pharyngitis, lymphocytosis, and fatigue. Primary EBV infection may occur during childhood, adolescence, or adulthood. Approximately 50% of all children have had such an infection before the age of five years and, in most of these children, the infection is subclinical. When this infection occurs in adolescents and adults, it may be either subclinical or it may be recognized as infectious mononucleosis. Once infected with the virus, persons remain asymptomatically infected for life, and the virus is shed intermittently from the oropharynx. The route of transmission for this infection is, therefore, by oropharyngeal contact (usually kissing) between an uninfected and a healthy EBV-seropositive individual who is asymptomatically shedding the virus.

The virus, after having been acquired, first binds to and infects the nasopharyngeal cells and then the B-lymphocytes. Circulating B-lymphocytes carry the virus throughout the body, producing a generalized infection of lymphoid tissues. The activated B-cells stimulate the proliferation of specific killer T-cells, giving rise to an atypical lymphocytosis associated with primary EBV infection. These killer T-lymphocytes destroy virally infected B-cells. Another type of T-cells released are the suppressor T-cells which inhibit the B-cell production of immunoglobulins.[1]

The onset of this disease is marked by malaise lasting from a few days to a week followed by fever, pharyngitis (which may be severe) and adenopathy. In other cases, enlargement of a solitary lymph node or a group of nodes may be the sole clinical manifestation. Splenomegaly due to hyperplasia of the red pulp is observed in about 50%

---

[1] Immunoglobulins are a group of closely related but not identical proteins which act as antibodies. Thus, all antibodies are immunoglobulins. However, the reverse may not be true. Researchers have not yet determined if all immunoglobulins are antibodies.

of cases. Because of the risk of splenic rupture, heavy lifting and contact sports should be avoided for two months after presentation, even if there is no lasting splenomegaly.

Complications, though rare, may be of a severe nature. Complications include CNS involvement (meningitis, encephalitis), hematologic complications (splenic rupture, thrombocytopenia, hemolytic anemia), pulmonary complications (airway obstruction, interstitial pulmonary infiltration), and hepatic complications (hepatitis).

Infectious mononucleosis is usually self-limiting with an acute phase of about two weeks and, in a few patients, intermittent fatigue of moderate intensity for months. Western medical treatment of this condition is supportive. Acetaminophen (as an antipyretic and analgesic), corticosteroids (to reduce inflammation and relieve pharyngitis), and oral or IV acyclovir (to decrease oropharyngeal shedding of EBV) are sometimes used. However, apart from acetaminophen, there is no convincing evidence that the use of the above drugs is warranted for uncomplicated cases.

Chinese medical disease explanation:

In Chinese medicine, infectious mononucleosis corresponds to the disease category of warm heat diseases (*wen re bing*). Transmission of warm evils follows the four divisions pattern discrimination, moving from the defensive to the qi division, from the qi to the constructive division, and from the constructive to the blood division.

If heat lodges in the lungs and causes upward flaming of lung heat, then there may be pulmonary complications characterized by difficulty breathing, cough, and panting. If the assailing disease evil is or transforms into damp heat, it may obstruct the gallbladder, thus leading to jaundice. This corresponds to hepatic complications. If the disease evil transmits to the constructive and blood divisions, symptoms of spirit clouding, such as deranged speech and vexation and agitation, occur. This corresponds to the complication of CNS involvement.

The Chinese medical treatment of infectious mononucleosis is based upon the pattern discrimination of the current stage of disease. Although not commonly mentioned in Chinese sources when discussing this disease but obvious from its formulas' ingredients, the lymphadenopathy in this disease corresponds to phlegm nodulation. Therefore, formulas always include hardness-softening and nodulation-scattering medicinals.

Treatment based on pattern discrimination:

1. Heat toxins invading the upper (part of the body) pattern

Main symptoms: Fever, painful, red, swollen throat, swollen, engorged tonsils, engorged uvula, swollen submandibular lymph nodes which are painful to the touch. If severe, there is fever with simultaneous chills, a yellow-white secretion covering the swollen tonsils, enlarged lymph nodes throughout the body, and red macules and papules whose color diminishes upon pressure. The tongue is red with white or yellowish white fur, and the pulse is floating and rapid.

Treatment principles: Clear heat and resolve toxins, transform stasis and scatter nodulation

Chinese medicinal formula:

JIE DU SAN JIE TANG (**Resolve Toxins & Scatter Nodulation Decoction**)
   Folium Daqingye (*Da Qing Ye*), Rhizoma Paridis Polyphyllae (*Zao Xiu*), Spica Prunellae Vulgaris (*Xia Ku Cao*), Fructus Forsythiae Suspensae (*Lian Qiao*), Radix Scrophulariae Ningpoensis (*Xuan Shen*), Radix Salviae Miltiorrhizae (*Dan Shen*), Radix Platycodi Grandiflori (*Jie Geng*), Radix Glycyrrhizae (*Gan Cao*)

2. Lung heat flaming upward pattern (pulmonary complications)

Main symptoms: Fever, cough, panting, nasal flaring; if severe, cyanosis of the lips. This pattern is seen more commonly in infants. Furthermore, it has a tendency to linger after the acute stage is over and residual symptoms may thus stay unresolved for many months.

Treatment principles: Resolve toxins and clear the lungs, quiet cough and stop panting

Chinese medicinal formula:

XIE BAI JIE DU TANG (**Drain the White & Resolve Toxins Decoction**)
   Flos Lonicerae Japonicae (*Jin Yin Hua*), Fructus Forsythiae Suspensae (*Lian Qiao*), Folium Daqingye (*Da Qing Ye*), Rhizoma Paridis Polyphyllae (*Zao Xiu*), Spica Prunellae Vulgaris (*Xia Ku Cao*), bile-processed Rhizoma Arisaematis (*Dan Nan Xing*), Bombyx Batryticatus (*Jiang Can*, taken as powder), Radix Scrophulariae Ningpoensis (*Xuan Shen*), uncooked Radix Rehmanniae (*Sheng Di*), Tuber

Ophiopogonis Japonici (*Mai Dong*), Semen Plantaginis (*Che Qian Zi*), Radix Platycodi Grandiflori (*Jie Geng*), Radix Glycyrrhizae (*Gan Cao*)

Additions & subtractions: For pronounced bronchial spasms with wheezing, add Herba Ephedrae (*Ma Huang*), Lumbricus (*Di Long*), Periostracum Cicadae (*Chan Tui*), and Semen Pruni Armeniacae (*Xing Ren*). For pronounced coughing, add Radix Stemonae (*Bai Bu*), Exocarpium Citri Erythrocarpae (*Ju Hong*), and Caulis Bambusae In Taeniis (*Zhu Ru*). For non-abating high fever with vexation and agitation, add Rhizoma Coptidis Chinensis (*Huang Lian*), Cortex Phellodendri (*Huang Bai*), Radix Scutellariae Baicalensis (*Huang Qin*), and Fructus Gardeniae Jasminoidis (*Zhi Zi*). For pneumonia with accompanying heart failure[2], add Buthus Martensis tail (*Xie Wei*) and Rhizoma Polygonati Odorati (*Yu Zhu*), and increase the dosages of *Sheng Di, Mai Dong*, and *Che Qian Zi*.

3. Damp heat smoldering internally pattern (hepatic complications)

Main symptoms: Fever, nausea, vomiting, reduced appetite, jaundiced skin and membranes, yellow urine, an enlarged liver, a red tongue with yellow fur, and a floating, rapid pulse. This pattern corresponds to infectious hepatitis and is marked by elevated/abnormal liver enzymes.

Treatment principles: Clear heat and disinhibit dampness, disinhibit the gallbladder and recede jaundice

Chinese medicinal formula:

QING RE TUI HUANG TANG (**Clear Heat & Abate Yellowing Decoction**)
Herba Lysimachiae Seu Desmodii Styracifolii (*Jin Qian Cao*), Herba Artemisiae Capillaris (*Yin Chen Hao*), Fructus Gardeniae Jasminoidis (*Zhi Zi*), Radix Et Rhizoma Rhei (*Da Huang*), Spica Prunellae Vulgaris (*Xia Ku Cao*), Rhizoma Atractylodis Macrocephalae (*Bai Zhu*), Sclerotium Poriae Cocos (*Fu Ling*), Radix Auklandiae Lappae (*Mu Xiang*), Massa Medica Fermentata (*Shen Qu*), Semen Plantaginis (*Che Qian Zi*), Caulis Akebiae (*Mu Tong*), Radix Glycyrrhizae (*Gan Cao*)

Additions & subtractions: For pronounced nausea and vomiting, add Caulis Bambusae In Taeniis (*Zhu Ru*) and Pericarpium Citri Reticulatae (*Chen Pi*). For reduced appetite and marked abdominal distention, add Endothelium Corneum Gigeriae Galli (*Ji Nei Jin*) and Semen Dolichoris Lablab (*Bai Bian Dou*). For non-abating high fever accompanied by vexation and agitation, add Ramulus Uncariae Cum Uncis (*Gou Teng*), Periostracum

---

[2]   It is imperative that such patients also receive emergency Western medical attention.

Cicadae (*Chan Tui*), Lumbricus (*Di Long*), and Bombyx Batryticatus (*Jiang Can*). For pronounced abdominal pain or aching and pain over the liver area, add Rhizoma Corydalis Yanhusuo (*Yan Hu Suo*), Radix Bupleuri (*Chai Hu*), and Herba Asari Cum Radice (*Xi Xin*).

4. Constructive & blood division pattern (CNS complications)

Main symptoms: This pattern usually develops 2-4 weeks after the initial onset of disease and presents mainly with neurologic manifestations. Initial symptoms are headache, dizziness, spirit clouding, deranged speech, and vexation and agitation. In severe cases, there are convulsions and spasms of the limbs. The tongue is a deep crimson color and has yellowish-brown fur, while the pulse is bowstring and rapid.

Treatment principles: Clear heat and resolve toxins, enrich yin and cool the blood, level the liver and extinguish wind

Chinese medicinal formulas:

JIA WEI QING WEN BAI DU YIN (**Added Flavors Clear Warmth & Resolve Toxins Drink**)
   Folium Daqingye (*Da Qing Ye*), Rhizoma Paridis Polyphyllae (*Zao Xiu*), Gypsum Fibrosum (*Shi Gao*), Fructus Gardeniae Jasminoidis (*Zhi Zi*), Rhizoma Coptidis Chinensis (*Huang Lian*), Radix Scutellariae Baicalensis (*Huang Qin*), Cornu Bubali (*Shui Niu Jiao*), uncooked Radix Rehmanniae (*Sheng Di*), Radix Anemarrhenae Asphodeloidis (*Zhi Mu*), Radix Scrophulariae Ningpoensis (*Xuan Shen*), Radix Rubrus Paeoniae Lactiflorae (*Chi Shao*), Radix Platycodi Grandiflori (*Jie Geng*), Fructus Forsythiae Suspensae (*Lian Qiao*), Semen Plantaginis (*Che Qian Zi*), Radix Glycyrrhizae (*Gan Cao*), Cortex Radicis Moutan (*Dan Pi*), Folium Bambusae (*Zhu Ye*)

This formula should be accompanied by *An Gong Niu Huang Wan* (Peaceful Palace Bezoar Pills).

KANG RE ZHEN LIANG SAN (**Combating Heat Settling & Cooling Powder**)
   Bile-processed Bombyx Batryticatus (*Jiang Can*), Rhizoma Coptidis Chinensis (*Huang Lian*), Fructus Gardeniae Jasminoidis (*Zhi Zi*), synthetic Calculus Bovis (*Niu Huang*), Cornu Bubali (*Shui Niu Jiao*), Secretio Moschi Moschiferi (*She Xiang*), Scolopendra Subspinipes (*Wu Gong*), Buthus Martensis (*Quan Xie*), Concretio Silicea Bambusae (*Tian Zhu Huang*), Borneolum (*Bing Pian*)

2 Eosinophilia

Eosinophils are a type of white blood cells which account for 1-4% of all leukocytes and belong to the granular type which stem from the myeloblast. Although they perform several functions, their most important role is to lead the counterattack against parasitic worms that are too large to be phagocytized, such as roundworms and flatworms. When eosinophils encounter parasitic worms, they gather around them and release enzymes from their cytoplasmic granules onto the parasite's surface, thus digesting it away. Eosinophils also have the function to destroy immune complexes (antigen-antibody complexes) and to inactivate allergy mediators, such as histamine and leukotrienes, released by mast cells.

Eosinophilia refers to a pathological increase in the peripheral blood count of eosinophils ($>350/mm^3$). It occurs mostly along with allergic/atopic diseases. Most commonly, the allergy involves the respiratory or integumentary systems. Furthermore, almost any parasitic invasion of the body tissues can elicit eosinophilia. Other conditions that may cause an elevation of eosinophils in the peripheral blood are infections (cat-scratch disease, infectious lymphocytosis, infectious monocytosis), neoplastic diseases (Hodgkin's disease, ovarian cancer), connective tissue disorders with increased circulating immune complexes and vasculitis, as well as both acquired and congenital immune disorders (hyperimmunoglobulinemia E, selective IgA deficiency, graft-versus-host disease). More recently, an epidemic of several hundred patients with an eosinophilia-myalgic syndrome has been identified in people using large quantities of L-tryptophan for sedation or psychotropic support. The symptom complex of this syndrome consists of severe muscle pain, tenosynovitis, muscle edema, and skin rashes lasting weeks to months, with several deaths having been reported.

Eosinophilia is divided into two types: primary and secondary. The second type is called secondary because it occurs secondary to some other disease. Thus, its Western medical treatment focuses on the underlying cause leading to the increase in eosinophil counts. The primary type of this disease is called idiopathic hypereosinophilic syndrome if the eosinophil count is sustained at $>1500/mm^3$ for more than six months in the absence of underlying parasitic infestations or other causes and manifesting with organ system involvement or dysfunction not attributable to any other disease cause. The clinical manifestations for this syndrome follow two broad patterns: 1) a myeloproliferative disorder with splenomegaly, thrombocytopenia, elevated serum vitamin B_{12} levels, and hypogranular or vacuolated eosinophils, and 2) a hypersensitivity type illness with angioedema, hypergammaglobulinemia, elevated serum IgE, and circulating immune complexes. The pathologic lesion in the affected organs is due to tissue infiltration by eosinophils or the release of their content. Western medical therapy thus focuses on the reduction of such eosinophil accumulations. Corticosteroids are effective in about 50% of patients responding to treatment. Cytotoxic therapy is effective for another 33%. Prior to advancement of treatment for this disorder, prognosis was poor and less than 20% of patients survived two years. With more modern treatments, the overall survival has increased to more than 85%.

Chinese medical disease explanation:

The Western medical disease category of eosinophilia does not correspond to any single or even any small group of traditional Chinese diseases. That being said, eosinophilia most commonly manifests as allergies of the respiratory or integumentary system. The lungs govern the defensive qi, the exterior, and the skin and body hair. If wind evils assail the lungs and the lung qi cannot diffuse and perform its function of depurative downbearing, cough and asthma may arise. The Chinese medical disease category in these cases is coughing and panting (*ke chuan*). Furthermore, if fire and heat are pronounced, the exterior and skin may be affected, leading to the engenderment of wind papules (*feng zhen*). The treatment principles in both of these two Chinese disease categories is to course wind, diffuse the lungs, and stop coughing if there is coughing, or to clear heat and stop itching if the skin is affected.

If parasites are the cause of the elevated eosinophil count, intestinal worms (*chong*) are believed to be involved. Treatment thus focuses on killing worms, and formulas for this purpose commonly contain harsh worm-killing medicinals. In this case, it is important that, after the worms are killed, supplementing formulas are administered to fortify the spleen and nourish yin.

Another commonly seen mechanism in those with eosinophilia also associated with intestinal worms is a disruption in the body's water metabolism with an accumulation and collection of damp qi in the body. If such damp evils encumber the spleen, water swelling, abdominal distention, and loose stools may arise. The treatment principles in that case is to fortify the spleen and disinhibit dampness.

In idiopathic hypereosinophilic syndrome, there is no discernible underlying disease pathology, such as respiratory infections or parasitic infestations. However, this fact does not present the same to practitioners of Chinese medicine as it does to practitioners of Western medicine since, in Chinese medicine, treatment is based on the patient's pattern which is, in turn, based on the patient's clinical signs and symptoms. Once the pattern has been discriminated, the treatment principles for this type of eosinophilia are whatever the pattern logically demands. In that case, one of the following formulas can be selected and modified so as to fit that patient's personal pattern. Because idiopathic hypereosinophilic syndrome is defined as an eosinophil count >1500/mm^3 *as well as* manifestations of organ system involvement or dysfunction not attributable to any other disease cause, there will always be clinical signs and symptoms on which to base a pattern discrimination.

Treatment based on pattern discrimination:

1. Intestinal & stomach worm accumulation pattern

Main symptoms: Intermittent abdominal pain, periumbilical pain, indigestion, no appetite, emaciation, loose stools, slight fever, a sallow facial complexion, nausea, vomiting, and a forceless pulse

Treatment principles: Fortify the spleen, expel worms, and astringe the intestines

Chinese medicinal formula:

WU MEI TANG (Mume Decoction)
Fructus Pruni Mume (*Wu Mei*), Fructus Meliae Toosendan (*Chuan Lian Zi*), Rhizoma Atractylodis Macrocephalae (*Bai Zhu*), cooked Radix Rehmanniae (*Shu Di*), Fructus Schisandrae Chinensis (*Wu Wei Zi*), Radix Dioscoreae Oppositae (*Shan Yao*), Semen Myristicae Fragrantis (*Rou Dou Kou*), Fructus Crataegi (*Shan Zha*)

2. Wind heat evils assailing the lungs pattern

Main symptoms: Cough, panting, sore throat, a raspy voice, dry throat, thick, sticky phlegm or thick, yellow phlegm, fever, stuffy nose, thirst, possible aversion to wind, wind papules, a red tongue with thin, yellow fur, and a floating, rapid pulse

Treatment principles: Clear heat, course wind, and diffuse the lungs

Chinese medicinal formulas:

SHU FENG XUAN FEI TANG (Course Wind & Diffuse the Lungs Decoction)
Fructus Arctii Lappae (*Niu Bang Zi*), Cortex Radicis Mori Albi (*Sang Bai Pi*), Folium Mori Albi (*Sang Ye*), Rhizoma Anemarrhenae Asphodeloidis (*Zhi Mu*), Bulbus Fritillariae Thunbergii (*Zhe Bei Mu*), mix-fried Radix Stemonae (*Bai Bu*), Radix Peucedani (*Qian Hu*), Radix Glycyrrhizae (*Gan Cao*), Radix Platycodi Grandiflori (*Jie*

Geng), Radix Adenophorae Strictae (*Nan Sha Shen*), Radix Glehniae Littoralis (*Bei Sha Shen*)

This formula courses wind and moistens dryness, diffuses the lungs and downbears the qi.

Additions & subtractions: For aversion to wind but less severe coughing, remove *Jie Geng* and *Nan Sha Shen*. For red and itchy papules on the four limbs, add Periostracum Cicadae (*Chan Tui*), Radix Rubrus Paeoniae Lactiflorae (*Chi Shao*), Radix Ledebouriellae Divaricatae (*Fang Feng*), and Herba Asari Cum Radice (*Xi Xin*). If roundworm eggs can be found, simply use Fructus Pruni Mume (*Wu Mei*), mix-fried Radix Stemonae (*Bai Bu*), Fructus Meliae Toosendan (*Chuan Lian Zi*), and Semen Arecae Catechu (*Bing Lang*). Once the illness turns for the better, then nourish yin and fortify the spleen.

CHAI LOU JIANG LI TANG (**Bupleurum & Trichosanthes Downbearing & Rectifying Decoction**)

Radix Bupleuri (*Chai Hu*), Radix Scutellariae Baicalensis (*Huang Qin*), processed Rhizoma Pinelliae Ternatae (*Ban Xia*), Radix Peucedani (*Qian Hu*), Radix Platycodi Grandiflori (*Jie Geng*), Fructus Citri Aurantii (*Zhi Ke*), Rhizoma Coptidis Chinensis (*Huang Lian*), Fructus Trichosanthis Kirlowii (*Gua Lou*), Flos Inulae Racemosae (*Xuan Fu Hua*, wrapped), Cortex Magnoliae Officinalis (*Hou Po*), Radix Glycyrrhizae (*Gan Cao*)

This formula harmonizes the constructive and defensive, resolves the exterior and clears heat, diffuses the lungs and transforms phlegm.

Additions & subtractions: For scanty intake with nausea and vomiting, add Caulis Bambusae In Taeniis (*Zhu Ru*). For hasty breathing and coughing, add Semen Pruni Armeniacae (*Xing Ren*). For thick, sticky yellow phlegm, add Ramulus Phragmitis Communis (*Wei Jing*) and Folium Eryobotryae Japonicae (*Pi Pa Ye*).

3. Liver-lung depressive heat pattern

Main symptoms: Fever, cough, panting, thick, sticky, blood-streaked phlegm, difficult to expectorate phlegm, a bitter taste in the mouth, vexation and agitation, rib-side pain, irascibility, constipation, a red tongue with yellow fur, and a rapid, bowstring pulse

Treatment principles: Clear the liver and diffuse the lungs

Chinese medicinal formula:

QING GAN XIE FEI TANG **(Liver-clearing, Lung-draining Decoction)**
Conchae Cyclinae Meretricis (*Hai Ge Ke*), Herba Houttuyniae Cordatae Cum Radice (*Yu Xing Cao*), Pulvis Indigonis (*Qing Dai*), Radix Scutellariae Baicalensis (*Huang Qin*), Cortex Radicis Mori Albi (*Sang Bai Pi*), Cortex Radicis Lycii Chinensis (*Di Gu Pi*), Radix Albus Paeoniae Lactiflorae (*Bai Shao*), mix-fried Radix Glycyrrhizae (*Gan Cao*)

Additions & subtractions: For rib-side pain, add Tuber Curcumae (*Yu Jin*) and Fructus Meliae Toosendan (*Chuan Lian Zi*). For hacking of blood, add Herba Agrimoniae Pilosae (*Xian He Cao*) and Nodus Nelumbinis Nuciferae (*Ou Jie*). For severe coughing and panting, add Succus Bambusae (*Zhu Li*) and Concretio Silicea Bambusae (*Tian Zhu Huang*). If the eosinophil count cannot be lowered, add Fructus Pruni Mume (*Wu Mei*).

4. Spleen-kidney dual vacuity pattern

Main symptoms: Fatigue, lack of strength, no appetite, loose stools, cockcrow diarrhea, long, clear urination, generalized edema, dizziness, low back and lower leg aching and limpness, fear of cold, cold hands and feet, decreased sexual desire, a pale and/or dark, enlarged tongue with slimy, white fur, and a deep, forceless pulse

Treatment principles: Warm and supplement the spleen and kidneys, replenish the essence and supplement the blood

Chinese medicinal formula:

SHEN LU BIE TANG **(Ginseng, Deer [Antler] & [Carapax] Amydae Decoction)**
Radix Panacis Ginseng (*Ren Shen*), Cervi Cornu (*Lu Jiao*), Carapax Amydae Sinensis (*Bie Jia*), Fructus Lycii Chinensis (*Gou Qi Zi*), Radix Codonopsitis Pilosulae (*Dang Shen*), Rhizoma Atractylodis Macrocephalae (*Bai Zhu*), Radix Morindae Officinalis (*Ba Ji Tian*), Fructus Psoraleae Corylifoliae (*Bu Gu Zhi*), Radix Angelicae Sinensis (*Dang Gui*), Radix Ligustici Wallichii (*Chuan Xiong*), Radix Albus Paeoniae Lactiflorae (*Bai Shao*), uncooked Radix Rehmanniae (*Sheng Di*), Radix Lateralis Praeparatus Aconiti Carmichaeli (*Fu Zi*)

Additions & subtractions: For central duct glomus and oppression with scanty intake, reduce the amount of *Bie Jia* and *Lu Jiao* and remove *Dang Gui* and *Sheng Di*.

3 Leukopenia

Leukopenia is a reduction of the circulating white blood cell count to less than 4000/mm^3. Leukopenia is most commonly due to a reduced number of neutrophils, in which case it is called neutropenia, although reduced lymphocytes, monocytes, eosinophils, or basophils may also contribute to the decreased total cell count. Since neutrophils can be referred to as granulocytes, if this condition is due to a granulocyte decrease, it can also be called granulocytopenia or agranulocytosis. Neutropenia is caused by either decreased and/or ineffective production or increased destruction of neutrophils. The most common cause of impaired neutrophil production are drugs. Some antineoplastic drugs, for example, cause neutropenia as a predictable side effect. Other causes of impaired production are rare hereditary diseases, marrow replacement or involvement (*e.g.*, malignancies, myelofibrosis), and severe vitamin B$_{12}$ and folic acid deficiency. Increased margination may be the cause during the acute phase of some infections, certain autoimmune disorders (*e.g.*, SLE, RA), and in certain conditions associated with splenomegaly. Many cases of neutropenia are asymptomatic and unexplained, a condition called chronic benign neutropenia.

Neutropenia has no specific manifestations except those of current infections, which generally depend upon the severity, duration, and cause of the neutropenia. In acute neutropenia, fever, painful mucosal ulcers of the mouth and perirectal area, and bacterial pneumonia are common. Bacteremia and septic shock are consequences in untreated cases. Chronic neutropenia has a far more benign outlook, particularly when other immune functions are intact.

The Western medical treatment of acute leukopenia focuses on removal of the cause (such as the discontinuation of drugs if they impair white blood cell production) and treatment of infections with antibiotics. In very severe cases, antibiotics may not be strong enough, and granulocyte transfusions are necessary. Chronic leukopenia is usually left untreated, with the patient being told to seek prompt medical attention in case of an infection.

Chinese medical disease explanation:

In Chinese medicine, leukopenia corresponds to the categories of qi and blood vacuity (*qi xue xu*) and vacuity taxation (*xu lao*). Chinese medicine holds that, "If evils encroach, the qi must be vacuous." Furthermore, qi vacuity is very closely related to debilitation of the former and latter heaven roots, *i.e.*, the spleen and kidneys. If the spleen is vacuous, then movement and transformation lose their power and the engenderment and transformation of qi and blood have no source. If the kidneys become vacuous, then essence and marrow are insufficient and blood becomes debilitated. Thus, the defensive qi is weak and the body is easily invaded by wind toxins and damp heat evils.

During the chronic benign stage of leukopenia, no acute infections are present. The manifestations are, therefore, indicative of qi, blood, yin, and/or yang vacuities with no evils present. Thus, the following five patterns are differentiated during the chronic benign stage of leukopenia: 1) qi and blood insufficiency with non-fortification of the spleen, 2) spleen and stomach vacuity weakness, 3) spleen and kidney vacuity, 4) liver and kidney yin vacuity, and 5) qi and blood insufficiency, essence depletion, and blood stasis. The presence of static blood in the last pattern is based on the saying, "Enduring diseases lead to blood stasis." In keeping with the above differentiation of patterns, the treatment principles for chronic leukopenia are to boost the qi and nourish the blood, invigorate yang and enrich yin, fortify the spleen and supplement the liver and kidneys as well as quicken the blood and transform stasis.

The acute phase of leukopenia is characterized by infections and, therefore, the presence of replete evils. Two main patterns are recognized: 1) defensive qi vacuity with toxic heat flaming and exuberant and 2) spleen and lung qi weakness with lingering disease evils. The former pattern is characterized by evil exuberance and thus by symptoms of repletion, such as vigorous fever, thirst for cold drinks, and even delirium. The second pattern describes a mutual struggle between righteous and evil qi. In this case, the righteous qi has no strength to expel the evils, but the evils also have no strength to penetrate any deeper into the body. Thus, the disease becomes lingering and there are symptoms of both qi vacuity and evil contraction. In addition, these two patterns may mutually transform into each other. If evils become exuberant and flare up, then the second pattern may turn into the first one. On the other hand, if the righteous qi becomes exhausted secondary to evil exuberance and evils cannot be expelled, they may become lingering, thus giving rise to pattern #2.

It should also be pointed out that, during the acute stage of leukopenia, one can base treatment on warm disease (*wen bing*) pattern discrimination. Commonly used treatment principles are to clear heat and resolve toxins, boost the qi and quicken the blood, and support the righteous and dispel evils.

Treatment based on pattern discrimination:

A. Chronic phase

1. Qi & blood insufficiency with non-fortification of the spleen pattern

Main symptoms: A lusterless facial complexion, dizziness, shortage of qi, fatigue, reduced appetite, abdominal distention, a pale tongue, and a fine, weak pulse

Treatment principles: Boost the qi, nourish the blood, and fortify the spleen

Chinese medicinal formulas:

GUI SHAO SHEN QI TANG (**Dang Gui, Peony, Codonopsis & Astragalus Decoction**)
Radix Astragali Membranacei (*Huang Qi*), Radix Codonopsitis Pilosulae (*Dang Shen*), Rhizoma Atractylodis Macrocephalae (*Bai Zhu*), Radix Albus Paeoniae Lactiflorae (*Bai Shao*), Radix Angelicae Sinensis (*Dang Gui*), Ramulus Cinnamomi Cassiae (*Gui Zhi*), Fructus Ligustri Lucidi (*Nu Zhen Zi*), Fructus Schisandrae Chinensis (*Wu Wei Zi*)

GUI ZHI JIA HUANG QI TANG (**Cinnamon Twig Plus Astragalus Decoction**)
Radix Astragali Membranacei (*Huang Qi*), Ramulus Cinnamomi Cassiae (*Gui Zhi*), Radix Albus Paeonia Lactiflorae (*Bai Shao*), uncooked Rhizoma Zingiberis (*Sheng Jiang*), Fructus Zizyphi Jujubae (*Da Zao*), Radix Glycyrrhizae (*Gan Cao*)

YU PING FENG SAN (**Jade Wind-screen Powder**)
Radix Astragali Membranacei (*Huang Qi*), Rhizoma Atractylodis Macrocephalae (*Bai Zhu*), uncooked Rhizoma Zingiberis (*Sheng Jiang*), Radix Ledebouriellae Divaricatae (*Fang Feng*)

The above two formulas are particularly indicated if there are frequent common colds and spontaneous perspiration.

DA BU YUAN JIAN (**Major Origin-supplementing Brew**)
Radix Panacis Ginseng (*Ren Shen*), cooked Radix Rehmanniae (*Shu Di*), Cortex Eucommiae Ulmoidis (*Du Zhong*), Radix Dioscoreae Oppositae (*Shan Yao*), Radix Angelicae Sinensis (*Dang Gui*), Fructus Corni Officinalis (*Shan Zhu Yu*), Fructus Lycii Chinensis (*Gou Qi Zi*), Radix Glycyrrhizae (*Gan Cao*)

This formula treats more severe blood vacuity with such additional symptoms as heart palpitations, fearful throbbing, and a somber white facial complexion.

SHEN QI TENG WEI TANG **(Codonopsis, Astragalus, Milletia & Pyrrosia Decoction)**
  Radix Astragali Membranacei (*Huang Qi*), Radix Codonopsitis Pilosulae (*Dang Shen*), Folium Pyrrosiae (*Shi Wei*), Caulis Milletiae Seu Spatholobi (*Ji Xue Teng*), Fructus Zizyphi Jujubae (*Da Zao*)

This formula is particularly indicated if qi and blood vacuity is due to radiation or chemotherapy. In addition to the above symptoms, the patient may also suffer from heart palpitations, profuse dreams, and insomnia.

2. Spleen-stomach vacuity weakness pattern

Main symptoms: Shortage of qi, laziness to speak, cumbersome and fatigued limbs, a weak body, scanty appetite, no taste for food and drink, inability to endure work (*i.e.*, very tired and exhausted), shortness of breath aggravated by activity, a pale tongue with white fur, and a vacuous or weak pulse

Treatment principles: Warm the qi and upbear yang, harmonize the stomach and supplement the spleen

Chinese medicinal formulas:

BU ZHONG YI QI TANG **(Supplement the Center & Boost the Qi Decoction)**
  Radix Panacis Ginseng (*Ren Shen*), Rhizoma Atractylodis Macrocephalae (*Bai Zhu*), Radix Astragali Membranacei (*Huang Qi*), Rhizoma Cimicifugae (*Sheng Ma*), Radix Bupleuri (*Chai Hu*), Pericarpium Citri Reticulatae (*Chen Pi*), Radix Angelicae Sinensis (*Dang Gui*), mix-fried Radix Glycyrrhizae (*Gan Cao*)

SI JUN ZI TANG **(Four Gentlemen Decoction)**
  Radix Panacis Ginseng (*Ren Shen*), Rhizoma Atractylodis Macrocephalae (*Bai Zhu*), Sclerotium Poriae Cocos (*Fu Ling*), mix-fried Radix Glycyrrhizae (*Gan Cao*)

LI ZHONG TANG **(Rectify the Center Decoction)**
  Radix Panacis Ginseng (*Ren Shen*), Rhizoma Atractylodis Macrocephalae (*Bai Zhu*), dry Rhizoma Zingiberis (*Gan Jiang*), mix-fried Radix Glycyrrhizae (*Gan Cao*)

This formula is indicated if there is middle burner cold with such additional manifestations as cold limbs, abdominal distention, and loose stools.

WEN DAN TANG (**Warm the Gallbladder Decoction**)

Caulis Bambusae In Taeniis (*Zhu Ru*), Fructus Immaturus Citri Aurantii (*Zhi Shi*), Rhizoma Pinelliae Ternatae (*Ban Xia*), Pericarpium Citri Reticulatae (*Chen Pi*), Sclerotium Poriae Cocos (*Fu Ling*), Radix Glycyrrhizae (*Gan Cao*), uncooked Rhizoma Zingiberis (*Sheng Jiang*)

This formula can be used if loss of movement and transformation of the spleen and stomach leads to damp turbidity brewing and obstructing with such manifestations as severe dizziness, chest oppression, a bland taste in the mouth, torpid intake, loose stools, slimy, yellow tongue fur, and a soggy, moderate (*i.e.*, slightly slow) pulse.

SHEN JIANG TANG (**Ginseng & Ginger Decoction**)

Radix Panacis Ginseng (*Ren Shen*), dry Rhizoma Zingiberis (*Gan Jiang*), Semen Myristicae Fragrantis (*Rou Dou Kou*), Caulis Akebiae (*Mu Tong*), Radix Scutellariae Baicalensis (*Huang Qin*), Cortex Magnoliae Officinalis (*Hou Po*), Herba Agastachis Seu Pogostemi (*Huo Xiang*), Cortex Sclerotii Poriae Cocos (*Fu Ling Pi*), Rhizoma Cyperi Rotundi (*Xiang Fu*), Radix Ligustici Wallichii (*Chuan Xiong*), Tuber Curcumae (*Yu Jin*), Talcum (*Hua Shi*)

This formula is for accumulation of dampness and turbidity due to a weak spleen and stomach not being able to perform their duty of moving and transforming the food. Indications for the use of this formula are chest oppression, nausea and vomiting, belching and eructation, cumbersome limbs, a heavy body, slimy, white tongue fur, and a soggy pulse.

Additions & subtractions: If the leukocyte count increases only slowly, add Radix Angelicae Sinensis (*Dang Gui*), Caulis Milletiae Seu Spatholobi (*Ji Xue Teng*), and Radix Salviae Miltiorrhizae (*Dan Shen*).

3. Spleen-kidney dual vacuity pattern

Main symptoms: Dizziness with flowery vision, lumbar aching, tinnitus, bodily fatigue and lack of strength, scanty food intake, loose stools, a lusterless yellow facial complexion, lumbar aching, knee limpness, a pale tongue, and a weak pulse

Treatment principles: Boost the qi and nourish the blood, enrich and supplement the kidneys, fortify the spleen and harmonize the middle

Chinese medicinal formulas:

SHENG BAI TIAO BU TANG **(White [Blood Cell] Engendering, Regulating & Supplementing Decoction)**

Radix Astragali Membranacei (*Huang Qi*), Radix Codonopsitis Pilosulae (*Dang Shen*), Radix Polygoni Multiflori (*He Shou Wu*), Fructus Germinatus Hordei Vulgaris (*Mai Ya*), Caulis Milletiae Seu Spatholobi (*Ji Xue Teng*), Rhizoma Drynariae (*Gu Sui Bu*), Fructus Ligustri Lucidi (*Nu Zhen Zi*), Fructus Citri Sarcodactylis (*Fo Shou*)

ER HUANG YI REN TANG **(Two Yellows & Coix Decoction)**

Radix Astragali Membranacei (*Huang Qi*), Rhizoma Polygonati (*Huang Jing*), Semen Coicis Lachryma-jobi (*Yi Yi Ren*), Fructus Lycii Chinensis (*Gou Qi Zi*), mix-fried Radix Glycyrrhizae (*Gan Cao*)

WEN SHEN TANG **(Warm the Kidneys Decoction)**

Herba Epimedii (*Yin Yang Huo*), Fructus Psoraleae Corylifoliae (*Bu Gu Zhi*), Semen Cuscutae Chinensis (*Tu Si Zi*), Radix Dioscoreae Oppositae (*Shan Yao*), Fructus Lycii Chinensis (*Gou Qi Zi*), Radix Angelicae Sinensis (*Dang Gui*), Caulis Milletiae Seu Spatholobi (*Ji Xue Teng*), Radix Astragali Membranacei (*Huang Qi*), Cortex Cinnamomi Cassiae (*Rou Gui*), mix-fried Radix Glycyrrhizae (*Gan Cao*)

SHENG BAI TANG JIANG **(White [Blood Cell] Engendering Syrup)**

Radix Astragali Membranacei (*Huang Qi*), Radix Codonopsitis Pilosulae (*Dang Shen*), Radix Salviae Miltiorrhizae (*Dan Shen*), Fructus Corni Officinalis (*Shan Zhu Yu*), Fructus Psoraleae Officinalis (*Bu Gu Zhi*), Radix Polygoni Multiflori (*He Shou Wu*), Caulis Milletiae Seu Spatholobi (*Ji Xue Teng*), Radix Angelicae Sinensis (*Dang Gui*), Radix Rubiae Cordifoliae (*Qian Cao Gen*), scorched Fructus Crataegi (*Shan Zha*)

YOU GUI WAN **(Restore the Right [Kidney] Pills)**

Radix Lateralis Praeparatus Aconiti Carmichaeli (*Fu Zi*), Cortex Eucommiae Ulmoidis (*Du Zhong*), Cortex Cinnamomi Cassiae (*Rou Gui*), cooked Radix Rehmanniae (*Shu Di*), Radix Dioscoreae Oppositae (*Shan Yao*), Fructus Corni Officinalis (*Shan Zhu Yu*), Semen Cuscutae Chinensis (*Tu Si Zi*), Radix Angelicae Sinensis (*Dang Gui*), Gelatinum Cornu Cervi (*Lu Jiao Jiao*)

This formula is especially indicated if there are, in addition to the above manifestations, cold hands and feet.

4. Liver-kidney yin vacuity pattern

Main symptoms: Dizziness, tinnitus, fatigue, emaciation, vexation and agitation, heart palpitations, insomnia, clouding of the head, a red tongue with scanty fur, and a fine, rapid pulse

Treatment principles: Enrich and supplement the kidneys and liver, and, in case of flaring up of vacuity fire, clear and downbear vacuity fire

Chinese medicinal formulas:

ZI SHEN TANG (Enrich the Kidneys Decoction)

Fructus Ligustri Lucidi (*Nu Zhen Zi*), Herba Ecliptae Prostratae (*Han Lian Cao*), Radix Polygoni Multiflori (*He Shou Wu*), Radix Salviae Miltiorrhizae (*Dan Shen*), Caulis Milletiae Seu Spatholobi (*Ji Xue Teng*), Radix Dioscoreae Oppositae (*Shan Yao*), Radix Angelicae Sinensis (*Dang Gui*), uncooked Radix Rehmanniae (*Sheng Di*), Pericarpium Citri Reticulatae (*Chen Pi*), mix-fried Radix Glycyrrhizae (*Gan Cao*)

YI HAO YU SHEN SHENG XUE TANG (Number One Foster the Kidney & Engender the Blood Decoction)

Frostbitten Folium Kaki (*Shuang Shi Ye*)[1], Conchae Ostreae (*Mu Li*), Plastrum Testudinis (*Gui Ban*), Carapax Amydae Sinensis (*Bie Jia*), Radix Anemarrhenae Asphodeloidis (*Zhi Mu*), Cortex Phellodendri (*Huang Bai*), Fructus Ligustri Lucidi (*Nu Zhen Zi*), Cortex Radicis Lycii Chinensis (*Di Gu Pi*), Fructus Lycii Chinensis (*Gou Qi Zi*), Rhizoma Polygoni Cuspidati (*Hu Zhang*), Radix Albus Paeoniae Lactiflorae (*Bai Shao*), Radix Scrophulariae Ningpoensis (*Xuan Shen*)

This formula is indicated if there is upward flaming of vacuity heat.

SHENG XUE TANG (Upbear the Blood Decoction)

Radix Albus Paeoniae Lactiflorae (*Bai Shao*), Radix Astragali Membranacei (*Huang Qi*), Radix Angelicae Sinensis (*Dang Gui*), Radix Polygoni Multiflori (*He Shou Wu*), Caulis Milletiae Seu Spatholobi (*Ji Xue Teng*), Herba Epimedii (*Xian Ling Pi*), Os Suis (*Zhu Gu*), Fructus Psoraleae Corylifoliae (*Bu Gu Zhi*), Gelatinum Cornu Cervi (*Lu Jiao Jiao*), Cortex Radicis Lycii Chinensis (*Di Gu Pi*)

This formula is particularly indicated if the leukopenia is due to anti-thyroid drugs and manifests a pattern of qi and yin dual vacuity with such additional symptoms as irascibility and spontaneous sweating. A report in the *Hei Long Jiang Zhong Yi Yao (Heilongjiang Journal of Chinese Medicine & Medicinals)*[2] noted that, in a clinical trial of 32 cases suffering from anti-thyroid drug induced leukopenia, the efficacy rate after

---

[1] Folium Kaki (*Shi Ye*) is bitter and cold in nature and enters the lung channel. It principally treats cough with panting, lung qi distention, and any type of internal swelling with bleeding. Recommended dosage is 5-15 grams.

[2] *Hei Long Jiang Zhong Yi Yao (Heilongjiang Journal of Chinese Medicine & Medicinals)*, #3, 1984, p. 17

two treatment courses with the above formula (time length of one treatment course not specified) was 96.6%.

5. Qi & blood insufficiency, essence depletion, and blood stasis pattern

Main symptoms: A lusterless facial complexion, dizziness, fatigue, lack of strength, lumbar aching, tinnitus, a pale white tongue with static macules, and a weak, choppy pulse

Treatment principles: Supplement the qi and boost the essence, nourish and quicken the blood

Chinese medicinal formulas:

DA ZAO JI XUE TENG TANG (Red Date & Milletia Decoction)
Fructus Zizyphi Jujubae (*Da Zao*), Caulis Milletiae Seu Spatholobi (*Ji Xue Teng*), Radix Astragali Membranacei (*Huang Qi*), Rhizoma Polygonati (*Huang Jing*), Fructus Ligustri Lucidi (*Nu Zhen Zi*), Radix Salviae Miltiorrhizae (*Dan Shen*)

SHENG XUE HE JI (Engender the Blood Mixture)
Fructus Corni Officinalis (*Shan Zhu Yu*), Rhizoma Polygoni Multiflori (*He Shou Wu*), Fructus Ligustri Lucidi (*Nu Zhen Zi*), Herba Epimedii (*Yin Yang Huo*), Radix Salviae Miltiorrhizae (*Dan Shen*), blast-fried Squama Manitis Pentadactylis (*Chuan Shan Jia*), Caulis Milletiae Seu Spatholobi (*Ji Xue Teng*), Cortex Magnoliae Officinalis (*Hou Po*)

This formula is indicated if leukopenia is due to chemotherapy and presents with blood stasis and kidney vacuity. Additional symptoms include withered, scanty hair, a withered or bright white, lusterless facial complexion, laziness to speak, lassitude of the spirit, and a weak pulse which is forceless especially when pressed deep.

B. Acute phase

1. Defensive qi vacuity with toxic heat flaming & exuberant pattern

Main symptoms: Oral ulcers, blood-engorged, swollen throat and tonsils, pneumonia, bronchitis, swollen lymph nodes all over the body, vigorous fever, vexation and agitation, thirst for cold liquids, headache, body aches, a dry mouth and throat, a somber white facial complexion, a red tongue with yellow fur, and a rapid pulse. If severe, there is spirit clouding and deranged speech.

Treatment principles: Clear heat and resolve toxins, boost the qi and quicken the blood

Chinese medicinal formulas:

ZENG BAI TANG (Increase White [Blood Cell] Decoction)
Flos Lonicerae Japonicae (*Jin Yin Hua*), Fructus Forsythiae Suspensae (*Lian Qiao*), Herba Taraxaci Mongolici Cum Radice (*Pu Gong Ying*), Herba Viola Yedoensitis Cum Radice (*Zi Hua Di Ding*), Radix Scutellariae Baicalensis (*Huang Qin*), Rhizoma Coptidis Chinensis (*Huang Lian*), Massa Medica Fermentata (*Shen Qu*), Radix Platycodi Grandiflori (*Jie Geng*), Radix Astragali Membranacei (*Huang Qi*), Radix Salviae Miltiorrhizae (*Dan Shen*), blast-fried Squama Manitis Pentadactylis (*Chuan Shan Jia*), Spica Prunellae Vulgaris (*Xia Ku Cao*), Radix Scrophulariae Ningpoensis (*Yuan Shen*), Radix Glycyrrhizae (*Gan Cao*)

Additions & subtractions: For bronchial pneumonia with marked coughing and panting, add Herba Ephedrae (*Ma Huang*), Herba Asari Cum Radice (*Xi Xin*), Bulbus Lilii (*Bai He*), and Bulbus Fritillariae Cirrhosae (*Chuan Bei Mu*). If there is accompanying vexation and agitation and, if severe, fright reversal and other signs of nervous system involvement, add Ramulus Uncariae Cum Uncis (*Gou Teng*), Periostracum Cicadae (*Chan Tui*), Scolopendra Subspinipes (*Wu Gong*), and Buthus Martensis (*Quan Xie*). For accompanying urinary frequency and pain, add Cortex Phellodendri (*Huang Bai*), Caulis Akebiae (*Mu Tong*), and Semen Plantaginis (*Che Qian Zi*).

PU JI XIAO DU YIN (Universal Salvation Disperse Toxins Drink)
Radix Scutellariae Baicalensis (*Huang Qin*), Rhizoma Coptidis Chinensis (*Huang Lian*), Exocarpium Citri Erythrocarpae (*Ju Hong*), Radix Scrophulariae Ningpoensis (*Xuan Shen*), Radix Glycyrrhizae (*Gan Cao*), Fructus Forsythiae Suspensae (*Lian Qiao*), Fructus Arctii Lappae (*Niu Bang Zi*), Rhizoma Imperatae Cylindricae (*Bai Mao Gen*), Fructificatio Lasiospherae (*Ma Bo*), Bombyx Batryticatus (*Bai Jiang Can*), Rhizoma Cimicifugae (*Sheng Ma*), Radix Bupleuri (*Chai Hu*), Folium Mentha Haplocalycis (*Bo He Ye*), Radix Platycodi Grandiflori (*Jie Geng*)

YIN QIAO SAN (Lonicera & Forsythia Powder)
Fructus Forsythiae Suspensae (*Lian Qiao*), Flos Lonicerae Japonicae (*Jin Yin Hua*), Herba Menthae Haplocalycis (*Bo He*), Radix Platycodi Grandiflorii (*Jie Geng*), Fructus Arctii Lappae (*Niu Bang Zi*), Herba Lophatheri Gracilis (*Dan Zhu Ye*), Rhizoma Phragmitis Communis (*Lu Gen*), Herba Seu Flos Schizonepetae Tenuifoliae (*Jing Jie*), Semen Praeparatum Sojae (*Dan Dou Chi*), Radix Glycyrrhizae (*Gan Cao*)

This formula is indicated for the early stages of infections when there is fever with simultaneous aversion to cold.

2. Spleen-lung qi vacuity with lingering disease evils pattern

Main symptoms: No or low-grade fever, relatively light inflammation or ulceration of the throat and oral cavity, somewhat fatigued limbs and body, a long and slow disease course

Note: This pattern may turn into the one above if the evils become exuberant.

Treatment principles: Fortify the spleen and boost the lungs, support the righteous and dispel evils

Chinese medicinal formula:

HUANG QI JI XUE TANG **(Astragalus & Milletia Decoction)**
   Radix Astragali Membranacei (*Huang Qi*), Radix Codonopsitis Pilosulae (*Dang Shen*), Rhizoma Atractylodis Macrocephalae (*Bai Zhu*), Sclerotium Poriae Cocos (*Fu Ling*), Caulis Milletiae Seu Spatholobi (*Ji Xue Teng*), Radix Salviae Miltiorrhizae (*Dan Shen*), Radix Polygoni Multiflori (*He Shou Wu*), Radix Rubiae Cordifoliae (*Qian Cao Gen*), Fructus Psoraleae Corylifoliae (*Bu Gu Zhi*), Radix Scutellariae Baicalensis (*Huang Qin*), Flos Lonicerae Japonicae (*Jin Yin Hua*), Radix Anemarrhenae Asphodeloidis (*Zhi Mu*), Radix Glycyrrhizae (*Gan Cao*)

4 The Leukemias

Leukemias are malignant neoplasms of the hematopoietic (blood forming) tissue. The cause in humans is unidentified, although two viral associations have been made: one with the Epstein-Barr virus (which is the causative agent of infectious mononucleosis and a suspected cause of malignant lymphoma) and one with the human T-cell lymphotrophic virus (HTLV-1). Furthermore, exposure to ionizing radiation and certain chemicals (benzene and some antineoplastics) is associated with an increased risk of leukemia. Certain genetic defects (Down syndrome) and familial disorders (Fanconi's anemia) are also predisposing factors to leukemia.

What is interesting is that transformation to malignancy appears to occur in a single cell with subsequent proliferation and clonal expansion. This transformation may affect pluripotential stem cells or committed stem cells with a more limited capacity for differentiation. Once a cell has transformed into a leukemic cell, it tends to have longer cell cycles and smaller growth fractions than normal cells. Accumulations of leukemic cells defective in maturation and differentiation then lead to clonal growth advantage. Inhibitory factors produced by the defective (leukemic) cells or replacement of marrow space by leukemic cells may suppress normal hematopoiesis, with ensuing anemia, thrombocytopenia, and granulocytopenia. Organ infiltration by leukemic cells leads to enlargement of the liver, spleen, and lymph nodes. The kidneys and gonads may occasionally be involved. If the meninges are infiltrated, clinical features of increased intracranial pressure manifest.

Leukemias are classified into acute and chronic types according to cellular maturity. Acute leukemias are mostly non-differentiated cell populations whereas chronic leukemias are more mature cells. Leukemias are hematopoietic cancers and their Western medical treatment, therefore, primarily focuses on the use of systemic chemotherapy. Radiation therapy is used to eradicate localized accumulations of leukemic cells, but surgery is rarely used. However, bone marrow transplantation is sometimes indicated. The goal of treatment is the eradication of leukemic cell populations. In chronic leukemias, however, the risk of such harsh treatment is too great and does not show evident survival benefits. Thus, the limitation of the leukemic clone size and maintenance of the patient in the asymptomatic stage become the goals of treatment in chronic leukemia.

A. Chronic leukemias

There exist two distinct types of chronic leukemias: chronic myelocytic leukemia (CML) and chronic lymphocytic leukemia (CLL). Chronic melocytic leukemia is a clonal proliferation caused by the malignant transformation of a pluripotent stem cell with a striking overproduction of granulocytes. Chronic myelocytic leukemia constitutes about 20% of all leukemias in the West and occurs in either sex at any age. However, it is more common in the middle-aged and elderly, with the median age of onset at 50 years.

Patients suffering from CML have pronounced granulocytosis. However, since the neoplastic clone includes erythrocytes, megakaryocytes, and monocytes, anemia, thrombocytopenia, and basophilia are also present. The CML clone is genetically unstable. With loss of differentiation and maturation capacity of the granulocytic precursor cells, accumulation of blast cells in medullary and extramedullary tissues occurs. This is called a blast crisis and terminates the chronic stable phase of CML in two thirds of patients. Symptoms of early CML may be subclinical and discovered ony at a routine CBS. Insidious onset of such symptoms as fatigue, weakness, anorexia, weight loss, fever, night sweats, or a sense of abdominal fullness appear in other patients. Splenomegaly progresses from moderate to very severe throughout the stable phase of 2-8 years (with a mean of 3-4 years). With progression of the disease, manifestations such as pallor (anemia), bleeding (thrombocytopenia or qualitative platelet defects), fever, and marked lymphadenopathy may appear.

Chemotherapy and interferon-alpha are used in the treatment of CML. Good results have been obtained with bone marrow transplantation.

Chronic lymphocytic leukemia is characterized by clonal proliferation of immunologically immature and functionally incompetent small lymphocytes. The B-cell lineage is most commonly affected, and the resulting leukemia is then termed B-CLL. This type of leukemia is the most common one in Western countries and constitutes 30% of all leukemias.[1] It is 2-3 times more common in men than women, and the average age of onset is 60 years. The cause of B-CLL is unknown. Lymphocyte accumulation begins in the lymphnodes and spreads to other lymphoid tissues, such as the spleen and liver. Infiltration of the bone marrow and displacement of viable hemopoietic tissue leads to

---

[1]   All source material for the Chinese medical treatments in this book come from mainland China. Since B-CLL is rare in China and other Asian countries, the treatment formulas below are designed for CML. However, considering the similarity in symptomatology, I believe that B-CLL can be differentiated among the same patterns, and thus similar medicinal prescriptions, with certain modifications, should prove to be helpful in treatment. Moreover, even though CLL is rare in China, one of the sources used for this work clearly states that chronic leukemia includes CLL, thus confirming the validity of the above Chinese medical approach to this leukemia's pattern discrimination and treatment.

anemia, agranulocytopenia, and thrombocytopenia. Immuno-regulatory problems with hypogammaglobulinemia is a common manifestation and makes patients with CLL susceptible to autoimmune diseases, such as RA, immunohemolytic anemia, thyroiditis, and vasculitis, as well as second and even third malignancies.

Onset of CLL, similar to CML, is insidious and may manifest as asymptomatic adenopathy. Nonspecific complaints, such as fatigue, anorexia, weight loss, dyspnea on exertion, and a sense of abdominal fullness from an enlarging spleen, are common at an early stage. The course of disease is highly variable, with an overall mean survival rate of six years. In some patients, the disease progresses rapidly, leading to death in 2-3 years. Other patients remain asymptomatic for 10-20 years. Bacterial infections are a common complication due to hypogammaglobulinemia and granulocytopenia. These and other infections (*i.e.*, viral and fungal infections) are features of advancing CLL. Western medical therapy is not indicated for currently asymptomatic patients. For symptomatic patients, Western medical treatment is supportive for presenting symptoms and antineoplastic (irradiation, antineoplastic drugs). However, treatment does not prolong survival and may be associated with significant side effects. *The Merck Manual* points out that, "overtreatment is more dangerous than undertreatment."[2]

Chinese medical disease explanation:

In Chinese medicine, chronic leukemia (including CML and CLL), is classified according to presenting symptoms and signs. If the main manifestations are fatigue, lack of strength, shortness of breath, spontaneous perspiration and/or night sweats, torpid intake, and emaciation, the disease is classified as vacuity taxation (*xu lao*). If there is bleeding, it is classified as a bleeding condition (*xue zheng*). If enlargement of the spleen and/or liver is pronounced, it falls into the category of concretions and conglomerations, accumulations and gatherings (*zheng jia ji ju*).

Disease causes leading to the engenderment of chronic leukemia include depletion of the righteous qi, emotional repression and depression, and unregulated food and drink. In children, this disease is commonly related to former heaven insufficiency. Repression and depression of emotions can lead to qi stagnation and blood stasis. Unregulated food and drink damages the spleen and stomach leading to the accumulation of phlegm and turbidity. If the righteous qi becomes vacuous and depleted, nourishing and warming of the five viscera and six bowels loses its strength, and the qi of these viscera becomes weak. Therefore, protection against invading disease evils is weak and insufficient. Toxic evils may, therefore, take advantage of this vacuity and assail the channels and network vessels. Lodging of such toxic evils in the bone marrow may lead to disorders of blood

---

[2]   *The Merck Manual*, 16th ed., Merck Research Laboratories, Rahway, NJ, 1992, p. 1243

engenderment. Obstruction of blood movement in the channels and vessels by the evils may lead to stasis and bindings, with accumulations and gatherings developing in the liver and spleen.

Therefore, chronic leukemia presents clinically as a combination of vacuity and repletion, *i.e.*, a root vacuity with a branch repletion. It is also said of leukemia that, "Because of vacuity, there is disease, and because of disease, there is vacuity."

During the early stages of this disease, the righteous qi is only slightly vacuous and evil repletion is not yet severe. Symptoms at this stage include an accumulation lump (*i.e.*, splenomegaly) which is still relatively small and soft. Other signs are often not yet present or manifest only mildly. The middle stages are characterized by gradual debilitation of righteous qi with increasing strength of evil qi. Symptoms at this stage include an accumulation lump which has increased in size and become harder, fatigue, lack of strength, low-grade fever, copious sweating, the effusion of macules, spontaneous blood ejections, and emaciation. During the late stages, the righteous qi has become seriously depleted and greatly vacuous, while evil qi is fiercely replete. Manifestations include a large accumulation lump, a sallow yellow facial complexion, and an emaciated bodily form. Pain in the limbs and body, high fever, and bleeding may be present.

The bleeding manifestations in the middle and late stages are due to either of three reasons. Qi vacuity may allow evil toxins to invade the body and progress to the blood division, there causing frenetic movement of hot blood. Secondly, qi vacuity may simply not contain the blood within its vessels. Bleeding caused by either heat or qi vacuity then may precipitate the third mechanism of bleeding. Bleeding into the tissues blocks and obstructs the blood and network vessels. Such obstruction by malign, static blood backs up the blood flow and forces the blood to flow outside its vessels. Furthermore, obstruction by static blood also leads to the pain in the limbs and body which manifests in the late stages of this disease.

Chinese medical treatment of this disease, as in all others, is based on pattern discrimination. During the early stages, emphasis should be on attacking without much supplementation. In the middle stages, simultaneous supplementation and attacking are appropriate, while in the late stages, the focus is on supplementation of vacuity accompanied by dispelling of evils.

Chronic leukemia is broken down into two main patterns below. Pattern #1 is characteristic of the early and middle stages, while pattern #2 includes middle and late stages. Due to the simultaneous existence of vacuity and repletion in this condition, practitioners must differentiate the relative proportions of repletion and vacuity and select and modify the following formulas accordingly.

Treatment based on pattern discrimination:

1. Essence debilitation & marrow vacuity with static blood concretions & conglomerations pattern

Main symptoms: A vacuous form and weak body, lack of strength, emaciation, irregular low-grade fever, afternoon tidal fever, heat in the hands and feet, reduced appetite, torpid intake, abdominal fullness and distention, scrofula of the neck and nape of the neck, swelling of the liver and spleen, a withered white facial complexion, possible mouth and tongue sores, a red tongue with scanty fur, and a fine, rapid pulse

Treatment principles: Boost the essence and replenish the marrow, transform stasis and disperse conglomerations

Chinese medicinal formulas:

GUI DI BIE JIA TANG **(Tortoise Shell, Rehmannia & Carapax Amydae Decoction)** Cooked Radix Rehmanniae (*Shu Di*), Radix Polygoni Multiflori (*He Shou Wu*), Fructus Ligustri Lucidi (*Nu Zhen Zi*), Plastrum Testudinis (*Gui Ban*), Carapax Amydae Sinensis (*Bie Jia*), Rhizoma Curcumae Zedoariae (*E Zhu*), Rhizoma Spargani Stoloniferae (*San Leng*), Radix Astragali Membranacei (*Huang Qi*), Radix Salviae Miltiorrhizae (*Dan Shen*), Hirudo Seu Whitmania (*Shui Zhi*), Spica Prunellae Vulgaris (*Xia Ku Cao*), Herba Potentillae Discoloris (*Fan Bai Cao*)[3], Massa Medica Fermentata (*Shen Qu*), Radix Glycyrrhizae (*Gan Cao*)

Additions & subtractions: For accompanying infections with high fevers, add Folium Daqingye (*Da Qing Ye*), Fructus Forsythiae Suspensae (*Lian Qiao*), and Flos Lonicerae Japonicae (*Jin Yin Hua*). For an elevated platelet count, add Eupolyphagia Seu Opisthoplatia (*Tu Bie Chong*) and Lumbricus (*Di Long*). For decreased platelets, add uncooked Pollen Typhae (*Pu Huang*), Herba Agrimoniae Pilosae (*Xian He Cao*), and Radix Rubiae Cordifoliae (*Qian Cao Gen*).

---

[3] Herba Potentillae Discoloris (*Fan Bai Cao*) is sweet, bitter, and neutral in nature. It clears heat and resolves toxins, scatters nodulation and disperses swellings, and stops bleeding. Together with *Xia Ku Cao*, it inhibits the disease evils and resolves the scrofulous phlegm kernels, thereby reducing the swelling of the lymph nodes. Recommended dosage is 9-15 grams.

XIA YU XUE TANG (Precipitating Static Blood Decoction)
Radix Et Rhizoma Rhei (*Da Huang*), Semen Pruni Persicae (*Tao Ren*), Eupolyphagia Seu Opisthoplatia (*Zhe Chong*)

This formula is indicated when static blood is the main concern, or it can be added to other formulas to strengthen their blood-quickening function.

JIAN PI XIAO SHI FANG (Spleen-fortifying, Food-dispersing Formula)
Pericarpium Citri Reticulatae (*Chen Pi*), Fructus Citri Sarcodactylis (*Fo Shou*), Radix Glycyrrhizae (*Gan Cao*), ginger-processed Caulis Bambusae In Taeniis (*Jiang Zhu Ru*), Massa Medica Fermentata (*Shen Qu*), Herba Agastachis Seu Pogostemi (*Huo Xiang*), Fructus Germinatus Oryzae Sativae (*Gu Ya*), Fructus Germinatus Hordei Vulgaris (*Mai Ya*), Folium Perillae Frutescentis (*Su Ye*), Caulis Perillae Frutescentis (*Su Geng*)

This formula is particularly indicated if chronic leukemia is accompanied by a pronounced loss of appetite.

MAN XING SUI XING BAI XUE BING FANG (Chronic Marrow Leukemia Formula)
Radix Astragali Membranacei (*Huang Qi*), Caput Radicis Angelicae Sinensis (*Dang Gui Tou*), Cortex Radicis Moutan (*Dan Pi*), Lignum Sappan (*Su Mu*), Radix Codonopsitis Pilosulae (*Dang Shen*), Plastrum Testudinis (*Gui Ban*), Carapax Amydae Sinensis (*Bie Jia*), Concha Haliotidis (*Shi Jue Ming*), Cortex Radicis Lycii Chinensis (*Di Gu Pi*), uncooked Radix Rehmanniae (*Sheng Di*), Gelatinum Corii Asini (*E Jiao*), Depositum Praeparatum Urinae Hominis (*Qiu Shi*)

2. Qi & blood consumption & detriment with accumulation of exuberant evil toxins pattern

Main symptoms: A bright white facial complexion, shortness of breath, dizziness, heart palpitations, spontaneous blood ejection into the skin and membranes, progressive emaciation of the entire body, spontaneous perspiration, joint aches, continuously increasing swelling of the lymph nodes, spleen, and liver, mouth sores, fever, a red tongue with yellow fur, and a bowstring, fine, rapid pulse. This pattern corresponds to a late stage phase or even the blast crisis phase of chronic leukemia.

Treatment principles: Clear heat and resolve toxins, boost the qi to engender the blood

Chinese medicinal formulas:

QING RE YI QI TANG (Clear Heat & Boost the Qi Decoction)
Radix Isatidis Seu Baphicacanthi (*Ban Lan Gen*), Herba Potentillae Discoloris (*Fan Bai Cao*), Rhizoma Paridis Polyphyllae (*Qi Ye Yi Zhi Hua*), Spica Prunellae Vulgaris (*Xia Ku Cao*), Radix Astragali Membranacei (*Huang Qi*), Rhizoma Polygonati (*Huang Jing*), Radix Salviae Miltiorrhizae (*Dan Shen*), Herba Rubiae Cordifoliae (*Qian Cao Gen*), Caulis Milletiae Seu Spatholobi (*Ji Xue Teng*), Radix Glycyrrhizae (*Gan Cao*)

Additions & subtractions: For vexation and agitation, add Ramulus Uncariae Cum Uncis (*Gou Teng*), Periostracum Cicadae (*Chan Tui*), and Lumbricus (*Di Long*). For vigorous and non-abating fever accompanied by spirit clouding and deranged speech, add *An Gong Niu Huang Wan* (Peaceful Palace Bezoar Pills). For markedly decreased platelets with severe bleeding, add Herba Agrimoniae Pilosae (*Xian He Cao*), Gelatinum Corii Asini (*E Jiao*), Herba Euphorbiae Humifusae (*Di Jin Cao*)[4], and Radix Pseudoginseng (*San Qi*).

XIAO BAI SAN (Disperse the White Powder)
Gecko Swinhoana (*Bi Hu*)[5], Scolopendra Subspinipes (*Wu Gong*), Cinnabar (*Zhu Sha*), Alumen (*Ku Fan*), Pulvis Indigonis (*Qing Dai*), Radix Pseudoginseng (*San Qi*), Zaocys Dhumnades (*Wu She*), Herba Patriniae Heterophyllae Cum Radice (*Bai Jiang Cao*)

This formula is indicated if toxins and blood contend and bind with such symptoms as hard and large concretions and accumulations and a somber facial complexion.

QING GAN HUA YU FANG (Clear the Liver & Transform Stasis Formula)
Herba Artemesiae Apiaceae (*Qing Hao*), Fructus Gardeniae Jasminoidis (*Zhi Zi*), Cortex Radicis Lycii Chinensis (*Di Gu Pi*), Radix Rubrus Paeoniae Lactiflorae (*Chi Shao*), Cortex Radicis Moutan (*Dan Pi*), Herba Senecionis Integrifolii (*Gou She Cao*)[6], Rhizoma Curcumae Zedoariae (*E Zhu*), Rhizoma Spargani Stoloniferae (*San*

---

[4] Herba Euphorbiae Humifusae (*Di Jin Cao*) is acrid and neutral in nature. It clears heat and resolves toxins, quickens the blood and stops bleeding, disinhibits dampness and frees the flow of breast milk. Recommended dosage is 3-6 grams.

[5] Gecko Swinhoana (*Bi Hu*) is salty, cold, and slightly toxic in nature. It dispels wind and settles fright, scatters nodulation and resolves toxins. No dosage noted in the *Zhong Yao Da Ci Dian*.

[6] Herba Senecionis Integrifolii (*Gou She Cao*) is bitter, cold, and slightly toxic in nature. It clears heat, disinhibits water, and kills worms. Recommended dosage is 9-15 grams.

Leng), Herba Solani Lyrati (*Bai Mao Teng*)[7], Radix Salviae Miltiorrhizae (*Dan Shen*), Herba Leonuri Heterophylli (*Yi Mu Cao*), Herba Oldenlandiae Diffusae Cum Radice (*Bai Hua She She Cao*)

Because this formula specifically clears the liver, it is indicated in patients with a particularly bowstring pulse and rib-side distention and pain.

YI QI YANG YIN TANG (Boost the Qi & Nourish Yin Decoction)

Radix Astragali Membranacei (*Huang Qi*), Radix Codonopsitis Pilosulae (*Dang Shen*), Cortex Radicis Lycii Chinensis (*Di Gu Pi*), Radix Bupleuri (*Chai Hu*), Sclerotium Poriae Cocos (*Fu Ling*), Tuber Ophiopogonis Japonici (*Mai Dong*), Semen Nelumbinis Nuciferae (*Lian Zi*), Radix Scutellariae Baicalensis (*Huang Qin*), Semen Plantaginis (*Che Qian Zi*), Radix Glycyrrhizae (*Gan Cao*)

This formula is for pronounced qi and yin dual vacuity with accompanying heat and dampness but with relatively mild toxic evils.

B. Acute leukemias

Acute leukemias are rapidly progressing forms of leukemia characterized by replacement of normal bone marrow by blast cells of a clone arising from malignant transformation of a hemopoietic stem cell. Without treatment, they are rapidly fatal and patients die within approximately two months. Acute leukemias are divided into two groups: acute myelogenic leukemia (AML) and acute lymphocytic leukemia (ALL). Acute myelogenic leukemia constitutes 20% of all leukemias in Western countries. Acute lymphocytic leukemia comprises 10% of all leukemias in the West. However, whereas AML accounts for only 20% of childhood leukemias, ALL is the most common childhood malignancy, and 60% of ALL occurs in children. In the United States, ALL occurs twice as commonly in whites as in blacks, and the peak incidence rate is between 3-5 years of age. Acute lymphocytic leukemia also occurs in adolescents and less commonly in adults. Acute myelogenic leukemia occurs in all ages. It accounts for 20% of acute leukemia in childhood and for 85% in adults.

The causes for both types of acute leukemia are unknown. However, chemotherapeutic agents, irradiation, genetic abnormalities (most notably Down syndrome), and other hematopoietic diseases, such as MDS, AA, and PNH, are established risk factors. The pathogenesis is principally related to the accumulation of leukemic cells in the bone marrow which replace normal hematopoietic cells and spread to the liver, spleen, lymph

---

[7] Herba Solani Lyrati (*Bai Mao Teng*) is sweet and cold in nature. It clears heat and resolve toxins, disinhibits urination and expels wind.

nodes, CNS, kidneys, and gonads. Disruption of organ function is usually minimal except for involvement of the CNS and bone marrow. Meningeal infiltration results in increased intracranial pressure, and replacement of normal hematopoiesis in the bone marrow causes anemia, thrombocytopenia, and granulocytopenia. Infiltration of the liver, spleen, and lymph nodes leads to enlargement of these organs.

Signs and symptoms of acute leukemia are due to the consequences of failure of normal hematopoiesis: bleeding, pallor, and fever. Bleeding usually involves the skin and mucous membranes and uncommonly is associated with hematuria or gastrointestinal bleeding. Sometimes, bone and joint aching are present. Bacterial infections secondary to neutropenia may bring the patient to medical attention. Central nervous system involvement, presenting with initial headache, vomiting, and irritability, is common even in the early stages of disease. This complication is now prevented by prophylactic irradiation of the craniospinal axis. A more insidious onset of acute leukemia is associated with progressive weakness, lethargy, and pallor.

Modern aggressive chemotherapy is the treatment of choice in Western medicine and has dramatically altered the outlook of this disease. Clinical remissions and even complete cures are no longer rare in patients who used to die within a few months prior to the invention of chemotherapy.

Chinese medical disease explanation:

In Chinese medicine, acute leukemia corresponds to the disease categories of acute taxation (*ji lao*), heat taxation (*re lao*), and vacuity taxation (*xu lao*). Because bleeding symptoms as well as swelling of the spleen, liver, and lymph nodes sometimes also occur, it can also be classified as a bleeding condition (*xue zheng*) or concretions and conglomerations (*zheng jia*).

The disease mechanisms for acute leukemia are similar to chronic leukemia. In children, a congenital kidney essence insufficiency lies at its core. In older patients, internal vacuity detriment leads to kidney qi and essence vacuity. Because essence transforms into source qi, essence depletion leads to general qi vacuity. Thus, the warming and nourishing of the viscera and bowels of the entire body is debilitated, and transformation and engenderment of qi, blood, liquids, and humors is insufficient. As the righteous qi becomes vacuous and weak, the body's defensive function decreases and toxic evils assail the exterior and settle deeply into the body. When such evil toxins brew internally, blood becomes static and phlegm congeals. When toxic evils penetrate to the bone marrow, they consume the blood and damage marrow. This then leads to dysfunctional blood engenderment with immature white blood cells.

Thus, one can see that vacuity of the righteous qi always mixes with repletion of toxic evils in leukemia patterns. Therefore, according to the strength of the evils or the severity of the righteous vacuity, Chinese medical treatment focuses on supplementing the righteous and dispelling evils. The former includes supplementing and nourishing the qi and blood and harmonizing and supplementing yin and yang. The latter principles include clearing heat and resolving toxins, quickening the blood and transforming stasis, and softening the hard and scattering nodulation.

Evils can also enter the source spirit. According to Li Shi-zhen, the source spirit is housed in the brain and is responsible for consciousness, memory, thinking, vision, hearing, etc. Thus, in keeping with the viscera and bowel theory that all cognitive functions are attributed to the spirit and that the spirit is housed in the heart, evils entering the source spirit is the same as evils entering the pericardium. This pattern corresponds to what Western medicine calls leukemic infiltration of the CNS.

Patients suffering from acute leukemia are at risk for the often deadly complication of disseminated intravascular coagulation (DIC). Disseminated intravascular coagulation arises due to 1) evil toxins causing detriment and damage to the network vessels, 2) insufficient qi not strong enough to contain the blood, and 3) static blood obstructing the vessels and network vessels. Furthermore, it is said that an inability by the liver to store the blood contributes to DIC. Modern research has shown that the treatment principles of quickening the blood and transforming stasis are effective in the prevention of DIC and should, therefore, be added to the treatment of at-risk leukemia patients.[8]

It is interesting to note that modern research performed in the People's Republic of China has also confirmed that boosting and supplementing medicinals increase immune cells' function to more effectively recognize and kill leukemic cells.[9] The treatment principles are, therefore, to clear heat and resolve toxins, boost the qi and supplement the blood, enrich yin and invigorate yang, and quicken the blood and transform stasis.

Treatment based on pattern discrimination:

1. Accumulated exuberant evil toxins pattern

Main symptoms: High fever, vexation and agitation, somber white facial complexion, sweating, thirst, static macules, joint aching, pronounced sternal pain, reddish urination, dry stools, a red or pale red tongue body with yellowish-white fur, and a floating, rapid

---

[8] *Zhong Yi Er Ke Xue Ye Bing Zhen Liao Jing Yan (Experiences in the Diagnosis & Treatment of Pediatric Hematological Diseases)*, 3rd ed., Cai Hua-li, ed., People's Health & Hygiene Press, Beijing, 1996, p. 168

[9] *Ibid.*, p. 169

or bowstring, rapid pulse. This pattern is characteristic of acute leukemia accompanied by bacterial or viral infections.

Treatment principles: Clear heat and resolve toxins, boost the qi and quicken the blood

Chinese medicinal formulas:

SHE SHE CAO TANG (Oldenlandia Decoction)

Herba Oldenlandiae Diffusae Cum Radice (*Bai Hua She She Cao*), Herba Scutellariae Barbatae (*Ban Zhi Lian*), Spica Prunellae Vulgaris (*Xia Ku Cao*), Rhizoma Paridis Polyphyllae (*Qi Ye Yi Zhi Hua*), Flos Lonicerae Japonicae (*Jin Yin Hua*), Fructus Forsythiae Suspensae (*Lian Qiao*), Folium Daqingye (*Da Qing Ye*), uncooked Radix Rehmanniae (*Sheng Di*), Rhizoma Anemarrhenae Asphodeloidis (*Zhi Mu*), Radix Astragali Membranacei (*Huang Qi*), Radix Codonopsitis Pilosulae (*Dang Shen*), Sclerotium Polypori Umbellati (*Zhu Ling*), Radix Salviae Miltiorrhizae (*Dan Shen*), Radix Rubrus Paeoniae Lactiflorae (*Chi Shao*), Fructus Gardeniae Jasminoidis (*Zhi Zi*), Herba Patriniae Heterophyllae Cum Radice (*Bai Jiang Cao*), Radix Glycyrrhizae (*Gan Cao*)

Additions & subtractions: For constipation, add Radix Et Rhizoma Rhei (*Da Huang*). For accompanying nausea and vomiting, add Pericarpium Citri Reticulatae (*Chen Pi*) and Caulis Bambusae In Taeniis (*Zhu Ru*). If these additions are not effective, add Rhizoma Pinelliae Ternatae (*Ban Xia*) and Herba Asari Cum Radice (*Xi Xin*). For accompanying headache and dizziness which could be indicative of leukemic meningitis, add Buthus Martensis (*Quan Xie*) and Scolopendra Subspinipes (*Wu Gong*). If this does not cause the headache to abate, add Hirudo Seu Whitmania (*Shui Zhi*).

JIE DU HUA YU TANG (Resolve Toxins & Transform Stasis Decoction)

Herba Oldenlandiae Diffusae Cum Radice (*Bai Hua She She Cao*), Herba Scutellariae Barbatae (*Ban Zhi Lian*), Radix Salviae Miltiorrhizae (*Dan Shen*), Semen Coicis Lachryma-jobi (*Yi Yi Ren*), uncooked Radix Rehmanniae (*Sheng Di*), Herba Patriniae Heterophyllae Cum Radice (*Bai Jiang Cao*), Rhizoma Curcumae Zedoariae (*E Zhu*), Rhizoma Sparganii (*San Leng*), Endothelium Corneum Gigeriae Galli (*Ji Nei Jin*)

This formula is indicated when blood stasis signs, such as a markedly swollen liver and spleen, hard abdominal lumps, a pale, purplish tongue, and a bowstring, slippery pulse, are prominent.

DANG GUI LONG HUI WAN (Dang Gui, Gentiana & Aloe Pills)

Radix Angelicae Sinensis (*Dang Gui*), Radix Gentianae Scabrae (*Long Dan Cao*), Fructus Gardeniae Jasminoidis (*Zhi Zi*), Rhizoma Coptidis Chinensis (*Huang Lian*),

Cortex Phellodendri (*Huang Bai*), Radix Scutellariae Baicalensis (*Huang Qin*), Radix Et Rhizoma Rhei (*Da Huang*), Herba Aloes (*Lu Hui*), Pulvis Indigonis (*Qing Dai*), Radix Auklandiae Lappae (*Mu Xiang*), Secretio Moschi Moschiferi (*She Xiang*)

This formula is indicated when toxic evils are in the form of damp toxins with such additional symptoms as afternoon tidal fever, dizziness, watery, loose stools, slimy, yellow tongue fur, and a rapid, slippery pulse.

XIAO DU QING XUE TANG (Disperse Toxins & Clear the Blood Decoction)

Folium Daqingye (*Da Qing Ye*), Radix Isatidis Seu Baphicacanthi (*Ban Lan Gen*), Radix Lithospermi Seu Arnebiae (*Zi Cao*), Radix Rubrus Paeoniae Lactiflorae (*Chi Shao*), Cortex Radicis Moutan (*Dan Pi*), Cornu Bubali (*Shui Niu Jiao*), Periostracum Cicadae (*Chan Tui*), Realgar (*Xiong Huang*)

JIE DU YU NU JIAN (Toxin-resolving Jade Lady Brew)

Cornu Antelopis Saiga-tataricae (*Ling Yang Jiao*)[10], Radix Scrophulariae Ningpoensis (*Xuan Shen*), Gypsum Fibrosum (*Shi Gao*), uncooked Radix Rehmanniae (*Sheng Di*), Tuber Asparagi Cochinensis (*Tian Dong*), Flos Lonicerae Japonicae (*Jin Yin Hua*), Fructus Forsythiae Suspensae (*Lian Qiao*), Herba Taraxaci Mongolici Cum Radice (*Pu Gong Ying*), Rhizoma Anemarrhenae Asphodeloidis (*Zhi Mu*), Cortex Radicis Moutan (*Dan Pi*)

2. Accumulated exuberant evil toxins with stasis & stagnation pattern

Main symptoms: High fever, vexation and agitation, abdominal pain, bone pain, abdominal fullness, rib-side distention, pain, and swollen, hard lumps, non-free flowing stool, subcutaneous static macules, a dark purple tongue with many static macules, and a bowstring, choppy pulse

Treatment principles: Resolve toxins and transform stasis

Chinese medicinal formulas:

JIE DU HUO XUE TANG (Resolve Toxins & Quicken the Blood Decoction)

Flos Lonicerae Japonicae (*Jin Yin Hua*), Herba Taraxaci Mongolici Cum Radice (*Pu Gong Ying*), Herba Patriniae Heterophyllae Cum Radice (*Bai Jiang Cao*), uncooked Radix Rehmanniae (*Sheng Di*), Cortex Radicis Moutan (*Dan Pi*), Radix Rubrus Paeoniae Lactiflorae (*Chi Shao*), Flos Carthami Tinctorii (*Hong Hua*), Radix Salviae

---

[10] For ecological reasons, one should always substitute Cornu Caprae (*Shan Yang Jiao*) for *Ling Yang Jiao*.

Miltiorrhizae (*Dan Shen*), Spica Prunellae Vulgaris (*Xia Ku Cao*), Carapax Amydae Sinensis (*Bie Jia*), Radix Achyranthis Bidentatae (*Niu Xi*), Radix Pseudoginseng (*San Qi*)

DANG GUI CHUAN XIONG TANG (Dang Gui & Ligusticum Decoction)

Radix Angelicae Sinensis (*Dang Gui*), Radix Ligustici Wallichii (*Chuan Xiong*), Caulis Milletiae Seu Spatholobi (*Ji Xue Teng*), Radix Rubrus Paeoniae Lactiflorae (*Chi Shao*), Flos Carthami Tinctorii (*Hong Hua*), Radix Pseudoginseng (*San Qi*)

Additions & subtractions: For accompanying liver and kidney yin vacuity, add Fructus Lycii Chinensis (*Gou Qi Zi*), Fructus Ligustri Lucidi (*Nu Zhen Zi*), and Radix Polygoni Multiflori (*He Shou Wu*). For accompanying qi and blood dual vacuity, add Radix Codonopsitis Pilosulae (*Dang Shen*), Radix Astragali Membranacei (*Huang Qi*), Fructus Lycii Chinensis (*Gou Qi Zi*), Radix Polygoni Multiflori (*He Shou Wu*), cooked Radix Rehmanniae (*Shu Di*), Rhizoma Polygonati (*Huang Jing*), and Rhizoma Atractylodis Macrocephalae (*Bai Zhu*). For accumulation and exuberance of heat toxins, add Cornu Bubali (*Shui Niu Jiao*), uncooked Radix Rehmanniae (*Sheng Di*), Cortex Radix Moutan (*Dan Pi*), Radix Rubiae Cordifoliae (*Qian Cao Gen*), Rhizoma Paridis Polyphyllae (*Zao Xiu*), Flos Lonicerae Japonicae (*Jin Yin Hua*), Fructus Forsythiae Suspensae (*Lian Qiao*), Herba Taraxaci Mongolici Cum Radice (*Pu Gong Ying*), and Radix Isatidis Seu Baphicacanthi (*Ban Lan Gen*).

3. Phlegm fire exuberance pattern

Main symptoms: This pattern is very similar to either of the above. However, there is pronounced swelling of the spleen, liver, and lymph nodes, the tongue is red with thick slimy, yellow fur, and the pulse is slippery, replete, and bowstring.

Treatment principles: Transform phlegm and soften hardness, clear heat and resolve toxins

Chinese medicinal formulas:

XIA KU CAO GAO (Prunella Paste)

Spica Prunellae Vulgaris (*Xia Ku Cao*), Radix Angelicae Sinensis (*Dang Gui*), Radix Albus Paeoniae Lactiflorae (*Bai Shao*), Radix Scrophulariae Ningpoensis (*Hei Shen*), Radix Linderae Strychnifoliae (*Wu Yao*), Bulbus Fritillariae Thunbergi (*Zhe Bei Mu*), Bombyx Batryticatus (*Jiang Can*), Thallus Algae (*Kun Bu*), Radix Platycodi Grandiflori (*Jie Geng*), Pericarpium Citri Reticulatae (*Chen Pi*), Radix Ligustici

Wallichii (*Chuan Xiong*), Radix Glycyrrhizae (*Gan Cao*), Rhizoma Cyperi Rotundi (*Xiang Fu*), Flos Carthami Tinctorii (*Hong Hua*)

This formula also has a blood-nourishing and liver-coursing function and is, therefore, particularly indicated when there is concurrent blood vacuity with liver depression.

QING HUO DI TAN TANG (Clear Fire & Flush Phlegm Decoction)

Radix Salviae Miltiorrhizae (*Dan Shen*), Tuber Ophiopogonis Japonici (*Mai Dong*), Sclerotium Pararadicis Poriae Cocos (*Fu Shen*), Semen Biotae Orientalis (*Bai Zi Ren*), Bombyx Batryticatus (*Jiang Can*), Bulbus Fritillariae Thunbergi (*Zhe Bei Mu*), Exocarpium Citri Erythrocarpae (*Ju Hong*), Flos Chrysanthemi Morifolii (*Ju Hua*), Semen Pruni Armeniacae (*Xing Ren*), bile-processed Rhizoma Arisaematis (*Dan Nan Xing*), Herba Lophatheri Gracilis (*Dan Zhu Ye*), uncooked Rhizoma Zingiberis (*Sheng Jiang*)

4. Qi & yin dual vacuity pattern

Main symptoms: Irregular low-grade fever, a somber white facial complexion with a characteristic dark greyish hue, fever in the palms of the hands and soles of the feet, heart palpitations, hasty breathing, shortage of qi, laziness to speak, dizziness, thirst, occasional inflammation of the oral cavity and tongue, possible slight bleeding with static speckles of the skin and membranes, or possible swelling of the liver, spleen, and lymph nodes, a red tongue with yellowish-white fur, and a floating, rapid or fine, rapid pulse

Treatment principles: Boost the qi and enrich yin, transform stasis and scatter nodulation

Chinese medicinal formulas:

SI HUANG ZHI LIAN TANG (Four Yellows Scutellaria Barbata Decoction)

Radix Panacis Ginseng (*Ren Shen*), Radix Astragali Membranacei (*Huang Qi*), Rhizoma Polygonati (*Huang Jing*), uncooked Radix Rehmanniae (*Sheng Di*), cooked Radix Rehmanniae (*Shu Di*), Tuber Ophiopogonis Japonici (*Mai Dong*), Rhizoma Anemarrhenae Asphodeloidis (*Zhi Mu*), Caulis Milletiae Seu Spatholobi (*Ji Xue Teng*), Fructus Zizyphi Jujubae (*Da Zao*), Radix Salviae Miltiorrhizae (*Dan Shen*), Herba Scutellariae Barbatae (*Ban Zhi Lian*), Spica Prunellae Vulgaris (*Xia Ku Cao*), Radix Rhapontici Seu Echinopsis (*Lou Lu*), Eupolyphagia Seu Opistholoplatia (*Zhe Chong*), Herba Agrimoniae Pilosae (*Xian He Cao*), Radix Glycyrrhizae (*Gan Cao*)

Additions & subtractions: For accompanying nausea and vomiting, add Pericarpium Citri Reticulatae (*Chen Pi*) and Rhizoma Pinelliae Ternatae (*Ban Xia*). For decreased food intake, add Endothelium Corneum Gigeriae Galli (*Ji Nei Jin*), Massa Medica Fermentata (*Shen Qu*), and Fructus Crataegi (*Shan Zha*). For cough, add Radix Stemonae (*Bai Bu*), Radix Scutellariae Baicalensis (*Huang Qin*), and Bulbus Fritillariae Cirrhosae (*Chuan Bei Mu*). For vexation and agitation, add Ramulus Uncariae Cum Uncis (*Gou Teng*) and Sclerotium Pararadicis Poriae Cocos (*Fu Shen*)

SAN CAI FENG SUI DAN (Three Powers Envelope the Marrow Elixir)

Radix Pseudostellariae Heterophyllae (*Tai Zi Shen*), Bulbus Shancigu (*Shan Ci Gu*), uncooked Radix Rehmanniae (*Sheng Di*), cooked Radix Rehmanniae (*Shu Di*), Tuber Ophiopogonis Japonici (*Mai Dong*), Tuber Asparagi Cochinensis (*Tian Dong*), Fructus Amomi (*Sha Ren*), Cortex Phellodendri (*Huang Bai*), Radix Glycyrrhizae (*Gan Cao*), blackened Fructus Gardeniae Jasminoidis (*Zhi Zi*), Rhizoma Paridis Polyphyllae (*Zao Xiu*)

ZI YIN SHEN QI WAN (Enrich Yin Kidney Qi Pills)

Uncooked Radix Rehmanniae (*Sheng Di*), cooked Radix Rehmanniae (*Shu Di*), Cortex Radicis Moutan (*Dan Pi*), Rhizoma Alismatis (*Ze Xie*), Sclerotium Poriae Cocos (*Fu Ling*), Caput Radicis Angelicae Sinensis (*Dang Gui Tou*), Fructus Corni Officinalis (*Shan Zhu Yu*), Radix Bupleuri (*Chai Hu*), Fructus Schisandrae Chinensis (*Wu Wei Zi*), Radix Dioscoreae Oppositae (*Shan Yao*)

This formula focuses on nourishing yin and is, therefore, indicated when there is pronounced yin vacuity with only mild qi vacuity.

SHEN QI DI HUANG TANG (Ginseng, Astragalus & Rehmannia Decoction)

Radix Panacis Ginseng (*Ren Shen*), Radix Astragali Membranacei (*Huang Qi*), cooked Radix Rehmanniae (*Shu Di*), Cortex Radicis Moutan (*Dan Pi*), Sclerotium Poriae Cocos (*Fu Ling*), Fructus Corni Officinalis (*Shan Zhu Yu*), Radix Dioscoreae Oppositae (*Shan Yao*), uncooked Rhizoma Zingiberis (*Sheng Jiang*), Fructus Zizyphi Jujubae (*Da Zao*)

SHEN QI MAI WEI TANG (Codonopsis, Astragalus, Ophiopogon & Schisandra Decoction)

Radix Astragali Membranacei (*Huang Qi*), Radix Codonopsitis Pilosulae (*Dang Shen*), Rhizoma Polygonati (*Huang Jing*), Herba Oldenlandiae Diffusae Cum Radice (*Bai Hua She She Cao*), Herba Scutellariae Barbatae (*Ban Zhi Lian*), Radix Salviae Miltiorrhizae (*Dan Shen*), uncooked Radix Rehmanniae (*Sheng Di*), Rhizoma Curcumae Zedoariae (*E Zhu*), Sclerotium Poriae Cocos (*Fu Ling*), Tuber Ophiopogonis Japonici (*Mai Dong*), Tuber Asparagi Cochinensis (*Tian Dong*), Herba

Cephalanoploris Segeti (*Xiao Ji*), Radix Pseudoginseng (*San Qi*), Herba Taraxaci Mongolici Cum Radice (*Pu Gong Ying*), Radix Glycyrrhizae (*Gan Cao*)

5. Source spirit evil damage pattern

Main symptoms: Headache, dizziness, nausea, vomiting, somnolence, and delirium. Frequently, there is papilledema[11] with blurred vision, facial nerve paralysis, or paralysis of the limbs. Occasionally, there are tugging wind[12] and epilepsy-like spasms.

Treatment principles: Break stasis and eliminate evils, extinguish wind and quiet the spirit

Chinese medicinal formulas:

DAN ZHU TANG **(Salvia & Zedoaria Decoction)**
Radix Salviae Miltiorrhizae (*Dan Shen*), Rhizoma Curcumae Zedoariae (*E Zhu*), Caulis Milletiae Seu Spatholobi (*Ji Xue Teng*), Radix Rubrus Paeoniae Lactiflorae (*Chi Shao*), Radix Ligustici Wallichii (*Chuan Xiong*), Radix Astragali Membranacei (*Huang Qi*), Rhizoma Gastrodiae Elatae (*Tian Ma*), Ramulus Uncariae Cum Uncis (*Gou Teng*), Lumbricus (*Di Long*), Spica Prunellae Vulgaris (*Xia Ku Cao*), Herba Scutellariae Barbatae (*Ban Zhi Lian*), uncooked Radix Rehmanniae (*Sheng Di*), Radix Anemarrhenae Asphodeloidis (*Zhi Mu*), Radix Glycyrrhizae (*Gan Cao*), Buthus Martensis (*Quan Xie*), Scolopendra Subspinipes (*Wu Gong*), Bombyx Batryticatus (*Jiang Can*), Eupolyphagia Seu Opistholoplatia (*Zhe Chong*), Hirudo Seu Whitmania (*Shui Zhi*)

Additions & subtractions: For high fever with spirit clouding and deranged speech, administer *An Gong Niu Huang Wan* (Peaceful Palace Bezoar Pills) in addition to the above formula. For papilledema due to increased cranial pressure, add Sclerotium Poriae Cocos (*Fu Ling*), Caulis Akebiae (*Mu Tong*), Rhizoma Alismatis (*Ze Xie*), and Semen Plantaginis (*Che Qian Zi*).

---

[11] Papilledema refers to edema and inflammation of the optic nerve at its point of entrance into the eyeball and is due to increased intracranial pressure. If not treated immediately, it can lead to blindness.

[12] Tugging wind is a technical term and refers to alternating tensing and slackening of the sinews, *i.e.,* convulsions.

6. Blood stasis & vessel stagnation pattern

Main symptoms: Marked static spots and static macules on the skin and membranes, blood ejection, if severe, bloody stools, vomiting of blood, and hematuria

Treatment principles: Boost the qi and quicken the blood, transform stasis and stop bleeding

Chinese medicinal formulas:

HUO LUO YI QI TANG **(Quicken the Network Vessels & Boost the Qi Decoction)**
Radix Astragali Membranacei (*Huang Qi*), Radix Ligustici Wallichii (*Chuan Xiong*), uncooked Radix Rehmanniae (*Sheng Di*), Radix Rubrus Paeoniae Lactiflorae (*Chi Shao*), Flos Carthami Tinctorii (*Hong Hua*), Semen Pruni Persicae (*Tao Ren*), Radix Pseudoginseng (*San Qi*), Pollen Typhae (*Pu Huang*), Herba Agrimoniae Pilosae (*Xian He Cao*), Folium Callicarpae (*Zi Zhu Cao*), Rhizoma Paridis Polyphyllae (*Qi Ye Yi Zhi Hua*), Herba Scutellariae Barbatae (*Ban Zhi Lian*), Radix Glycyrrhizae (*Gan Cao*)

Additions & subtractions: For disseminated intravascular coagulation (DIC), add Hirudo Seu Whitmania (*Shui Zhi*) and increase the amount of *San Qi*. For severe bleeding secondary to viral or bacterial infections, add Flos Lonicaerae Japonicae (*Jin Yin Hua*), Folium Daqingye (*Da Qing Ye*), Herba Taraxaci Mongolici Cum Radice (*Pu Gong Ying*), and Herba Violae Yedoensitis Cum Radice (*Zi Hua Di Ding*).

QIAN GEN SAN **(Rubia Powder)**
Radix Rubiae Cordifoliae (*Qian Cao Gen*), Radix Sanguisorbae (*Di Yu*), Semen Iridis Pallasii (*Ma Lin Zi*)[13], Rhizoma Coptidis Chinensis (*Huang Lian*), Cortex Phellodendri (*Huang Bai*), Radix Scutellariae Baicalensis (*Huang Qin*), Radix Angelicae Sinensis (*Dang Gui*)

XI JIAO DI HUANG TANG JIA JIAN **(Rhinocerus Horn[14] & Rehmannia Decoction with Additions & Subtractions)**
Cornu Bubali (*Shui Niu Jiao*), Radix Rubrus Paeoniae Lactiflorae (*Chi Shao*), Cortex Radicis Moutan (*Dan Pi*), uncooked Radix Rehmanniae (*Sheng Di*)

---

[13] Semen Iridis Pallasii (*Ma Lin Zi*) is sweet and neutral in nature and enters the spleen and lung channels. It clears heat, disinhibits dampness, stops bleeding, and resolves toxins. Recommended dosage is 3-9 grams.

[14] This medicinal comes from a seriously endangered species and should always be substituted with Cornu Bubali *(Shui Niu Jiao)*.

Combining Chinese medicinals & chemotherapy

Patients suffering from acute leukemia need to receive Western chemotherapy. Chinese medicinals by themselves are not sufficient to treat this disease. However, Chinese medicine is extremely helpful in supporting patients undergoing chemotherapy.

Chemotherapy depresses the hemopoietic function of the marrow, leading to a decrease in the output of all formed elements of the blood. Further, it does not kill leukemic cells selectively but rather wipes out all white blood cells. This leaves the body very susceptible to bacterial and viral infections. Symptoms associated with these two adverse effects of chemotherapy are bleeding (thrombocytopenia) and fever (infections), with the fever tending to be high. This symptom complex corresponds to the Chinese medical pattern of toxic evils with blood heat.

Other common symptoms of patients undergoing chemotherapy are jaundice, nausea, vomiting, aversion to oily and greasy foods, torpid intake, epigastric and abdominal distention and oppression, pain in the hepatic area, visceral swelling, thick, slimy, yellow-white or gray tongue fur, and a bowstring, slippery pulse. The corresponding pattern in Chinese medicine for this symptom complex is damp heat smoldering and stagnating in the liver and gallbladder. Chinese medical treatment for this pattern focuses on clearing heat, resolving toxins, and dispelling dampness, coursing the liver and disinhibiting the gallbladder, and fortifying the spleen. Appropriate formulas which can be used are *Yin Chen Hao Tang* (Artemisia Capillaris Decoction) with the addition of *Dan Zhi Xiao Yao Er Chen Tang* (Moutan & Gardenia Rambling plus Two Aged [Ingredients] Decoction). For severe jaundice, add Herba Lysimachiae Seu Desmodii Styracifolii (*Jin Qian Cao*). For exuberant dampness, add Rhizoma Atractylodis (*Cang Zhu*) and Cortex Magnoliae Officinalis (*Hou Po*).

Because chemotherapy damages and causes detriment to the digestive system, common post-chemotherapy manifestations are decreased appetite, nausea, abdominal distention, fatigue, and thick, slimy, yellow-white or black-brown tongue fur. In other patients, there is lack of strength, night sweats and/or spontaneous perspiration, heart palpitations, abnormal sleep, and a pale tongue with thin fur. Post-chemotherapy manifestations are divided into five different patterns which are differentiated mainly according to the thickness and color of the tongue fur as well as the color of the tongue body.

1. Spleen vacuity with smoldering & stagnant damp heat pattern

Main symptoms: A selection of the above digestive complaints plus thick, slimy, yellow-white tongue fur

Treatment principles: Fortify the spleen, clear heat, and eliminate dampness

Chinese medicinal formula:

SI JUN ZI TANG HE PING WEI SAN JIA WEI (**Four Gentlemen Decoction plus Stomach-leveling Powder with Added Flavors**)
Rhizoma Atractylodis Macrocephalae (*Bai Zhu*), Sclerotium Poriae Cocos (*Fu Ling*), Radix Panacis Ginseng (*Ren Shen*), mix-fried Radix Glycyrrhizae (*Gan Cao*), Rhizoma Atractylodis (*Cang Zhu*), Cortex Magnoliae Officinalis (*Hou Po*), Fructus Zizyphi Jujubae (*Da Zao*), Pericarpium Citri Reticulatae (*Chen Pi*), uncooked Rhizoma Zingiberis (*Sheng Jiang*), Radix Scutellariae Baicalensis (*Huang Qin*), Rhizoma Coptidis Chinensis (*Huang Lian*)

2. Yin vacuity with accompanying damp heat pattern

Main symptoms: A selection of the above symptoms plus thick ash-black or brown tongue fur

Treatment principles: Nourish yin, clear heat, and eliminate dampness

Chinese medicinal formula:

ZENG YE TANG HE SI JUN ZI TANG JIA JIAN (**Humor-increasing Decoction plus Four Gentlemen Decoction & Stomach-leveling Powder**)
Rhizoma Atractylodis Macrocephalae (*Bai Zhu*), Sclerotium Poriae Cocos (*Fu Ling*), mix-fried Radix Glycyrrhizae (*Gan Cao*), Radix Panacis Ginseng (*Ren Shen*), Rhizoma Atractylodis (*Cang Zhu*), Cortex Magnoliae Officinalis (*Hou Po*), Fructus Zizyphi Jujubae (*Da Zao*), uncooked Rhizoma Zingiberis (*Sheng Jiang*), Pericarpium Citri Reticulatae (*Chen Pi*), Radix Scrophulariae Ningpoensis (*Xuan Shen*), Tuber Ophiopogonis Japonici (*Mai Dong*), uncooked Radix Rehmanniae (*Sheng Di*)

3. Heat accumulation with yin depletion & fluid exhaustion pattern

Main symptoms: Patients manifesting this pattern commonly suffer from a severe disease. They are very weak and are often critically ill. Their tongue is crimson red with prickles, and the fur is scorched, black, and rough.

Treatment principles: Enrich yin, clear heat, and cool the blood

Chinese medicinal formula:

ZENG YE TANG JIA WEI (**Fluid-increasing Decoction with Added Flavors**)
Radix Scrophulariae Ningpoensis (*Xuan Shen*), Tuber Ophiopogonis Japonici (*Mai Dong*), uncooked Radix Rehmanniae (*Sheng Di*), Flos Lonicerae Japonicae (*Jin Yin Hua*), Fructus Forsythiae Suspensae (*Lian Qiao*), Rhizoma Anemarrhenae Asphodeloidis (*Zhi Mu*), Cortex Radicis Moutan (*Dan Pi*), Radix Rubrus Paeoniae Lactiflorae (*Chi Shao*)

4. Qi & yin (blood) dual vacuity pattern

Main symptoms: A selection of the above symptoms plus a pale tongue with thin fur or a pale-red, fissured tongue with scanty fur

Treatment principles: Boost the qi and nourish yin (blood)

Chinese medicinal formula:

SHENG MAI SAN HE SI JUN ZI SI WU TANG (**Engender the Pulse Powder plus Four Gentlemen & Four Materials Decoction**)
Radix Panacis Ginseng (*Ren Shen*), Tuber Ophiopogonis Japonici (*Mai Dong*), Fructus Schisandrae Chinensis (*Wu Wei Zi*), Rhizoma Atractylodis Macrocephalae (*Bai Zhu*), Sclerotium Poriae Cocos (*Fu Ling*), Radix Angelicae Sinensis (*Dang Gui*), Radix Ligustici Wallichii (*Chuan Xiong*), cooked Radix Rehmanniae (*Shu Di*), Radix Albus Paeoniae Lactiflorae (*Bai Shao*), mix-fried Radix Glycyrrhizae (*Gan Cao*)

5. Spleen-kidney dual vacuity pattern

Main symptoms: Shortness of breath, lack of strength, lumbar aching, knee limpness, hair loss, decreased sexual desire, irregular menstruation, reduced appetite, uncomfortable stomach duct, abdominal distention, loose stools, white tongue fur, and a fine, weak pulse, especially in the cubit position

Treatment principles: Fortify the spleen and supplement the kidneys

Chinese medicinal formula:

HUANG QI XIAN MAO TANG (**Astragalus & Curculigo Decoction**)
Radix Codonopsitis Pilosulae (*Dang Shen*), Rhizoma Atractylodis Macrocephalae (*Bai Zhu*), Sclerotium Poriae Cocos (*Fu Ling*), Radix Astragali Membranacei (*Huang Qi*), Pericarpium Citri Reticulatae (*Chen Pi*), lime-processed Rhizoma Pinelliae Ternatae

(*Ban Xia*), cooked Radix Rehmanniae (*Shu Di*), Radix Angelicae Sinensis (*Dang Gui*), Radix Albus Paeoniae Lactiflorae (*Bai Shao*), Radix Achyranthis Bidentatae (*Niu Xi*), Rhizoma Curculiginis Orchioidis (*Xian Mao*), Herba Epimedii (*Yin Yang Huo*), Herba Leonuri Heterophylli (*Yi Mu Cao*), Gelatinum Corii Asini (*E Jiao*)

According to a study by Xiao Qian, physician at the Second Hospital of Nanjing in Jiangsu province, the group of leukemic patients treated only with chemotherapy had a total amelioration rate of 60.5%. The group treated with a combination of Chinese medicinals and chemotherapy, on the other hand, had a total amelioration rate of 86.8%. This remarkable difference clearly demonstrates the benefit of administering Chinese medicinals to patients suffering from acute leukemia and undergoing chemotherapy.[15]

Remission period treatment

According to research published in 1998 and conducted from 1992-1997 by Ma Rou *et al.* from the Department of Hematology at the Xi Yuan Hospital in Beijing, clinical remission can be drastically prolonged by the continuous taking of Chinese medicinals. The main form of treatment for acute leukemia is chemotherapy. Chemotherapy dispels evils. However, it also attacks the righteous qi and leaves the body weak and the qi vacuous. According to the statement in the *Su Wen (Simple Questions)* that, "If the qi recovers and returns, there is life; if qi does not return, there is death," treatment during the remission period should focus on supporting the righteous and banking the root. The formula below can be used for patients in clinical remission. It needs to be administered long-term. One treatment course needs to last approximately three months and anywhere from 2-12 courses should be administered.[16]

Chinese medicinal formula:

FU ZHEN KANG BAI CHONG JI (**Support the Righteous Anti-white [Blood Cell] Soluble Mixture**)
Radix Panacis Ginseng (*Ren Shen*), Radix Astragali Membranacei (*Huang Qi*), Radix Polygoni Multiflori (*He Shou Wu*), Herba Epimedii (*Yin Yang Huo*), Tuber Asparagi Cochinensis (*Tian Men Dong*), Fructus Psoraleae Corylifoliae (*Bu Gu Zhi*), Fructus

---

[15] Xiao Qian, "Treatment Effect Observations on the Treatment of 38 Cases of Acute Leukemia with a Combination of Chinese Medicinals & Chemotherapy," *Zhong Yi Za Zhi (Journal of Chinese Medicine)*, #5, 1998, p. 283-285

[16] Ma Rou *et al.*, "Clinical Study of the Effect of *Fu Zhen Kang Bai Chong Ji* (Support the Righteous Anti-white [Blood Cell] Soluble Mixture) on Long-term Survival of Patients with Acute Leukemia," *Zhong Guo Zhong Xi Yi Jie He Za Zhi (Chinese Journal of Integrated Chinese-Western Medicine)*, #5, 1998, p. 276-278

Ligustri Lucidi (*Nu Zhen Zi*), stir-fried Rhizoma Atractylodis Macrocephalae (*Bai Zhu*)

5 Lymphomas

Lymphomas are a heterogenous group of neoplasms arising in the reticuloendothelial and lymphatic systems. The two major types of lymphomas (and the ones discussed in this book) are Hodgkin's and non-Hodgkin's lymphomas.

Hodgkin's lymphoma, one and a half times more prevalent in men and most common at either age 15-34 or after 60, is a proliferation of lymph tissue of unknown origin. Besides involvement of the lymph nodes, the spleen, liver, and bone marrow are commonly affected. Hodgkin's lymphoma, also referred to as Hodgkin's disease (HD), is divided into four different histopathologic subtypes: 1) lymphocyte-predominant, 2) mixed cellularity, 3) lymphocyte depleted, and 4) nodular sclerosis. The lymphocyte predominant type is of indolent nature and often does not manifest with any other symptoms except for cervical or inguinal lymph node enlargement. Prognosis for this type is excellent. The mixed cellularity type has an intermediate prognosis, and half of all patients suffering from this type of HD manifest with so-called B signs (*i.e.*, low-grade fever which is occasionally cyclical, night sweats, and weight loss exceeding 10% of body weight in the six months preceding diagnosis). Lymphocyte-depleted HD is the most clinically aggressive type. B-signs as well as pancytopenia, fevers of unknown origin, and prominent involvement of the spleen, liver, and bone marrow are common. The cure rate for this type of lymphoma is low, and most patients die from immunodeficiency with secondary infections. Nodular sclerosis HD is most common in young adult women and usually presents as lower cervical, supraclavicular, and mediastinal adenopathy. B-signs occur in about 40% of cases. The prognosis for this type is good, with a cure rate of 80-85%.

Non-Hodgkin's lymphoma, also called malignant lymphoma, shares some clinical and pathologic features with HD. Malignant lymphomas constitute about 3% of all malignancies in Western countries. Etiologic factors involved in the arisal of this disease are unknown in most cases. However, two subtypes of this tumor are etiologically associated with the Epstein-Barr virus (EBV) and human T-cell leukemia/lymphoma virus (HTLV-1). Furthermore, congenital and acquired immunodeficiency disorders are particularly associated with an increased risk for the development of aggressive B-cell immunoblastic lymphomas.

Malignant lymphomas derive from the malignant transformation of a single lymphocyte which is arrested at a specific stage of B or T-lymphoid cell differentiation. Three subgroups, related to survival, are differentiated: 1) low-grade or clinically indolent, 2) intermediate, and 3) high-grade or clinically aggressive. Clinically, patients present with asymptomatic adenopathy involving the cervical or inguinal regions or both. The enlarged lymph nodes are rubbery and discrete and later become matted. Anemia is initially present in about 33% of patients and eventually develops in most. This may be due to bleeding from gastrointestinal involvement, low platelet levels, hemolysis due to hypersplenism, hemolytic anemia, bone marrow infiltration by the lymphoma, or marrow suppression by drugs and irradiation. A leukemic phase develops in 10-40% of lymphomas.

Western medical treatment for both Hodgkin's disease and malignant lymphomas consists of radiation and chemotherapy. As outlined above, success rate depends on the type of the lymphoma.

Chinese medical disease explanation:

In Chinese medicine, lymphoma belongs to the categories of loss of luxuriance (*shi rong*)[1], scrofula (*luo li*)[2], stone flat abscess (*shi ju*)[3], phlegm node (*tan he*)[4], malign node

---

[1]   Loss of luxuriance or loss of construction is a hard swelling on the neck. It starts with a slight swelling without change in skin color, and slowly grows and becomes hard as rock. It is firmly fixed and hard to move. In advanced stage, it becomes covered with purple patches and ulcerates to exude blood and water. At the same time, qi and blood become gradually debilitated and the patient becomes emaciated like a tree that has lost its splendor; hence the name.

[2]   This term is used here as a technical term of Chinese medicine and is not to be confused with the Western medical term scrofula which refers to tuberculosis of the lymph nodes. Scrofula are lumps beneath the skin down the side of the neck and under the armpits. Scrofula starts as bean-like lumps, associated with neither pain nor heat. Subsequently the lumps expand and assume a string-like formation, merge, and even bunch up into heaps. They are hard and do not move under pressure. In the latter stages, they may become slightly painful. They can rupture to exude a thin pus and sometimes contain matter that resembles bean curd dregs.

[3]   A flat abscess prior to the Song dynasty was a headless (*i.e.*, there was no superficial sore visible and, therefore, no head visible), deep, malign suppuration in the flesh, sinews, and even the bones attributed to toxic evils obstructing the qi and blood. From the Song dynasty on, it came to be used to denote certain superficial sores, and thus it is nowadays distinguished between headless and headed flat abscesses. Stone flat abscess means that it is hard like a rock.

[4]   Any lump below the skin that feels soft and slippery under the finger, is associated with no redness, pain, or swelling, and, unlike scrofula, does not suppurate.

(*e he*)[5], and yin flat abscess (*yin ju*).[6] Because one of the main manifestations of lymphoma is swelling of the lymph nodes, the engenderment of phlegm is at the very core of the disease mechanism. Basically, there are two main reasons for phlegm engenderment: cold dampness and fire. If cold dampness congeals, it can bind into phlegm. On the other hand, replete or vacuity fire or heat can brew the fluids and thus engender phlegm.

However, the reasons for the occurrence of cold dampness and fire are manifold. Eating dampening foods, such as wheat, sugar, and dairy products, quickly overwhelms the spleen and leads to the accumulation of dampness. Excessive thinking also damages the spleen and thus makes the accumulation of dampness very likely. Liver depression qi stagnation, often due to the socioeconomic stresses and constraints of Western society, obstructs the free flow of qi and fluids and thus may lead to the accumulation of phlegm and dampness. Liver depression qi stagnation may also transform into heat. Transformative heat may then stir fire which flames upward to invade the lungs and brew the fluids into phlegm.

Qi pushes and propels the blood through the entire body. Therefore, if qi becomes stagnant, blood is not moved and stasis is engendered. Phlegm, on the other hand, may obstruct the free flow of both qi and blood and lead to phlegm stasis (*i.e.,* phlegm accumulation mixed with blood stasis). Furthermore, prolonged accumulations of phlegm, dampness, and static blood lead to vacuity of the viscera and bowels, causing depletion and detriment of the liver and kidneys as well as depletion of the qi and blood.

Therefore, the patterns for malignant lymphoma are 1) cold phlegm congealing and binding, 2) qi depression with phlegm binding, 3) concretions and conglomerations of static blood, 4) mutual binding of stasis and heat, 5) liver fire invading the lungs, 6) yin depletion blood vacuity, and 7) qi and blood dual vacuity.

The Chinese medical treatment of this disease focuses on both supporting the righteous and dispelling any evils. If vacuity of the righteous is marked, then supporting the righteous is the primary treatment method. If evil repletion is severe and the righteous qi is not depleted or not obviously depleted, one can primarily use the method of attacking evils. Depending on the severity and acuteness of the disease and the individual patient's preferences for the overall treatment approach, this disease can be treated with pure Chinese medicine or with a combination of Chinese medicine and radiation and

---

[5] The term "malign" is used here to indicate that it is a sore which is severe and difficult to cure. This term is not to be confused with "malignant" as used in Western medicine.

[6] In this context, yin flat abscess means a flat abscess characterized by yin cold signs.

chemotherapy. In the latter case, Chinese medicinals are mainly used to reduce the toxic side effects of radiation and chemotherapy so as to protect the bone marrow and blood and maintain an adequately functioning immune system.

Treatment based on pattern discrimination:

1. Cold phlegm congealing & binding pattern

Main symptoms: Swelling of the lymphnodes in the neck and subauricular, subaxillary, and groin regions. The nodes are hard like rock, not itchy, and of a normal color. There is no accompanying fever, and the body and extremities feel cool, the facial complexion is lusterless, the spirit is fatigued, and there is lack of strength of the body. The tongue is pale, the fur thin and white, and the pulse is deep, fine, and weak.

Treatment principles: Warm yang and nourish the blood, scatter nodulation and free the flow of the channels

Chinese medicinal formula:

YANG HE TANG **(Harmonious Yang Decoction)**
   Cooked Radix Rehmanniae (*Shu Di*), Gelatinum Cornu Cervi (*Lu Jiao Jiao*), Cortex Cinnamomi Cassiae (*Rou Gui*), blast-fried Rhizoma Zingiberis (*Pao Jiang*), Semen Sinapis Albae (*Bai Jie Zi*), Herba Ephedrae (*Ma Huang*), Radix Glycyrrhizae (*Gan Cao*)

2. Qi depression & phlegm binding pattern

Main symptoms: Swelling of the lymph nodes in the neck and subauricular, subaxillary, and groin regions. There is no pain, itching, or change of skin color over the nodulations. There are also dizziness, tinnitus, a bitter taste in the mouth, a dry throat, vexation and agitation with irascibility, chest and abdominal oppression and distention, chest and rib-side pain, dry, bound stools, short, reddish urination, yellow tongue fur, and a bowstring, rapid pulse.

Treatment principles: Course the liver and move the qi, quicken the blood and stop pain, transform phlegm and soften hardness

Chinese medicinal formulas:

CHAI HU SHU GAN SAN JIA WEI (**Bupleurum Course the Liver Decoction with Added Flavors**)
Pericarpium Citri Reticulatae (*Chen Pi*), Radix Bupleuri (*Chai Hu*), Radix Albus Paeoniae Lactiflorae (*Bai Shao*), Fructus Citri Aurantii (*Zhi Ke*), mix-fried Radix Glycyrrhizae (*Gan Cao*), Radix Ligustici Wallichii (*Chuan Xiong*), Radix Cyperi Rotundi (*Xiang Fu*), Rhizoma Arisaematis (*Nan Xing*), lime-processed Rhizoma Pinelliae Ternatae (*Ban Xia*), Rhizoma Dioscoreae Bulbiferae (*Huang Yao Zi*), Thallus Algae (*Kun Bu*), Herba Sargassi (*Hai Zao*)

QING GAN LU HUI FANG (**Clear the Liver Aloe Formula**)
Radix Angelicae Sinensis (*Dang Gui*), Radix Ligustici Wallichii (*Chuan Xiong*), Radix Albus Paeoniae Lactiflorae (*Bai Shao*), Pericarpium Citri Reticulatae Viride (*Qing Pi*), Herba Aloes (*Lu Hui*), Thallus Algae (*Kun Bu*), Filamentum Notarchi (*Hai Fen*)[7], Radix Glycyrrhizae (*Gan Cao*), Fructus Parvus Gleditschiae Chinensis (*Ya Zao*)[8], Rhizoma Coptidis Chinensis (*Huang Lian*)

This formula is particularly indicated if, in addition to qi depression and phlegm binding, there are indications of a wind heat invasion with blood dryness, such as fever, aversion to cold, a dry mouth, and skin itching.

NEI XIAO LUO LI WAN (**Internally Dispersing Scrofula Pills**)
Spica Prunellae Vulgaris (*Xia Ku Cao*), Radix Scrophulariae Ningpoensis (*Xuan Shen*), Halitum (*Qing Yan*)[9], Herba Sargassi (*Hai Zao*), Bulbus Fritillariae Cirrhosae (*Chuan Bei Mu*), Herba Menthae Haplocalycis (*Bo He*), Radix Trichosanthis Kirilowii (*Tian Hua Fen*), Filamentum Notarchi (*Hai Fen*), Radix Ampelopsis (*Bai Lian*)[10], Fructus Forsythiae Suspensae (*Lian Qiao*), Radix Et Rhizoma Rhei (*Da Huang*), Radix Glycyrrhizae (*Gan Cao*), uncooked Radix Rehmanniae (*Sheng Di*), Radix Platycodi Grandiflori (*Jie Geng*), Fructus Citri Aurantii (*Zhi Ke*), Radix Angelicae Sinensis (*Dang Gui*), Talcum (*Hua Shi*)

---

[7] Filamentum Notarchi (*Hai Fen*) is sweet, salty, and cold in nature and enters the lung and liver channels. It clears heat and nourishes yin, softens hardness and disperses phlegm.

[8] Fructus Parvus Gleditschiae Chinensis (*Ya Zao*) is acrid, salty, warm, and toxic in nature and enters the lung, stomach, and large intestine channels. It frees the flow of the orifices, flushes phlegm, tracks wind, and kills worms. Recommended dosage is 1.5-3 grams.

[9] Halitum (*Qing Yan*), also called *Rong Yan*, is salty and cold in nature and enters the heart, kidney, and urinary bladder channels. It cools the blood and brightens the eyes. Recommended dosage is 3-5 pieces.

[10] Radix Ampelopsis (*Bai Lian*) is acrid, bitter, and slightly cold in nature and enters the spleen, stomach, liver, and heart channels. It astringes sores and toxic swellings, clears heat and resolves toxins, disperses tumors, stops pain, and engenders the flesh.

This formula is indicated if qi depression has given rise to transformative fire. Thus there may be fever present. This formula should be taken with alcohol.

KAI YU DAO QI TANG (Open Depression & Abduct the Qi Decoction)

Rhizoma Atractylodis (*Cang Zhu*), Rhizoma Cyperi Rotundi (*Xiang Fu*), Radix Ligustici Wallichii (*Chuang Xiong*), Radix Angelicae Dahuricae (*Bai Zhi*), Sclerotium Poriae Cocos (*Fu Ling*), Talcum (*Hua Shi*), Fructus Gardeniae Jasminoidis (*Zhi Zi*), Massa Medica Fermentata (*Shen Qu*), Pericarpium Citri Reticulatae (*Chen Pi*), dry Rhizoma Zingiberis (*Gan Jiang*), Radix Glycyrrhizae (*Gan Cao*)

This formula is particularly for retroperitoneal lymph node involvement with abdominal pain.

3. Static blood concretions & conglomerations pattern

Main symptoms: Emaciated body, binding lumps in the abdomen, abdominal distention and pain, torpid intake, nausea and vomiting, dry, bound and/or black stools, a dark tongue with possible static macules and yellow fur, and a bowstring, choppy pulse

Treatment principles: Quicken the blood and transform stasis assisted by resolving toxins and combatting cancer

Chinese medicinal formulas:

BIE JIA JIAN WAN (Carapax Amydae Brew Pills)

Carapax Amydae Sinensis (*Bie Jia*), Radix Bupleuri (*Chai Hu*), Radix Gentianae Macrophyllae (*Qin Jiao*), Herba Menthae Haplocalycis (*Bo He*), Herba Artemesiae Apiaceae (*Qing Hao*), uncooked Radix Rehmanniae (*Sheng Di*), uncooked Rhizoma Zingiberis (*Sheng Jiang*)

SHENG LI DAN (Overcoming & Disinhibiting Elixir)

Realgar (*Xiong Huang*), Resina Olibani (*Ru Xiang*), Gypsum Fibrosum (*Shi Gao*), Squama Manitis Pentadactylis (*Chuan Shan Jia*), Scolopendra Subspinipes (*Wu Gong*), Sanguis Draconis (*Xue Jie*), Buthus Martensis (*Quan Xie*), Eulota (*Wo Niu*)[11], Calomelas (*Qing Fen*), Cinnabar (*Zhu Sha*), Radix Angelicae Dahuricae (*Bai Zhi*), Borneolum (*Bing Pian*), Secretio Bufo Bufonis (*Chan Su*), Borax (*Peng Sha*), Secretio Moschi Moschiferi (*She Xiang*), Radix Et Rhizoma Rhei (*Da Huang*)

---

[11] Eulota (*Wo Niu*) is salty and cold in nature and enters the gallbladder and liver channels. It clears heat, resolves toxins, and disperses swellings.

DAN SHEN GAO (Salvia Paste)

Radix Salviae Miltiorrhizae (*Dan Shen*), Herba Seu Radix Sambuci (*Shuo Diao*)[12], Radix Cynanchi Atrati (*Bai Wei*), Flos Rhododendri Mollis (*Zhi Zhuo Hua*)[13], Flos Chrysanthemi Morifolii (*Ju Hua*), Radix Gentianae Macrophyllae (*Qin Jiao*), Radix Angelicae Pubescentis (*Du Huo*), Radix Aconiti (*Wu Tou*), Pericarpium Zanthoxyli Bungeani (*Chuan Jiao*), Fructus Forsythiae Suspensae (*Lian Qiao*), Cortex Radicis Mori Albi (*Sang Bai Pi*), Radix Achyranthis Bidentatae (*Niu Xi*)

These ingredients can be prepared into a paste and then either taken internally or applied externally.

BAI LIAN GAO (Ampelopsis Paste)

Radix Ampelopsis (*Bai Lian*), Radix Cynanchi Atrati (*Bai Wei*), Radix Scrophulariae Ningpoensis (*Xuan Shen*), Radix Auklandia Lappae (*Mu Xiang*), Radix Albus Paeoniae Lactiflorae (*Bai Shao*), Radix Et Rhizoma Rhei (*Da Huang*)

4. Mutual binding of stasis & heat pattern

Main symptoms: Hard and painful swellings, heart vexation, chest and abdominal oppression and distention, a reddish purple tongue and/or possible static macules, and a forceful, rapid pulse

Treatment principles: Quicken the blood and resolve toxins, soften hardness and scatter nodulation

Chinese medicinal formulas:

DA HUANG SAN (Rhubarb Powder)

Radix Et Rhizoma Rhei (*Da Huang*), Radix Angelicae Sinensis (*Dang Gui*), Mirabilitum (*Mang Xiao*), Pericarpium Semenis Glycinis Sojae (*Hei Dou Pi*), Fructus Citri Aurantii (*Zhi Ke*), Fructus Arctii Lappae (*Niu Bang Zi*), Radix Ligustici Wallichii (*Chuan Xiong*), Radix Glycyrrhizae (*Gan Cao*)

XUAN SHEN SAN (Scrophularia Powder)

Radix Scrophulariae Ningpoensis (*Xuan Shen*), Fructus Forsythiae Suspensae (*Lian Qiao*), Radix Anemarrhenae Asphodeloidis (*Zhi Mu*), Radix Angelicae Sinensis (*Dang*

---

[12] Herba Seu Radix Sambuci (*Shuo Diao*) is sweet, sour, and warm in nature and enters the liver channel. It dispels wind and eliminates dampness, quickens blood and scatters stasis. Recommended dosage is 6-12 grams.

[13] Flos Rhododendri Mollis (*Zhi Zhuo Hua*), also called *Nao Yang Hua*, is acrid and toxic in nature. It dispels wind, eliminates dampness, and settles pain. Recommended dosage is 0.3-0.6 grams.

Gui), Realgar (*Xiong Huang*), Semen Pharbiditis (*Qian Niu Zi*), Radix Scutellariae Baicalensis (*Huang Qin*), Cornu Bubali (*Shui Niu Jiao*), Radix Albus Paeoniae Lactiflorae (*Bai Shao*), Radix Rubrus Paeoniae Lactiflorae (*Chi Shao*), Azurite (*Kong Qin*)[14], Fructus Perillae Frutescentis (*Su Zi*), Alumen (*Fan Shi*), Herba Elephantopi (*Di Dan*)[15], Mylabris (*Ban Mao*)

LIN BA XIAN LIU FANG (Lymph Gland Tumor Formula)
Bulbus Fritillariae Cirrhosae (*Chuan Bei Mu*), Cortex Radicis Moutan (*Dan Pi*), Bulbus Fritillariae Thunbergi (*Zhe Bei Mu*), Radix Salviae Miltiorrhizae (*Dan Shen*), Bulbus Shancigu (*Shan Ci Gu*), Squama Manitis Pentadactylis (*Chuan Shan Jia*), Herba Sargassi (*Hai Zao*), Thallus Algae (*Kun Bu*), Tuber Curcumae (*Yu Jin*), Flos Lonicerae Japonicae (*Jin Yin Hua*), Caulis Lonicerae Japonicae (*Ren Dong Teng*), Herba Cephalanoploris Segeti (*Xiao Ji*), Semen Pruni Persicae (*Tao Ren*), Semen Pruni Armeniacae (*Xing Ren*), Fructus Arctii Lappae (*Niu Bang Zi*), Spina Gleditschiae Chinensis (*Zao Jiao Ci*), Radix Platycodi Grandiflori (*Jie Geng*), Radix Scrophulariae Ningpoensis (*Xuan Shen*), Spica Prunellae Vulgaris (*Xia Ku Cao*), Radix Pseudoginseng (*San Qi*, powdered and swallowed with the decoction)

5. Liver fire invading the lungs pattern

Main symptoms: Scorching phlegm in chest and rib-side, coughing, qi counterflow, chest oppression, shortness of breath, vexation and agitation, easy anger, heart palpitations, panting, a dry mouth and throat, dizziness, lack of strength, a red tongue with slightly yellow fur, and a bowstring, rapid pulse

Treatment principles: Clear the liver and drain the lungs, resolve depression and scatter evils

Chinese medicinal formula:

QING DAI GE KE SAN (Indigo & Clam Shell Powder)
Pulvis Indigonis (*Qing Dai*), Concha Cyclinae Meretricis (*Hai Ge Ke*), Cortex Radicis Mori Albi (*Sang Bai Pi*), Cortex Radicis Lycii Chinensis (*Di Gu Pi*), Radix Platycodi Grandiflori (*Jie Geng*), Radix Scutellariae Baicalensis (*Huang Qin*), Bulbus Fritillariae Thunbergii (*Zhe Bei Mu*), Thallus Algae (*Kun Bu*), Radix Scrophulariae

---

[14] Azurite (*Kong Qin*) is bitter and cold in nature and enters the liver channel. It brightens the eyes, eliminates eye screens, and disinhibits the orifices. Recommended dosage is 0.3-0.9 grams of powdered *Kong Qin*.

[15] Herba Elephantopi (*Di Dan*) is bitter, acrid, neutral, and cold in nature and enters the lung channel. It clears heat and drains fire, harmonizes water and disinhibits urination.

Ningpoensis (*Xuan Shen*), Spica Prunellae Vulgaris (*Xia Ku Cao*), Concha Ostreae (*Mu Li*), Bulbus Shancigu (*Shan Ci Gu*)

6. Yin depletion & blood vacuity pattern

Main symptoms: Rock-hard nodes in the neck, dizziness, tinnitus, a dry mouth and throat, vexatious heat in the five hearts, pain in both rib-sides, lumbar aching and knee limpness, seminal emission in men, menstrual irregularities in women, a red tongue with scanty fur, and a fine, rapid pulse

Treatment principles: Nourish the blood and enrich yin, clear fire and transform phlegm, soften hardness and scatter nodulations

Chinese medicinal formulas:

SI WU XIAO LUO TANG (**Four Materials Disperse Scrofula Decoction**)
  Radix Angelicae Sinensis (*Dang Gui*), Radix Ligustici Wallichii (*Chuan Xiong*), uncooked Radix Rehmanniae (*Sheng Di*), Radix Rubrus Paeoniae Lactiflorae (*Chi Shao*), Radix Scrophulariae Ningpoensis (*Xuan Shen*), Herba Sargassi (*Hai Zao*), Spica Prunellae Vulgaris (*Xia Ku Cao*), Concha Ostreae (*Mu Li*), Rhizoma Paridis Polyphyllae (*Zao Xiu*), Rhizoma Dioscoreae Bulbiferae (*Huang Yao Zi*)

ZI YIN SAN JIE TANG (**Enrich Yin & Scatter Nodulation Decoction**)
  Uncooked Radix Rehmanniae (*Sheng Di*), cooked Radix Rehmanniae (*Shu Di*), Radix Scrophulariae Ningpoensis (*Xuan Shen*), Rhizoma Atractylodis Macrocephalae (*Bai Zhu*), Cortex Radicis Moutan (*Dan Pi*), Fructus Lycii Chinensis (*Gou Qi Zi*), Plastrum Testudinis (*Gui Ban*), Fructus Ligustri Lucidi (*Nu Zhen Zi*), Herba Oldenlandiae Diffusae Cum Radice (*Bai Hua She She Cao*), Herba Scutellariae Barbatae (*Ban Zhi Lian*), Eupolyphagia Seu Opisthoplatia (*Tu Bie Chong*), Tuber Bolbostemmatis (*Tu Bei Mu*)[16]

7. Qi & blood dual vacuity pattern

Main symptoms: Swollen lymph nodes in the neck, fatigue, lack of strength, a bright white facial complexion, shortness of breath, heart palpitations, emaciated body, slimy, white tongue fur, and a fine, forceless pulse

---

[16] Tuber Bolbostemmatis (*Tu Bei Mu*) is bitter and cool in nature. It dissipates toxic bindings and disperses swollen abscesses. Recommended dosage is 10-30 grams.

Treatment principles: Boost the qi and nourish the blood, disperse swellings and soften hardness

Chinese medicinal formulas:

HE RONG SAN JIAN WAN (**Harmonize the Constructive & Scatter Hardness Pills**)
Radix Angelicae Sinensis (*Dang Gui*), cooked Radix Rehmanniae (*Shu Di*), Sclerotium Pararadicis Poriae Cocos (*Fu Shen*), Rhizoma Cyperi Rotundi (*Xiang Fu*), Radix Panacis Ginseng (*Ren Shen*), Rhizoma Atractylodis Macrocephalae (*Bai Zhu*), Exocarpium Citri Erythrocarpae (*Ju Hong*), Bulbus Fritillariae Thunbergii (*Zhe Bei Mu*), Rhizoma Arisaematis (*Tian Nan Xing*), Semen Zizyphi Spinosae (*Suan Zao Ren*), Radix Polygalae Tenuifoliae (*Yuan Zhi*), Semen Biotae Orientalis (*Bai Zi Ren*), Cortex Radicis Moutan (*Dan Pi*), Dens Draconis (*Long Chi*)

XIANG BAI YANG YING TANG (**Cyperus & Peony Nourish the Constructive Decoction**)
Radix Angelicae Sinensis (*Dang Gui*), cooked Radix Rehmanniae (*Shu Di*), Sclerotium Poriae Cocos (*Fu Ling*), Rhizoma Cyperi Rotundi (*Xiang Fu*), Radix Ligustici Wallichii (*Chuan Xiong*), Radix Panacis Ginseng (*Ren Shen*), Rhizoma Atractylodis Macrocephalae (*Bai Zhu*), Pericarpium Citri Reticulatae (*Chen Pi*), Radix Albus Paeoniae Lactiflorae (*Bai Shao*), Bulbus Fritillariae Thunbergii (*Zhe Bei Mu*), Radix Platycodi Grandiflori (*Jie Geng*), Radix Glycyrrhizae (*Gan Cao*)

Section III
Hemostatic Disorders

1 Idiopathic Thrombocytopenic Purpura

Idiopathic thrombocytopenic purpura (ITP) is a quantitative disorder of platelets caused by antibodies directed against platelet or megakaryocytic antigens. Two types of ITP are recognized: acute and chronic. The acute type usually occurs in children and is mostly due to viral antigen (Ag) triggering synthesis of antibody (Ab) that may react with viral Ag that has come down onto platelet surfaces or that may come down onto the platelet as viral Ag-Ab immune complexes. Chronic ITP, on the other hand, occurs in adults and usually stems from a development of antibodies directed against a structural platelet antigen (an auto-antigen).

Children with acute ITP manifest with sudden onset of petechia, purpura, and mucosal bleeding but no other symptoms. Chronic ITP in adults manifests such bleeding disorders as epistaxis, menorrhagia, and ecchymoses. Bleeding in both acute and chronic ITP may be minimal or extensive. Peripheral blood is normal except for a decreased platelet number varying from a few thousand to $100,000/\text{mm}^3$. Bone marrow aspiration usually reveals a compensatory increase in megakaryocytes (platelet precursors) in an otherwise healthy marrow.

Western medical treatment of chronic ITP focuses on the administration of heavy doses of corticosteroids which are slowly tapered off. Unfortunately, most patients do not respond adequately or relapse during tapering. Splenectomy is curative in 50-60% of such patients. The use of immunosuppressive therapy may be effective if both of the above two treatments fail. In children, acute ITP often spontaneously recovers within six months. If that is not the case, splenectomy is frequently curative.

If there is life-threatening bleeding in ITP patients, an attempt to quickly raise the number of platelets needs to be made. Although very costly, high doses of intravenous immune globulin (IGIV), have been shown to effectively and rapidly raise the platelet count. However, results only last 2-4 weeks. The ITP patient suffering from severe bleeding also needs to be given platelet concentrates.

Chinese medical disease explanation:

In Chinese medicine, ITP corresponds to the disease categories of vacuity taxation (*xu lao*), bleeding conditions (*xue zheng*), and purple macules (*zi ban*). It is commonly differentiated according to five basic patterns. However, similar to allergic purpura, bleeding is their common denominator, and all of the following patterns lead to bleeding through one of three Chinese mechanisms of bleeding: heat, qi vacuity, and/or stasis.

If the disease is acute and starts off with an externally contracted condition, bleeding is caused by external toxic heat evils entering the constructive and blood or latent heat toxins hidden in the constructive and blood leading to exuberant fire stirring the blood and scorching and damaging the vessels and network vessels. This corresponds to the childhood form of acute ITP following a viral infection and is, categorically, a repletion pattern. Over time, fire and heat evils damage qi and consume yin. If yin becomes vacuous, then vacuity fire may stir internally. Blood may then follow this stirring of the fire and frenetically moves outside the vessels and network vessels. In this case, however, blood heat has its origin in vacuity rather than repletion. One of qi's functions is to contain and control the blood. If qi becomes vacuous, then blood may not be contained but rather seeps outside of the vessels. In both of these vacuity patterns, *i.e.*, qi and yin vacuities, it is repletion heat from the above-mentioned repletion pattern which damages qi and consumes yin, thereby leading to the chronic vacuity stages of ITP. Thus, the vacuity patterns secondary to damage by replete heat correspond to recurrent and refractory ITP which neither recovers spontaneously nor responds to treatment.

On the other hand, if ITP is of chronic onset and not succeeding acute ITP (*i.e.*, the adult type), it most commonly corresponds to the pattern of spleen-kidney dual vacuity. A dual vacuity of the spleen and kidneys implies that the yang and qi of these two viscera are insufficient. As discussed above, if qi is vacuous, blood may not be contained properly. Furthermore, since kidney yang is the base of spleen yang qi, spleen disease may eventually reach the kidneys, thus resulting in spleen and kidney vacuity. This often occurs during aging where the spleen qi becomes vacuous and weak first and then leads to spleen qi and kidney yang vacuity. Because kidney qi is responsible for sealing and storing as well as governing the two yin orifices, the anus and urethra/vaginal meatus, spleen-kidney qi vacuity may result in hematuria, hemafecia, and/or meno-metrorrhagia.

For all of the above mechanisms, bleeding is the final result. In addition, blood can only flow freely if it remains inside its channels and vessels. Therefore, when blood leaves its vessels and network vessels and seeps into the surrounding tissue, it engenders blood stasis which further obstructs blood movement. Obstruction and blockage of the blood flow then causes bleeding in and of itself by forcing the blood to move outside its channels. Thus blood stasis often complicates the sequella of bleeding due to either heat evils or qi vacuity and further aggravates those mechanisms, making the bleeding either more severe or repetitive and/or incessant. In addition, because qi moves the blood, if the qi has been consumed by heat toxins or if qi is vacuous due to spleen-kidney dual vacuity, blood will not be moved properly and it may also become static.

Therefore, the treatment principles of quickening the blood and transforming stasis should accompany all of the above patterns in some way, but especially if the disease is chronic and recalcitrant. In the pattern differentiation below, blood stasis is listed as a single pattern for the sake of clarity. In actual clinical practice, however, patients' patterns are often a combination of two or more of the following single patterns. It is further very important to pay attention to the severity of qi vacuity. If blood is static due to qi vacuity, then simply applying the method of quickening the blood will damage the righteous qi even further and lead to an aggravation of the bleeding symptoms. On the other hand, boosting the qi without quickening the blood does not remove stasis and thus new blood cannot be engendered. Therefore, it is important to pay close attention to repletion and vacuity factors and base treatment upon this balance.

Treatment based on pattern discrimination:

1. Frenetic movement due to hot blood pattern

Main symptoms: Acute onset of disease, spontaneous bleeding of the flesh, fresh red-colored blood, epistaxis, bleeding gums, hemoptysis, hematemesis, hemafecia, hematuria, profuse menstruation, heart vexation, thirst, fever, a dry throat, yellow urine, constipation, a crimson red tongue with dry, yellow fur, and a slippery, rapid pulse

Treatment principles: Clear heat and resolve toxins, cool the blood and stop bleeding

Chinese medicinal formulas:

BAI XIAN XIAO DIAN TANG **(Dictamnus Disperse Spots Decoction)**
Cortex Radicis Dictamni Dasycarpi (*Bai Xian Pi*), Herba Galii (*Xue Jian Chou*)[1], Radix Rubiae Cordifoliae (*Qian Cao Gen*), Herba Agrimoniae Pilosae (*Xian He Cao*), Cortex Radicis Moutan (*Dan Pi*), carbonized Radix Sanguisorbae (*Di Yu*), carbonized uncooked Radix Rehmanniae (*Sheng Di*), Flos Lonicerae Japonicae (*Jin Yin Hua*), Radix Salviae Miltiorrhizae (*Dan Shen*), Radix Pseudoginseng (*San Qi*), Cornu Caprae (*Shan Yang Jiao*), Radix Lithospermi Seu Arnebiae (*Zi Cao*)

---

[1] Herba Galii (*Xue Jian Chou*) is sweet and neutral in nature. It stops bleeding and quickens the blood. Recommended dosage is 5-15 grams.

ER HAO QU DIAN HE JI (Spot-dispelling Mixture #2)
Uncooked Radix Rehmanniae (*Sheng Di*), Radix Rumicis Crispi (*Yang Ti Gen*)[2], Cortex Radicis Moutan (*Dan Pi*), Radix Rubrus Paeoniae Lactiflorae (*Bai Shao*), Cornu Bubali (*Shui Niu Jiao*), Depositum Praeparatum Urinae Hominis (*Qiu Shi*), carbonized Pollen Typhae (*Pu Huang*), Radix Achyranthis Bidentatae (*Huai Niu Xi*), mix-fried Radix Glycyrrhizae (*Gan Cao*)

LING YANG SAN HUANG TANG (Antelope Horn Three Yellows Decoction)
Cornu Caprae (*Shan Yang Jiao*), uncooked Radix Rehmanniae (*Sheng Di*), Cortex Phellodendri (*Huang Bai*), Rhizoma Coptidis Chinensis (*Huang Lian*), blackened Fructus Gardeniae Jasminoidis (*Zhi Zi*), Radix Albus Paeoniae Lactiflorae (*Bai Shao*), Flos Lonicerae Japonicae (*Jin Yin Hua*), Cortex Radicis Moutan (*Dan Pi*), Pericarpium Citri Reticulatae (*Chen Pi*), Rhizoma Imperatae Cylindricae (*Bai Mao Gen*), Radix Glycyrrhizae (*Gan Cao*), Gelatinum Corii Asini (*E Jiao*)

QING RE JIE DU HUO XUE TANG (Clear Heat, Resolve Toxins & Quicken the Blood Decoction)
Uncooked Radix Rehmanniae (*Sheng Di*), Radix Rubrus Paeoniae Lactiflorae (*Chi Shao*), Cortex Radicis Moutan (*Dan Pi*), Radix Scrophulariae Ningpoensis (*Xuan Shen*), Radix Isatidis Seu Baphicacanthi (*Ban Lan Gen*), Fructus Forsythiae Suspensae (*Lian Qiao*), Radix Glycyrrhizae (*Gan Cao*), Caulis Akebiae (*Mu Tong*), Radix Lithospermi Seu Arnebiae (*Zi Cao*), Rhizoma Imperatae Cylindricae (*Bai Mao Gen*)

QING RE JIE DU TANG (Clear Heat & Resolve Toxins Decoction)
Rhizoma Cimicifugae (*Sheng Ma*), Radix Puerariae (*Gan Ge*), Fructus Forsythiae Suspensae (*Lian Qiao*), uncooked Radix Rehmanniae (*Sheng Di*), Radix Rubrus Paeoniae Lactiflorae (*Chi Shao*), Cortex Radicis Moutan (*Dan Pi*), Cortex Phellodendri (*Huang Bai*), Rhizoma Coptidis Chinensis (*Huang Lian*), Fructus Gardeniae Jasminoidis (*Zhi Zi*), Radix Scutellariae Baicalensis (*Huang Qin*), Radix Platycodi Grandiflori (*Jie Geng*), Radix Glycyrrhizae (*Gan Cao*)

JIE DU HUA BAN TANG (Resolve Toxins & Transform Macules Decoction)
Uncooked Radix Rehmanniae (*Sheng Di*), Caulis Akebiae (*Mu Tong*), Cortex Radicis Moutan (*Dan Pi*), Radix Angelicae Sinensis (*Dang Gui*), Cornu Bubali (*Shui Niu Jiao*), Radix Lithospermi Seu Arnebiae (*Zi Cao*), Fructus Arctii Lappae (*Niu Bang Zi*), Radix Rubiae Cordifoliae (*Qian Cao Gen*), Radix Glycyrrhizae (*Gan Cao*), Squama Manitis Pentadactylis (*Chuan Shan Jia*)

---

[2] Radix Rumicis Crispi (*Yang Ti Gen*) is bitter, cold, and slightly toxic in nature and enters the heart channel. It clears heat, frees the flow of the stools, disinhibits water, stops bleeding, and kills worms. Recommended dosage is 15-25 grams.

DAI MAO HUA BAN TANG (**Erethmochelyos Transform Macules Decoction**)
Carapax Erethmochelyos (*Dai Mao*), Fructus Ligustri Lucidi (*Nu Zhen Zi*), Herba Ecliptae Prostratae (*Han Lian Cao*), Radix Et Rhizoma Rhei (*Da Huang*), Rhizoma Dioscoreae Bulbiferae (*Huang Yao Zi*), Radix Sophorae Subprostratae (*Shan Dou Gen*), uncooked Radix Rehmanniae (*Sheng Di*), Cortex Radicis Moutan (*Dan Pi*), Radix Angelicae Sinensis (*Dang Gui*), Radix Rubiae Cordifoliae (*Qian Cao Gen*), Radix Lithospermi Seu Arnebiae (*Zi Cao*), Herba Agrimoniae Pilosulae (*Xian He Cao*)

QING YE SAN HUANG TANG (**Daqingye Three Yellows Decoction**)
Folium Daqingye (*Da Qing Ye*), Rhizoma Coptidis Chinensis (*Huang Lian*), Radix Et Rhizoma Rhei (*Da Huang*), Fructus Gardeniae Jasminoidis (*Zhi Zi*), Cortex Radicis Moutan (*Dan Pi*), Radix Lithospermi Seu Arnebiae (*Zi Cao*), Cacumen Biotae Orientalis (*Ce Bai Ye*), Herba Agrimoniae Pilosae (*Xian He Cao*), Radix Sanguisorbae (*Di Yu*), powdered Radix Pseudoginseng (*San Qi,* swallowed with the decoction), uncooked Radix Rehmanniae (*Sheng Di*), Carapax Amydae Sinensis (*Bie Jia*), Fructus Psoraleae Corylifoliae (*Bu Gu Zhi*), Semen Cuscutae Chinensis (*Tu Si Zi*), uncooked Radix Glycyrrhizae (*Gan Cao*)

This formula not only focuses on cooling the blood and stopping bleeding but also enriches the kidneys and supplements yin. Furthermore, it contains anti-viral medicinals. For this reason, it is a good formula in the treatment of acute pediatric ITP when the bleeding is preceded and precipitated by a viral infection.

2. Qi & yin dual vacuity pattern

Main symptoms: Chronic purpura, dizziness, lack of strength, a lusterless facial complexion, blood macules dispersed all over the body, heart palpitations, shortness of breath, spontaneous perspiration and/or night sweats, a pale tongue with thin, yellow fur, and a fine, rapid pulse

Treatment principles: Boost the qi and nourish yin, cool the blood and stop bleeding

Chinese medicinal formulas:

YI QI YANG YIN TANG (**Boost the Qi & Nourish Yin Decoction**)
Radix Pseudostellariae Heterophyllae (*Tai Zi Shen*), Radix Astragali Membranacei (*Huang Qi*), Rhizoma Polygonati (*Huang Jing*), Rhizoma Atractylodis Macrocephalae (*Bai Zhu*), Sclerotium Poriae Cocos (*Fu Ling*), uncooked Radix Rehmanniae (*Sheng Di*), Tuber Asparagi Cochinensis (*Tian Men Dong*), Tuber Ophiopogonis Japonici (*Mai Dong*), Fructus Lycii Chinensis (*Gou Qi Zi*), Herba Chinese Cephalanoploris

Segeti (*Xiao Ji*), Radix Angelicae Sinensis (*Dang Gui*), Herba Ecliptae Prostratae (*Han Lian Cao*), Radix Glycyrrhizae (*Gan Cao*)

ZHI ZI SHENG DI TANG (Gardenia & Uncooked Rehmannia Decoction)
Blackened Fructus Gardeniae Jasminoidis (*Zhi Zi*), uncooked Radix Rehmanniae (*Sheng Di*), Cortex Radicis Moutan (*Dan Pi*), Radix Rubrus Paeoniae Lactiflorae (*Chi Shao*), Radix Angelicae Sinensis (*Dang Gui*), Radix Astragali Membranacei (*Huang Qi*)

Additions & subtractions: For severe bleeding, add Folium Callicarpae (*Zi Zhu Cao*), Radix Rubiae Cordifoliae (*Qian Cao*), and Herba Agrimoniae Pilosae (*Xian He Cao*). For accompanying anemia, add Gelatinum Corii Asini (*E Jiao*), Caulis Milletiae Seu Spatholobi (*Ji Xue Teng*), and Radix Polygoni Multiflori (*He Shou Wu*). For pronounced yin vacuity, add Radix Glehniae Littoralis (*Sha Shen*), Tuber Ophiopogonis Japonici (*Mai Dong*), and Rhizoma Imperatae Cylindricae (*Bai Mao Gen*). For pronounced qi vacuity, add Radix Codonopsitis Pilosulae (*Dang Shen*), Rhizoma Atractylodis Macrocephalae (*Bai Zhu*), Sclerotium Poriae Cocos (*Fu Ling*), and Radix Dioscoreae Oppositae (*Shan Yao*).

ZI YIN YI QI LIANG XUE TANG (Enrich Yin, Boost the Qi & Cool the Blood Decoction)
Uncooked Radix Rehmanniae (*Sheng Di*), Rhizoma Imperatae Cylindricae (*Bai Mao Gen*), Cortex Radicis Mori Albi (*Sang Bai Pi*), Radix Codonopsitis Pilosulae (*Dang Shen*), Radix Rumicis Patientiae (*Niu Xi Xi*)[3]

PING DIAN TANG (Level Spots Decoction)
Radix Astragali Membranacei (*Huang Qi*), Rhizoma Bletillae Striatae (*Bai Ji*), Rhizoma Polygonati (*Huang Jing*), Radix Glycyrrhizae (*Gan Cao*), Cortex Radicis Moutan (*Dan Pi*), Gelatinum Corii Asini (*E Jiao*), Radix Rubrus Paeoniae Lactiflorae (*Chi Shao*), Fructus Forsythiae Suspensae (*Lian Qiao*), Rhizoma Imperatae Cylindricae (*Bai Mao Gen*), Radix Salviae Miltiorrhizae (*Dan Shen*), Herba Agrimoniae Pilosulae (*Xian He Cao*)

Additions & subtractions: For accompanying blood heat, add Radix Scutellariae Baicalensis (*Huang Qin*) and Radix Lithospermi Seu Arnebiae (*Zi Cao*). For severe qi vacuity, add Radix Codonopsitis Pilosulae (*Dang Shen*) and Fructus Zizyphi Jujubae (*Da*

---

[3] Radix Rumicis Patientiae (*Niu Xi Xi*) is bitter, sour, and cold in nature. It clears heat and resolves toxins, quickens the blood and stops bleeding, frees the flow of the stools and kills worms. Recommended dosage is 15-25 grams.

Zao). For pronounced yin vacuity, add Cortex Radicis Lycii Chinensis (*Di Gu Pi*). For obvious blood stasis, add powdered Radix Pseudoginseng (*San Qi*).

SAN HAO QU DIAN HE JI (Spot-dispelling Mixture #3)

Cooked Radix Rehmanniae (*Shu Di*), Radix Angelicae Sinensis (*Dang Gui*), Radix Astragali Membranacei (*Huang Qi*), Fructus Corni Officinalis (*Shan Zhu Yu*), Cervi Cornu (*Lu Jiao*), Gelatinum Corii Asini (*E Jiao*), Fructus Psoraleae Corylifoliae (*Bu Gu Zhi*), Pericarpium Citri Reticulatae (*Chen Pi*), Fructus Zizyphi Jujubae (*Hong Zao*), mix-fried Radix Glycyrrhizae (*Gan Cao*).

This formula also addresses essence vacuity and is, therefore, indicated if there are such additional manifestations as lumbar aching and knee limpness.

DI HUANG QI XING XUE TANG (Rehmannia & Astragalus Move the Blood Decoction)

Radix Astragali Membranacei (*Huang Qi*), Radix Codonopsitis Pilosulae (*Dang Shen*), Rhizoma Atractylodis Macrocephalae (*Bai Zhu*), Sclerotium Poriae Cocos (*Fu Ling*), Radix Salviae Miltiorrhizae (*Dan Shen*), Pollen Typhae (*Pu Huang*), Flos Carthami Tinctorii (*Hong Hua*), Gelatinum Corii Asini (*E Jiao*), uncooked Radix Rehmanniae (*Sheng Di*), Carapax Amydae Sinensis (*Bie Jia*), Radix Angelicae Sinensis (*Dang Gui*), Bombyx Batryticatus (*Bai Jiang Can*), Radix Glycyrrhizae (*Gan Cao*)

Additions & subtractions: For accompanying abdominal distention or decreased appetite, add Radix Aucklandiae Lappae (*Mu Xiang*), Fructus Amomi (*Sha Ren*), Massa Medica Fermentata (*Shen Qu*), and Endothelium Corneum Gigeriae Galli (*Ji Nei Jin*). For accompanying nausea, add Rhizoma Pinelliae Ternatae (*Ban Xia*) and Pericarpium Citri Reticulatae (*Chen Pi*). For upper respiratory infections with fever, sore throat, and cough, add Flos Lonicerae Japonicae (*Jin Yin Hua*), Fructus Forsythiae Suspensae (*Lian Qiao*), Radix Stemonae (*Bai Bu*), Bulbus Fritillariae Cirrhosae (*Chuan Bei Mu*), and Radix Scutellariae Baicalensis (*Huang Qin*).

This formula also moves the blood and is particularly indicated if, in addition to the symptoms above, there are signs of blood stasis, such as a swollen spleen.

3. Liver-kidney yin vacuity with internal heat pattern

Main symptoms: Profuse bleeding which is fresh red in color, tidal reddening, heart vexation, heat in the palms of the hands and soles of the feet, night sweats, scorching hot flesh and skin, thirst without a desire to drink water, dizziness, tinnitus, impaired memory, lumbar aching, knee limpness, a dry tongue with red sides and scanty fur, and a fine, rapid pulse

Treatment principles: Enrich yin and clear heat, cool the blood and quiet the network vessels

Chinese medicinal formulas:

XIAO RE ZI YIN TANG (Disperse Heat & Enrich Yin Decoction)
Radix Angelicae Sinensis (*Dang Gui*), Radix Ligustici Wallichii (*Chuan Xiong*), uncooked Radix Rehmanniae (*Sheng Di*), Cortex Phellodendri (*Huang Bai*), Rhizoma Anemarrhenae Asphodeloidis (*Zhi Mu*), Pericarpium Citri Reticulatae (*Chen Pi*), Rhizoma Atractylodis Macrocephalae (*Bai Zhu*), Tuber Ophiopogonis Japonici (*Mai Dong*), Cortex Radicis Moutan (*Dan Pi*), Radix Rubrus Paeoniae Lactiflorae (*Chi Shao*), Radix Scrophulariae Ningpoensis (*Xuan Shen*), Fructus Gardenia Jasminoidis (*Zhi Zi*), Radix Glycyrrhizae (*Gan Cao*)

ZI DIAN TANG (Purple Spots Decoction)
Uncooked Radix Rehmanniae (*Sheng Di*), Rhizoma Imperatae Cylindricae (*Bai Mao Gen*), Herba Agrimoniae Pilosulae (*Xian He Cao*), Cortex Radicis Moutan (*Dan Pi*), Fructus Gardenia Jasminoidis (*Zhi Zi*), Radix Albus Paeoniae Lactiflorae (*Bai Shao*), Herba Cephalanoploris Segeti (*Xiao Ji*), Nodus Nelumbinis Nuciferae (*Ou Jie*), Flos Lonicerae Japonicae (*Jin Yin Hua*), Folium Artemesiae Argyii (*Ai Ye*), Plastrum Testudinis (*Gui Ban*), powdered Radix Pseudoginseng (*San Qi*, swallowed with the decoction)

OU JIE DI HUANG TANG (Lotus Node & Rehmannia Decoction)
Uncooked Radix Rehmanniae (*Sheng Di*), Nodus Nelumbinis Nuciferae (*Ou Jie*), Tuber Ophiopogonis Japonici (*Mai Dong*), Radix Scrophulariae Ningpoensis (*Xuan Shen*), Radix Glycyrrhizae (*Gan Cao*)

Additions & subtractions: For enduring disease with severe yin depletion and exuberance of heat, add Radix Albus Paeoniae Lactiflorae (*Bai Shao*), Cortex Radicis Moutan (*Dan Pi*), Radix Scutellariae Baicalensis (*Huang Qin*), and blackened Fructus Gardeniae Jasminoidis (*Zhi Zi*). For simple yin depletion after prolonged diseases, add Os Draconis (*Long Gu*), Concha Ostreae (*Mu Li*), Herba Cephalanoploris Segeti (*Xiao Ji*), and Herba Cirsii Japonici (*Da Ji*).

YU YIN HUA BAN TANG **(Foster Yin & Transform Macules Decoction)**
Cooked Radix Rehmanniae (*Shu Di*), uncooked Radix Rehmanniae (*Sheng Di*), Cortex Radicis Moutan (*Dan Pi*), Fructus Ligustri Lucidi (*Nu Zhen Zi*), Herba Ecliptae Prostratae (*Han Lian Cao*), Fructus Lycii Chinensis (*Gou Qi Zi*), Gelatinum Corii Asini (*E Jiao*), Radix Rubrus Paeoniae Lactiflorae (*Chi Shao*), Radix Albus Paeoniae Lactiflorae (*Bai Shao*), Caulis Milletiae Seu Spatholobi (*Ji Xue Teng*), Radix Rubiae Cordifoliae (*Qian Cao*), Nodus Nelumbinis Nuciferae (*Ou Jie*)

DAN PI SHENG DI TANG **(Moutan & Uncooked Rehmannia Decoction)**
Rhizoma Polygonati (*Huang Jing*), uncooked Radix Rehmanniae (*Sheng Di*), Fructus Ligustri Lucidi (*Nu Zhen Zi*), Radix Scutellariae Baicalensis (*Huang Qin*), Folium Daqingye (*Da Qing Ye*), Cortex Radicis Moutan (*Dan Pi*), Radix Rubiae Cordifoliae (*Qian Cao Gen*), Folium Callicarpae (*Zi Zhu Cao*), Herba Galii (*Xue Jian Chou*), Herba Agrimoniae Pilosae (*Xian He Cao*), Pollen Typhae (*Pu Huang*), Bombyx Batryticatus (*Bai Jiang Can*), Massa Medica Fermentata (*Shen Qu*), Radix Glycyrrhizae (*Gan Cao*)

Additions & subtractions: For dry stools, add Radix Et Rhizoma Rhei (*Da Huang*). For accompanying cough, add Radix Stemonae (*Bai Bu*), Bulbus Fritillariae Cirrhosae (*Chuan Bei Mu*), Herba Ephedrae (*Ma Huang*), Periostracum Cicadae (*Chan Tui*), and Herba Asari Cum Radice (*Xi Xin*). For recurring common colds, add Radix Astragali Membranacei (*Huang Qi*) and Radix Albus Paeoniae Lactiflorae (*Bai Shao*).

4. Spleen-kidney dual vacuity pattern

Main symptoms: Pale-colored purpura, fatigued spirit, no thought of food and drink, aversion to cold, cold limbs, a pale tongue with white fur, and a deep, fine, weak pulse

Treatment principles: Fortify the spleen and warm the kidneys

Chinese medicinal formulas:

SHUANG BU TANG **(Double Supplementing Decoction)**
Radix Panacis Ginseng (*Ren Shen*), Radix Dioscoreae Oppositae (*Shan Yao*), Sclerotium Poriae Cocos (*Fu Ling*), Semen Nelumbinis Nuciferae (*Lian Zi*), Fructus Psoraleae Corylifoliae (*Bu Gu Zhi*), Herba Cistanchis Deserticolae (*Cong Rong*), Fructus Corni Officinalis (*Shan Zhu Yu*), Fructus Schisandrae Chinensis (*Wu Wei Zi*), Radix Morindae Officinalis (*Ba Ji Tian*), Semen Cuscutae Chinensis (*Tu Si Zi*), Fructus Rubi Chingii (*Fu Pen Zi*)

WEN BU PI SHEN TANG (**Warm the Spleen & Supplement the Kidneys Decoction**)
  Radix Lateralis Praeparatus Aconiti Carmichaeli (*Fu Zi*), Semen Cuscutae Chinensis (*Tu Si Zi*), Rhizoma Atractylodis Macrocephalae (*Bai Zhu*), Sclerotium Poriae Cocos (*Fu Ling*), Fructus Rosae Laevigatae (*Jin Ying Zi*), Caulis Milletiae Seu Spatholobi (*Ji Xue Teng*)

SUO YANG TANG (**Cynomorium Decoction**)
  Radix Morindae Officinalis (*Ba Ji Tian*), Herba Cynomorii Songarici (*Suo Yang*), Herba Cistanchis Deserticolae (*Rou Cong Rong*), Radix Lateralis Praeparatus Aconiti Carmichaeli (*Fu Zi*), Radix Codonopsitis Pilosulae (*Dang Shen*), Rhizoma Dioscoreae Oppositae (*Shan Yao*)

5. Blood stasis pattern

Main symptoms: Dark-colored, recurrent purpura, swelling of the liver and spleen, fixed location abdominal pain, a dark and/or purple tongue or possible static macules or spots with thin fur, and a fine, choppy, or bowstring pulse

Treatment principles: Quicken the blood and free the flow of the network vessels

Chinese medicinal formulas:

JIA WEI SI WU TANG (**Added Flavors Four Materials Decoction**)
  Radix Angelicae Sinensis (*Dang Gui*), Radix Ligustici Wallichii (*Chuang Xiong*), cooked Radix Rehmanniae (*Shu Di*), Radix Rubrus Paeoniae Lactiflorae (*Chi Shao*), Semen Pruni Persicae (*Tao Ren*), Flos Carthami Tinctorii (*Hong Hua*)

QU YU HUA BAN TANG (**Dispel Stasis & Transform Macules Decoction**)
  Radix Angelicae Sinensis (*Dang Gui*), Radix Ligustici Wallichii (*Chuang Xiong*), Radix Rubrus Paeoniae Lactiflorae (*Chi Shao*), Caulis Milletiae Seu Spatholobi (*Ji Xue Teng*), Herba Leonuri Heterophylli (*Yi Mu Cao*), Pollen Typhae (*Pu Huang*), Feces Trogopterori Seu Pteromi (*Wu Ling Zhi*), Semen Pruni Persicae (*Tao Ren*), Flos Carthami Tinctorii (*Hong Hua*), Rhizoma Cyperi Rotundi (*Xiang Fu*), mix-fried Radix Astragali Membranacei (*Huang Qi*)

HUO XUE HUA YU TANG (**Quicken the Blood & Transform Stasis Decoction**)
  Radix Angelicae Sinensis (*Dang Gui*), Radix Ligustici Wallichii (*Chuang Xiong*), Flos Carthami Tinctorii (*Hong Hua*), Radix Rubrus Paeoniae Lactiflorae (*Chi Shao Yao*), Herba Leonuri Heterophylli (*Yi Mu Cao*), Caulis Milletiae Seu Spatholobi (*Ji Xue Teng*), Radix Astragali Membranacei (*Huang Qi*), Radix Codonopsitis Pilosulae (*Dang Shen*)

2 Primary Thrombocythemia

Primary or essential thrombocythemia is a disease characterized by an increased platelet count, megakaryocytic hyperplasia, and a hemorrhagic or thrombotic tendency. Platelets derive from the hemocytoblast stem cell and the megakaryoblast precursor. Similar to other chronic myeloproliferative syndromes (*i.e.,* polycythemia vera and chronic myelogenous leukemia), primary thrombocythemia is due to clonal abnormality of a multipotent hematopoietic stem cell. However, besides the megakaryocyte, no other blood elements are affected and thus, in order to establish the diagnosis of primary thrombocythemia, the RBC mass must be normal, Philadelphia chromosome (present in myelogenous leukemia) must be absent, and teardrop RBCs or significant increase in bone marrow fibrosis (indicative of idiopathic myelofibrosis) must also be absent. The thrombocyte count is usually more than one million per microliter ($1 \times 10^6 /mm^3$), and the thrombocytes are abnormally shaped.

Average age at onset is 50-70 years, and males are slightly more commonly affected than females (1.2:1). Common symptoms of primary thrombocythemia include bodily weakness, hemorrhage, nonspecific headaches, and dizziness. Bleeding is usually mild, manifesting as epistaxis, easy bruising, or gastrointestinal bleeding. However, in older patients, increased platelet numbers combined with degenerative vascular diseases may lead to serious bleeding or thrombosis. Paresthesia[1] of the hands and feet or digital ischemia may be seen. Splenomegaly and/or hepatomegaly may be found in about half the patients.

Western medical treatment is indicated if the platelet count is over one million and if hemorrhage or thrombotic complications manifest. Myelosuppressive medications are commonly the drugs of choice. Because myelosuppressive drugs tend to work rather slowly, plateletpheresis[2] can be used for immediate reduction in the platelet count in such emergency cases as serious hemorrhage or thrombosis or before an emergency surgical procedure.

---

[1] Paresthesia is a sensation of numbness, prickling, or tingling and is experienced in central and peripheral nerve lesions and in locomotor ataxia. It occurs in this disease due to a lack of blood supply to the peripheral nervous tissue.

[2] Plateletpheresis refers to the treatment of donor blood to remove platelets and then returning the blood to the donor.

Thrombocythemia may also be secondary to causes such as chronic inflammatory disorders, acute infection, hemorrhage, iron deficiency, hemolysis, neoplasms, and post-operative splenectomy. In these cases, Western medical treatment focuses on the underlying cause.

Chinese medical disease explanation:

In Chinese medicine, primary thrombocythemia corresponds to the disease category of bleeding conditions (*xue zheng*). The two viscera most involved in its disease mechanisms are the liver and kidneys. The kidneys store the essence, govern the bones, engender marrow, and nourish the liver. The liver stores blood. Enduring diseases lead to kidney essence depletion and detriment and liver yin consumption and dryness. This then causes the accumulation of vacuity fire internally which stirs the blood. If the liver loses control over its function of coursing and discharging, then there will be qi stagnation and blood stasis. Blood stasis internally congests and obstructs the network vessels' free flow; this leads to concretions and accumulations. If there is already phlegm and blood obstructing the channels and vessels, new blood cannot flow as smoothly and quietly as it should. This also leads to bleeding due to the blood being forced outside its vessels.

In clinical practice, essentially every case of primary thrombocytopenia involves blood stasis. Depending on whether this blood stasis is complicated by qi stagnation, qi and blood vacuity, yin vacuity, or vacuity heat, several mixed patterns of this disease are discriminated.

Treatment based on pattern discrimination:

1. Qi & blood stasis & stagnation pattern

Main symptoms: Fixed and piercing headache, purple macules, nose-bleeding with dark-colored blood, enlarged spleen and liver, rib-side pain, numbness in the limbs, purple nails, possible pain in the abdomen, a purple tongue with possible static spots or macules, and a bowstring pulse

Treatment principles: Move the qi, quicken the blood, and dispel stasis

Chinese medicinal formulas:

SHUI ZHI TANG **(Hirudo Decoction)**
Hirudo Seu Whitmania (*Shui Zhi*), Tabanus (*Meng Chong*)[3], Eupolyphaga Seu Opisthoplatia (*Di Bie Chong*), Semen Pruni Persicae (*Tao Ren*), Cortex Radicis Moutan (*Dan Pi*), Radix Rubrus Paeoniae Lactiflorae (*Chi Shao*), uncooked Radix Rehmanniae (*Sheng Di*), Pollen Typhae (*Pu Huang*), Feces Trogopterori Seu Pteromi (*Wu Ling Zhi*)

This formula breaks and cools the blood. It is especially indicated to treat thrombocythemia due to splenectomy of an enlarged spleen secondary to portal vein hypertension.

SHU GAN HUO XUE TANG **(Course the Liver & Quicken the Blood Decoction)**
Radix Bupleuri (*Chai Hu*), Radix Angelicae Sinensis (*Dang Gui*), Tuber Curcumae (*Yu Jin*), Radix Linderae Strychnifoliae (*Wu Yao*), Fructus Citri Aurantii (*Zhi Ke*), Semen Pruni Persicae (*Tao Ren*), Cortex Radicis Moutan (*Dan Pi*), Radix Rubrus Paeoniae Lactiflorae (*Chi Shao*), Radix Ligustici Wallichii (*Chuan Xiong*), Flos Carthami Tinctorii (*Hong Hua*)

This formula courses the liver and rectifies the qi as well as quickens the blood.

2. Blood stasis complicated by qi & blood vacuity pattern

Main symptoms: Fatigue, weakness, nose-bleeding, purple macules, numbness and tingling of the limbs, possible enlarged spleen and liver, headache, a pale purple tongue with possible static spots or macules, and a choppy, forceless pulse

Treatment principles: Disperse stasis and scatter nodulation, boost the qi, nourish the blood, and clear heat

Chinese medicinal formula:

XIAO ZHENG HUA YU TANG **(Disperse Concretions & Transform Stasis Decoction)**
Radix Salviae Miltiorrhizae (*Dan Shen*), Semen Pruni Persicae (*Tao Ren*), Radix Rubrus Paeoniae Lactiflorae (*Chi Shao*), Flos Carthami Tinctorii (*Hong Hua*), Radix Angelicae Sinensis (*Dang Gui*), Carapax Amydae Sinensis (*Bie Jia*), Rhizoma Sparganii (*San Leng*), Rhizoma Curcumae Zedoariae (*E Zhu*), Radix Et Rhizoma Rhei

---

[3] Tabanus (*Meng Chong*) is bitter, cool, and toxic in nature and enters the liver channel. It dispels stasis, breaks accumulations, and frees the flow of the channels. Recommended dosage is 1.5-3 grams.

(*Da Huang*), Pericarpium Citri Reticulatae Viride (*Qing Pi*), Herba Lycopi Lucidi (*Ze Lan*), Radix Astragali Membranacei (*Huang Qi*), Herba Artemisiae Apiaceae (*Qing Hao*)

Additions & subtractions: For strengthening heat-clearing, nodulation-scattering, and hardness-softening, add Fructus Forsythiae Suspensae (*Lian Qiao*), Radix Scrophulariae Ningpoensis (*Xuan Shen*), Rhizoma Dioscoreae Bulbiferae (*Huang Yao Zi*), and Hirudo Seu Whitmania (*Shui Zhi*). In order to supplement vacuity, add Radix Codonopsitis Pilosulae (*Dang Shen*), cooked Radix Rehmanniae (*Shu Di*), and Gelatinum Piscis Vesicae Acris (*Yu Biao Jiao*).[4]

3. Stasis heat pattern

Main symptoms: Vexation and agitation, nose-bleeding, purple macules, hemafecia with fresh red blood and clots, possible enlarged liver and spleen, fever worsening at night, a dry, crimson tongue, and a fine, bowstring, rapid pulse

Treatment principles: Clear heat, cool the blood, and dispel stasis

Chinese medicinal formula:

XI DI TAO REN TANG JIA JIAN **(Rhinoceros, Rehmannia & Persica Decoction with Additions & Subtractions)**
   Cornu Bubali (*Shui Niu Fen*), Cortex Radicis Moutan (*Dan Pi*), uncooked Radix Rehmanniae (*Sheng Di*), Radix Albus Paeoniae Lactiflorae (*Bai Shao*), Semen Pruni Persicae (*Tao Ren*), Flos Carthami Tonctorii (*Hong Hua*), Semen Coicis Lachrymae-jobi (*Yi Yi Ren*), Radix Lithospermi Seu Arnebiae (*Zi Cao*)

Additions & subtractions: For leg pain, small itchy papules on the entire body, and headache, add Radix Ligustici Wallichii (*Chuan Xiong*), Herba Pycnostelmae (*Xu Chang Qing*)[5], stir-fried Semen Zizyphi Spinosae (*Suan Zao Ren*), and Radix Angelicae Dahuricae (*Bai Zhi*).

---

[4] Gelatinum Piscis Vesicae Acris (*Yu Biao Jiao*) is sweet and neutral in nature, and enters the kidney channel. It supplements the kidneys, boosts essence, enriches and nourishes the sinews and vessels, stops bleeding, scatters stasis, and disperses swellings. Recommended dosage is 9-15 grams.

[5] Herba Pycnostelmae (*Xu Chang Qing*) is acrid and warm in nature and enters the spleen, stomach, and kidney channels. It dispels wind and eliminates dampness, alleviates pain, resolves toxins, and disperses swellings.

4. Blood stasis & kidney yin vacuity pattern

Main symptoms: Bodily weakness, evening heat, night sweats, dry skin, numbness of the limbs, dizziness, tinnitus, nose-bleeding, purple macules, early or erratic menses, possible enlarged spleen and liver, a red tongue with possible static macules or spots and scanty, possibly yellow fur, and a fine, rapid pulse

Treatment principles: Enrich and nourish kidney yin as well as cool the blood and transform stasis

Chinese medicinal formulas:

ZI SHEN HUO XUE FANG (**Enrich the Kidneys & Quicken the Blood Formula**)
Uncooked Radix Rehmanniae (*Sheng Di*), Radix Scrophulariae Ningpoensis (*Xuan Shen*), Radix Ligustici Wallichii (*Chuan Xiong*), Radix Rubrus Paeoniae Lactiflorae (*Chi Shao*), Flos Carthami Tinctorii (*Hong Hua*), Rhizoma Sparganii (*San Leng*), Semen Pruni Persicae (*Tao Ren*), Hirudo Seu Whitmania (*Shui Zhi*)

Additions & subtractions: For severe damp heat, add Herba Artemesiae Capillaris (*Yin Chen Hao*), Radix Scutellariae Baicalensis (*Huang Qin*), Fructus Gardeniae Jasminoidis (*Zhi Zi*), Cortex Magnoliae Officinalis (*Hou Po*), and Flos Lonicerae Japonicae (*Jin Yin Hua*). For yin vacuity with fire effulgence, add Rhizoma Anemarrhenae Asphodeloidis (*Zhi Mu*), Cortex Radicis Moutan (*Dan Pi*), and Cortex Phellodendri (*Huang Bai*). To strengthen blood-quickening and stasis-transforming, add Radix Salviae Miltiorrhizae (*Dan Shen*), Herba Leonuri Heterophylli (*Yi Mu Cao*), and Radix Lithospermi Seu Arnebiae (*Zi Cao*). For a dry mouth, add Radix Puerariae (*Ge Gen*). For chest oppression, add Lignum Dalbergiae Odoriferae (*Jiang Xiang*). For aching and limpness of the four limbs, add Herba Lycopodii (*Shen Jin Cao*)[6] and Ramulus Loranthi Seu Visci (*Sang Ji Sheng*).

JIANG BAN TANG (**Thrombocyte-downbearing Decoction**)
Caulis Lonicerae Japonicae (*Ren Dong Ten*), Flos Lonicerae Japonicae (*Lian Qiao*), Radix Bupleuri (*Chai Hu*), Cortex Radicis Moutan (*Dan Pi*), Spica Prunellae Vulgaris (*Xia Ku Cao*), Radix Angelicae Sinensis (*Dang Gui*), Radix Ligustici Wallichii (*Chuan Xiong*), uncooked Radix Rehmanniae (*Sheng Di*), Radix Albus Paeoniae Lactiflorae (*Bai Shao*), Cortex Radicis Lycii Chinensis (*Di Gu Pi*), Rhizoma Anemarrhenae Asphodeloidis (*Zhi Mu*), Radix Glycyrrhizae (*Gan Cao*), Carapax

---

[6] Herba Lycopodii (*Shen Jin Cao*) is bitter, acrid, and warm in nature and enters the liver channel. It expels wind, dispels cold, and eliminates dampness, relaxes the sinews and muscles, frees the flow of the channels, and nourishes the blood.

Amydae Sinensis (*Bie Jia*), Cornu Bubali (*Shui Niu Jiao*, powdered and swallowed with the decoction)

This formula enriches yin and clears the liver, dispels stasis and frees the flow of the network vessels.

3 Allergic Purpura

Allergic purpura is an acute or chronic vasculitis primarily affecting the small vessels of the skin, joints, gastrointestinal tract, and kidneys. The disease is most common in young children but can also occur in older children or adults. In young children in a majority of cases, an acute respiratory infection precedes the purpura. A variety of Western drugs is another initiating factor.

The disease begins abruptly with the sudden appearance of a purpuric skin rash primarily involving the extensor surfaces of the feet and legs, a strip across the buttocks, and the extensor surfaces of the arms. Lesions may start as small areas of urticaria that progress to become indurated, palpable, purpuric spots. Crops of new lesions may appear over several days to several weeks. Because of bleeding into the joints, most patients also manifest with polyarthralgias and periarticular tenderness. Bleeding into the gastrointestinal tract gives rise to abdominal tenderness and colicky abdominal pain as well as melena or occult blood in the stools. Hematuria and proteinuria secondary to renal involvement develops in 25-50% of all patients. Fever and edema of the hands and feet are present in most patients. The disease usually remits after approximately four weeks but often recurs one or more times after a disease-free interval of several weeks. Although not common, renal lesions in some patients may progress to chronic renal failure.

The Western medical treatment of this disease is primarily symptomatic. If a drug is the initiating factor of the purpura, the drug is eliminated. Corticosteroids may help to control edema, joint pain, and abdominal pain by reducing the inflammatory reaction. However, they do not have any effect upon the course of acute renal involvement.

Chinese medical disease explanation:

In Chinese medicine, this disease corresponds to the categories of spontaneous bleeding of the flesh (*ji nu*), warm toxin macular eruptions (*wen du fa ban*), grape epidemic (*pu tao yi*), and purple patch wind (*zi dian feng*). Bleeding is the underlying factor leading to the arisal of the disease. However, four distinct mechanisms of engendering bleeding are differentiated.

First, if the exterior defensive is not secure, warm heat toxic evils may invade the exterior and muscles where they become depressed. Such depressed heat evils may then scorch and damage the vessels and network vessels and lead to frenetic movement of the blood. Blood thus seeps into the skin and flesh and purple patches arise.

Secondly, if eating and drinking are unregulated, the spleen and stomach may be damaged and movement and transformation may become disturbed. In some patients, this causes damp heat to brew internally. Just as depressed heat may force the blood to move frentically outside its channels, so may the heat of damp heat, thus resulting in blood seeping into the skin and flesh. Thus, purpura may arise.

Third, if yin is vacuous, yang may become hyperactive and vacuity fire may stir internally. This vacuity heat may also lead to frenetic movement of the blood, with the blood spilling outside the vessels and into the skin and flesh. Thus, again, purple patches may arise.

And fourth, because the spleen qi contains the blood, if, due to any reason, the spleen becomes vacuous and weak, the spleen's function of containing the blood may be insufficient. Hence blood seeps outside the vessels and purple patches may arise.

The fact that this disease is more common in young children is explained in Chinese medicine by the facts that A) children's bodies are pure yang and, therefore, engender heat quickly, and B) their spleen and stomach as well as their kidneys are inherently insufficient and weak. Therefore, blood containment has no strength and the exterior defensive is not secure. Thus the body is invaded by exterior evils more rapidly and more frequently than in adults. This leads to a greater likelihood of the engenderment of evil heat and, therefore, bleeding and the arisal of purpura.

Because this disease not only attacks the skin and flesh but also the joints, intestines, kidneys, and brain[1], the Chinese medical literature uses a second system of differentiation according to the location of bleeding. According to this system, detriment and damage by wind evils and heat toxins of the following five different body areas are differentiated: 1) the skin network vessels, 2) the intestinal network vessels, 3) the joints, 4) the kidney network vessels, and 5) the brain network vessels. This second system of differentiation focuses on the acute attack of the disease and corresponds to the first of the five patterns discriminated below (i.e., frenetic movement due to hot blood). When this second system of differentiation is used to treat patients suffering from allergic

---

[1]   There is no mention in the Western medical literature that this disease leads to intercranial bleeding. However, in *Zhong Yi Er Ke Xue Ye Bing Zhen Liao Jing Yan, op. cit.*, neurological disorders secondary to either intercranial bleeding or intercranial blood stasis are discussed and are given below for reference.

purpura, it is important to modify the formulas according to pattern discrimination, *e.g.*, yin vacuity, damp heat, spleen vacuity, or fire heat.

Treatment based on pattern discrimination:

1. Wind heat & fire toxins damaging the network vessels and leading to frenetic movement of hot blood pattern

Main symptoms: Acute onset of disease, fever, slight aversion to wind, copious effusion of purple patches on the four limbs which are more severe on the lower limbs, fresh red-colored macules, the macules may combine into patches, itchy skin, nausea and vomiting, abdominal pain, hemafecia, joint swelling and pain, a red tongue with slightly yellow fur, and a floating, rapid pulse

Treatment principles: Course wind and clear heat, cool the blood and dispel stasis

Chinese medicinal formulas:

XIAO FENG QING RE YIN (Disperse Wind & Clear Heat Drink)
Herba Seu Flos Schizonepetae Tenuifoliae (*Jing Jie*), Radix Ledebouriellae Divaricatae (*Fang Feng*), Herba Lemnae Seu Spirodelae (*Fu Ping*), Periostracum Cicadae (*Chan Tui*), Radix Angelicae Sinensis (*Dang Gui*), Radix Rubrus Paeoniae Lactiflorae (*Chi Shao*), Folium Daqingye (*Da Qing Ye*), Radix Scutellariae Baicalensis (*Huang Qin*)

KANG ZI DIAN FANG (Combatting Purple Patches [*i.e.*, Purpura] Formula)
Flos Lonicerae Japonicae (*Jin Yin Hua*), Herba Taraxaci Mongolici Cum Radice (*Pu Gong Ying*), Herba Viola Yedoensitis Cum Radice (*Zi Hua Di Ding*), Rhizoma Smilacis Glabrae (*Tu Fu Ling*), Cortex Radicis Dictamni Dasycarpi (*Bai Xian Pi*), Fructus Kochiae Scopariae (*Di Fu Zi*), Rhizoma Dioscoreae Hypoglaucae (*Bei Xie*), Radix Salviae Miltiorrhizae (*Dan Shen*), Radix Rubrus Paeoniae Lactiflorae (*Chi Shao*), Periostracum Cicadae (*Chan Tui*), Radix Ledebouriellae Divaricatae (*Fang Feng*), Rhizoma Alismatis (*Ze Xie*), Radix Angelicae Dahuricae (*Bai Zhi*), Radix Glycyrrhizae (*Gan Cao*)

2. Damp heat obstruction pattern

Main symptoms: Fever, purple patches, painful, scorching hot, swollen, and distended joints, heavy limbs, abdominal pain, diarrhea and dysentery, hematuria, vexatious heat in the chest and stomach duct, thirst, panting, sweating, a red tongue with yellow fur, and a rapid pulse. This pattern corresponds to allergic purpura predominantly affecting the intestines.

Treatment principles: Clear heat and disinhibit dampness, transform stasis and free the flow of the network vessels

Chinese medicinal formulas:

SI MIAO WAN **(Four Wonders Pills)**
Rhizoma Atractylodis (*Cang Zhu*), Cortex Phellodendri (*Huang Bai*), Radix Achyranthis Bidentatae (*Niu Xi*), Semen Coicis Lachrymae-jobi (*Yi Yi Ren*)

GE GEN QIN LIAN TANG **(Pueraria, Scutellaria & Coptis Decoction)**
Radix Puerariae (*Ge Gen*), Radix Scutellariae Baicalensis (*Huang Qin*), Rhizoma Coptidis Chinensis (*Huang Lian*), Radix Glycyrrhizae (*Gan Cao*)

3. Yin vacuity-yang hyperactivity pattern

Main symptoms: Purple patches that come and go, dizziness, tinnitus, vexatious heat in the five hearts, afternoon low-grade fever, night sweats, a dry mouth and throat, lumbar aching, knee limpness, a red tongue with static spots, and a fine, rapid or choppy pulse

Treatment principles: Clear heat and enrich the kidneys, cool the blood and stop bleeding

Chinese medicinal formula:

ZI YIN BA WEI JIAN **(Yin-enriching Eight Flavors Brew)**
Radix Dioscoreae Oppositae (*Shan Yao*), Cortex Radicis Moutan (*Dan Pi*), Sclerotium Poriae Cocos (*Fu Ling*), Fructus Corni Officinalis (*Shan Zhu Yu*), Rhizoma Alismatis (*Ze Xie*), Cortex Phellodendri (*Huang Bai*), cooked Radix Rehmanniae (*Shu Di*), Radix Anemarrhenae Asphodeloidis (*Zhi Mu*)

Additions & subtractions: For chronic, recurrent allergic purpura or for enduring disease without a cure which has damaged and consumed yin fluids, subtract *Huang Bai* and *Zhi Mu*, and add Tuber Ophiopogonis Japonici (*Mai Dong*) and Fructus Schisandrae Chinensis (*Wu Wei Zi*).

4. Spleen vacuity non-containment of blood pattern

Main symptoms: Pale-colored purple macules, a bright white facial complexion, decreased intake (*i.e.,* lack of appetite), loose and/or black stools, fatigued limbs, lack of strength, a swollen, enlarged tongue, and a fine, forceless pulse

Treatment principles: Fortify the spleen and nourish and contain the blood

Chinese medicinal formula:

GUI PI TANG (Return the Spleen Decoction)
Radix Astragali Membranacei (*Huang Qi*), Radix Panacis Ginseng (*Ren Shen*), Rhizoma Atractylodis Macrocephalae (*Bai Zhu*), Sclerotium Pararadicis Poriae Cocos (*Fu Shen*), Radix Angelicae Sinensis (*Dang Gui*), Semen Zizyphi Spinosae (*Suan Zao Ren*), Radix Polygalae Tenuifoliae (*Yuan Zhi*), Arillus Euphoriae Longanae (*Long Yan Rou*), Radix Auklandiae Lappae (*Mu Xiang*), Radix Glycyrrhizae (*Gan Cao*), uncooked Rhizoma Zingiberis (*Sheng Jiang*), Fructus Zizyphi Jujubae (*Da Zao*)

Differentiation according to location:

1. Wind evils & heat toxins causing detriment & damage to the network vessels of the skin

Main symptoms: Itchy, purple skin papules predominantly distributed on the four limbs and the buttocks, most often on the lower limbs and crowded around the ankles, possibly pronounced angioneurotic edema with itching, puffy swelling of the face and eyelids[2], irregular low- to medium-grade fever, a red tongue with yellowish white fur, and a floating, rapid pulse

Treatment principles: Dispel wind and soothe the network vessels, transform stasis and disperse patches

Chinese medicinal formula:

SHU LUO JIE DU MA HUANG TANG (Soothe the Network Vessels & Resolve Toxins Ephedra Decoction)
Caulis Milletiae Seu Spatholobi (*Ji Xue Teng*), Radix Salviae Miltiorrhizae (*Dan Shen*), Radix Ligustici Wallichii (*Chuan Xiong*), Flos Carthami Tinctorii (*Hong Hua*), Semen Pruni Persicae (*Tao Ren*), uncooked Radix Rehmanniae (*Sheng Di*), Radix

---

[2] Puffy face (*mian fu*), also called puffy swelling of the face and eyelids, refers to non-pitting facial edema. Puffy face is a species of qi swelling caused by qi vacuity due to lung and/or spleen vacuity.

Rubrus Paeoniae Lactiflorae (*Chi Shao*), Radix Ledebouriellae Divaricatae (*Fang Feng*), Radix Angelicae Pubescentis (*Du Huo*), Herba Ephedrae (*Ma Huang*), Lumbricus (*Di Long*), Herba Asari Cum Radice (*Xi Xin*), Radix Achyranthis Bidentatae (*Niu Xi*), Flos Lonicerae Japonicae (*Jin Yin Hua*), Radix Glycyrrhizae (*Gan Cao*), Radix Scutellariae Baicalensis (*Huang Qin*)

Additions & subtractions: If urticaria or angioneurotic edema is severe or if there is swelling of the throat with a hoarse voice, add Periostracum Cicadae (*Chan Tui*) and Rhizoma Paridis Polyphyllae (*Qi Ye Yi Zhi Hua*) and increase the amount of *Ma Huang*.

2. Wind evils & heat toxins causing detriment & damage to the intestinal network vessels

Main symptoms: This pattern is differentiated into two types. The first type is characterized by skin purpura with accompanying abdominal pain and occult blood in the stools or bloody stools. The second type is characterized by initial abdominal pain with occult blood in the stools or bloody stools and subsequent effusion of skin purpura. Frequently, both types are also accompanied by nausea and, if severe, vomiting.

Treatment principles: Quicken the blood and transform stasis, fortify the spleen and disinhibit urination

Chinese medicinal formula:

SHU LUO JIE DU MU XIANG TANG (**Soothe the Network Vessels & Resolve Toxins Auklandia Decoction**)
Radix Salviae Miltiorrhizae (*Dan Shen*), Rhizoma Curcumae Zedoariae (*E Zhu*), Rhizoma Corydalis Yanhusuo (*Yan Hu Suo*), Rhizoma Atractylodis Macrocephalae (*Bai Zhu*), Sclerotium Poriae Cocos (*Fu Ling*), Semen Plantaginis (*Che Qian Zi*), Radix Auklandiae Lappae (*Mu Xiang*), Radix Et Rhizoma Rhei (*Da Huang*), Herba Ephedrae (*Ma Huang*), Herba Asari Cum Radice (*Xi Xin*), Periostracum Cicadae (*Chan Tui*), Lumbricus (*Di Long*), Radix Glycyrrhizae (*Gan Cao*)

Additions & subtractions: If there are nausea and vomiting, add ginger stir-fried Radix Pinelliae Ternatae (*Ban Xia*) and Pericarpium Citri Reticulatae (*Chen Pi*). If there is abdominal distention, add Fructus Cardamomi (*Bai Dou Kou*). For accompanying fever, add Radix Scutellariae Baicalensis (*Huang Qin*), Rhizoma Coptidis Chinensis (*Huang Lian*), and Flos Lonicerae Japonicae (*Jin Yin Hua*).

3. Wind evils & heat toxins causing detriment & damage to the joints

Main symptoms: Joint pain is the prominent sign in this pattern. The main joints involved are the knees, ankles, wrists, and elbows. The joints are swollen and aching and movement is limited. The pain is wandering in nature. There are also accompanying skin purpura, a somber white facial complexion, a red tongue with thin, white or yellowish white fur, and a floating, rapid or bowstring, tight pulse.

Treatment principles: Dispel wind and quicken the network vessels, transform stasis and alleviate impediment

Chinese medicinal formula:

SHU LUO JIE DU DU HUO TANG (Soothe the Network Vessels & Resolve Toxins Angelica Pubescens Decoction)
Radix Angelicae Pubescentis (*Du Huo*), Radix Ledebouriellae Divaricatae (*Fang Feng*), Radix Aconiti Carmichaeli (*Chuan Wu*), Herba Ephedrae (*Ma Huang*), Herba Asari Cum Radice (*Xi Xin*), Periostracum Cicadae (*Chan Tui*), Lumbricus (*Di Long*), Caulis Milletiae Seu Spatholobi (*Ji Xue Teng*), Radix Salviae Miltiorrhizae (*Dan Shen*), Radix Ligustici Wallichii (*Chuan Xiong*), Flos Carthami Tinctorii (*Hong Hua*), Radix Achyranthis Bidentatae (*Niu Xi*), Radix Astragali Membranacei (*Huang Qi*), powdered Bombyx Batryticatus (*Bai Jiang Can*, swallowed with the decoction), Radix Glycyrrhizae (*Gan Cao*)

Additions & subtractions: For accompanying fever, add Radix Scutellariae Baicalensis (*Huang Qin*), Rhizoma Coptidis Chinensis (*Huang Lian*), and Radix Gentianae Macrophyllae (*Qin Jiao*). For severe joint swelling and pain with inhibited movement, add powdered Agkistrodon Seu Bungarus (*Bai Hua She*, swallowed with the decoction).

4. Wind evils & heat toxins causing detriment & damage to the kidney network vessels

Main symptoms: If evil toxins gather and lie deeply and stagnate in the kidney network vessels, the network vessels' blood circulation is inhibited. If the blood cannot circulate, it seeps outside the vessels and percolates into the urine. Thus, there is gross hematuria or microscopic hematuria. Puffy swelling is generally not marked, but, in severe cases, there may be puffy swelling of the face as well as elevated blood pressure.

Treatment principles: Transform stasis and disperse macules, warm and free the flow of the network vessels of the kidneys

Chinese medicinal formulas:

SHU LUO JIE DU DA HUANG TANG (Soothe the Network Vessels & Resolve Toxins Rhubarb Decoction)

Radix Salviae Miltiorrhizae (*Dan Shen*), Radix Ligustici Wallichii (*Chuan Xiong*), Radix Rubrus Paeoniae Lactiflorae (*Chi Shao*), Hirudo Seu Whitmania (*Shui Zhi*), Lumbricus (*Di Long*), quick-fried Carapax Amydae Sinensis (*Bie Jia*), Radix Lateralis Praeparatus Aconiti Carmichaeli (*Fu Zi*), Herba Epimedii (*Xian Ling Pi*), Herba Asari Cum Radice (*Xi Xin*), Cortex Rhizomatis Zingiberis (*Jiang Pi*), Radix Et Rhizoma Rhei (*Da Huang*), Radix Achyranthis Bidentatae (*Niu Xi*), Semen Plantaginis (*Che Qian Zi*), Radix Glycyrrhizae (*Gan Cao*)

Additions & subtractions: For accompanying proteinuria, add Radix Astragali Membranacei (*Huang Qi*) and Periostracum Cicadae (*Chan Tui*). For an accompanying increase in blood cholesterol, add Rhizoma Alismatis (*Ze Xie*) and Semen Cassiae Torae (*Cao Jue Ming*). Fever is rarely seen in nephrotic purpura. However, if there is fever, add Flos Lonicerae Japonicae (*Jin Yin Hua*) and Herba Taraxaci Mongolici Cum Radice (*Pu Gong Ying*).

WU SHAO SHE TANG (Zaocys Decoction)

Zaocys Dhumnades (*Wu Shao She*), Cordyceps Chinensis (*Dong Chong Xia Cao*), Lumbricus (*Di Long*), Bombyx Batryticatus (*Bai Jiang Can*), Radix Lateralis Praeparatus Aconiti Carmichaeli (*Fu Zi*), Herba Ephedrae (*Ma Huang*), Herba Asari Cum Radice (*Xi Xin*), uncooked Pollen Typhae (*Pu Huang*), Hirudo Seu Whitmania (*Shui Zhi*), Eupolyphaga Seu Opistholoplatia (*Zhe Chong*), Radix Et Rhizoma Rhei (*Da Huang*), Radix Glycyrrhizae (*Gan Cao*)

ZHI ZI DIAN XING SHEN YAN FANG (Nephrotic Allergic Purpura Treatment Formula)

Uncooked Radix Rehmanniae (*Sheng Di*), Radix Et Rhizoma Rhei (*Da Huang*), Fructus Crataegi (*Sheng Shan Zha*), Herba Evolvuli (*Lu Han Cao*)[3], Radix Lithospermi Seu Arnebiae (*Zi Cao*), Radix Glycyrrhizae (*Gan Cao*), Radix Ledebouriellae Divaricatae (*Fang Feng*)

QING ZI HE JI (Purple Mixture)

Pulvis Indigonis (*Qing Dai*), Rhizoma Imperatae Cylindricae (*Bai Mao Gen*), Radix Salviae Miltiorrhizae (*Dan Shen*), Herba Cephalanoploris Segeti (*Xiao Ji*), Herba

---

[3] Herba Evolvuli (*Lu Han Cao*) is also called *Tu Ding Gui* and is bitter, acrid, and cool in nature and enters the liver, spleen, and kidney channels. It clears heat and disinhibits dampness. Recommended dosage is 5-15 grams.

Cirsii Japonici (*Da Ji*), Cortex Radicis Moutan (*Dan Pi*), Radix Rubrus Paeoniae Lactiflorae (*Chi Shao*), Semen Coicis Lachryma-jobi (*Yi Yi Ren*), Herba Pteridis (*Feng Wei Cao*)[4], Herba Achyranthis Asperae (*Dao Kou Cao*), Radix Clematidis Chinensis (*Wei Ling Xian*), uncooked Radix Rehmanniae (*Sheng Di*)

5. Wind evils & heat toxins causing detriment & damage to the brain network vessels

If allergic purpura is accompanied by neurological symptoms, the brain is involved. This then is subdivided into two patterns: A) seeping of blood from the brain network vessels and B) stasis and stagnation of the brain network vessels. The first of these is due to wind evils and heat toxins accumulating in and damaging the brain's network vessels. Thus the blood within the brain's network vessels becomes static and forces the blood to flow outside these vessels, thus seeping into the brain. In the second of these two sub-patterns, the blood in the brain network vessels is static but does not seep outside the vessels. Hence the brain is insufficiently nourished due to slow blood flow. In addition, this obstruction and blockage leads to an increase in intracranial pressure and thus distention and pain.

A. Seeping of blood from the brain's network vessels pattern

Main symptoms: Intense headaches, dizziness, vomiting, vexation and agitation, and, if severe, spirit clouding with deranged speech, convulsions, and paralysis of the limbs

Treatment principles: Transform stasis and stop bleeding, level the liver and extinguish wind

Chinese medicinal formula:

HUA YU XI FENG TANG (**Transform Stasis & Extinguish Wind Decoction**)
Radix Astragali Membranacei (*Huang Qi*), Radix Ligustici Wallichii (*Chuan Xiong*), Radix Salviae Miltiorrhizae (*Dan Shen*), Periostracum Cicadae (*Chan Tui*), Radix Rubrus Paeoniae Lactiflorae (*Chi Shao*), Lumbricus (*Di Long*), uncooked Radix Rehmanniae (*Sheng Di*), Flos Carthami Tinctorii (*Hong Hua*), Semen Pruni Persicae (*Tao Ren*), Rhizoma Gastrodia Elatae (*Tian Ma*), Ramulus Uncariae Cum Uncis (*Gou Teng*), Periostracum Cicadae (*Chan Tui*), Tuber Curcumae (*Yu Jin*), Caulis Akebiae (*Mu Tong*), Semen Plantaginis (*Che Qian Zi*), Radix Glycyrrhizae (*Gan Cao*)

---

[4] Herba Pteridis (*Feng Wei Cao*) is sweet, bitter, and cold in nature and enters the lung and large intestine channels. It clears heat and cools the blood, disinhibits urination and astringes diarrhea.

If the neurological symptoms are severe, this formula can be combined with the following formula:

Fructus Gardeniae Jasminoidis (*Zhi Zi*), Radix Et Rhizoma Rhei (*Da Huang*), synthetic Calculus Bovis (*Niu Huang*), Periostracum Cicadae (*Chan Tui*), Scolopendra Subspinipes (*Wu Gong*), Bombyx Batryticatus (*Bai Jiang Can*), Agkistrodon Seu Bungarus (*Bai Hua She*), Concretio Silicea Bambusae (*Tian Zhu Huang*), and Radix Glycyrrhizae (*Gan Cao*). Prepare this as a powder and take with the decoction.

B. Stagnation of the brain network vessels pattern

Main symptoms: Headache, nausea, vexation and agitation, insomnia or somnolence. There may be accompanying dizziness. However, there are no convulsions, paralysis, or spirit clouding. If this pattern is very severe, it may lead to pattern A.

Treatment principles: Transform stasis and remove wind, course and free the flow of the brain's network vessels

Chinese medicinal formulas:

SAN CHONG TANG (Three Worms Decoction)
Lumbricus (*Di Long*), Hirudo Seu Whitmania (*Shui Zhi*), Radix Et Rhizoma Rhei (*Da Huang*), Caulis Milletiae Seu Spatholobi (*Ji Xue Teng*), Radix Ligustici Wallichii (*Chuan Xiong*), Periostracum Cicadae (*Chan Tui*), Herba Asari Cum Radice (*Xi Xin*), Radix Ligustici Sinensis (*Gao Ben*), Semen Plantaginis (*Che Qian Zi*), Radix Glycyrrhizae (*Gan Cao*)

Addendum: Much research is currently being done in China on the treatment of allergic purpura with Chinese medicinals. Below are a few formulas which, with the correct additions and subtractions, can be used to treat any type of allergic purpura. All these formulas have been proven through clinical research to benefit recovery of this disease and decrease the susceptibility to its recurrence.

XIAO DIAN JIE DU TANG (Disperse Patches & Resolve Toxins Decoction)
Radix Lithospermi Seu Arnebiae (*Zi Cao*), Semen Plantaginis (*Che Qian Zi*), Radix Et Rhizoma Rhei (*Da Huang*), Lumbricus (*Di Long*), Herba Agrimoniae Pilosae (*Xian He Cao*), uncooked Radix Rehmanniae (*Sheng Di*), Radix Salviae Miltiorrhizae (*Dan Shen*), Periostracum Cicadae (*Chan Tui*)

Additions & subtractions: For pronounced fever, add Rhizoma Coptidis Chinensis (*Huang Lian*) and Herba Lophatheri Gracilis (*Dan Zhu Ye*). For joint swelling, add Radix

Clematidis Chinensis (*Wei Ling Xian*) and Caulis Lonicerae Japonicae (*Ren Dong Teng*). For abdominal pain and hemafecia, add Radix Albus Paeoniae Lactiflorae (*Bai Shao*), Radix Corydalis Yanhusuo (*Yan Hu Suo*), and carbonized Radix Sanguisorbae (*Di Yu*). For involvement of the kidneys with water swelling and hematuria, add Rhizoma Imperatae Cylindricae (*Bai Mao Gen*) and Rhizoma Alismatis (*Ze Xie*).

QING ZAO TANG (Indigo & Lithospermum Decoction)

Pulvis Indigonis (*Qing Dai*), Radix Lithospermi Seu Arnebiae (*Zi Cao*), Resina Olibani (*Ru Xiang*), Fructus Tribuli Terrestris (*Bai Ji Li*)

This formula is very small and needs to be modified according to the presenting pattern.

QING DAI ZI CAO RU XIANG TANG (Indigo, Lithospermum & Frankincense Decoction)

Pulvis Indigonis (*Qing Dai*), Radix Lithospermi Seu Arnebiae (*Zi Cao*), Resina Olibani (*Ru Xiang*), Radix Salviae Miltiorrhizae (*Dan Shen*), Rhizoma Imperatae Cylindricae (*Bai Mao Gen*), Radix Clematidis Chinensis (*Wei Ling Xian*), Cortex Radicis Moutan (*Dan Pi*), uncooked Radix Rehmanniae (*Sheng Di*), Radix Auklandiae Lappae (*Mu Xiang*), scorched Fructus Crataegi (*Shan Zha*)

Additions & subtractions: For swollen and painful joints, add Fasciculus Vascularis Luffae Cylindricae (*Si Gua Luo*), Radix Achyranthis Bidentatae (*Niu Xi*), and Flos Carthami Tinctorii (*Hong Hua*). For abdominal pain, add Fructus Citri Aurantii (*Zhi Ke*), Radix Corydalis Yanhusuo (*Yan Hu Suo*), Radix Rubrus Paeoniae Lactiflorae (*Chi Shao*), and Radix Glycyrrhizae (*Gan Cao*). For nephritic involvement, add Herba Cephalanoploris Segeti (*Xiao Ji*), Herba Cirsii Japonici (*Da Ji*), Semen Coicis Lachryma-jobi (*Yi Yi Ren*), Herba Pteridis (*Feng Wei Cao*), and Herba Achyranthis Asperae (*Dao Kou Cao*).

LIANG XUE JIE DU TANG (Cool the Blood & Resolve Toxins Decoction)

Fructus Forsythiae Suspensae (*Lian Qiao*), Radix Lithospermi Seu Arnebiae (*Zi Cao*), Flos Immaturus Sophorae Japonicae (*Huai Hua Mi*), Herba Pycnostelmae (*Xu Chang Qing*)[5], Fructus Zizyphi Jujubae (*Da Zao*), Radix Glycyrrhizae (*Gan Cao*)

Additions & subtractions: For nausea and vomiting, add Rhizoma Pinelliae Ternatae (*Ban Xia*) and Caulis Bambusae In Taeniis (*Zhu Ru*). For abdominal pain, add Radix Albus Paeoniae Lactiflorae (*Bai Shao*). For hemafecia, add stir-fried Radix Sanguisorbae (*Di Yu*). For joint pain, add Semen Coicis Lachryma-jobi (*Yi Yi Ren*) and Radix

---

[5] Herba Pycnostelmae (*Xu Chang Qing*) is acrid and warm in nature and enters the spleen, stomach, and kidney channels. It dispels wind, eliminates dampness, and stops pain as well as resolves toxins and scatters nodulation.

Ledebouriellae Divaricatae (*Fang Feng*). For nephritic symptoms, add Sclerotium Poriae Cocos (*Fu Ling*), Radix Astragali Membranacei (*Huang Qi*), and Radix Dioscoreae Oppositae (*Shan Yao*). For an increased WBC count, add Herba Taraxaci Mongolici Cum Radice (*Pu Gong Ying*). For RBCs in the urine, add Rhizoma Imperatae Cylindricae (*Bai Mao Gen*).

ZI DIAN TANG (Purple Patches Decoction)

Herba Galli (*Xue Jian Chou*), Rhizoma Coptidis Chinensis (*Huang Lian*), uncooked Radix Rehmanniae (*Sheng Di*), Cacumen Biotae Orientalis (*Ce Bai Ye*), Fructus Quisqualis Indicae (*Shi Jun Zi*), Fructus Gardeniae Jasminoidis (*Zhi Zi*), Rhizoma Atractylodis (*Cang Zhu*), Acacia Seu Uncaria (*Er Cha*), Periostracum Cicadae (*Chan Tui*)

4 Hemophilia

Hemophilia is the most common of all bleeding disorders and is due to an X-linked recessive hereditary clotting factor deficiency.[1] Depending on which of the clotting factors is deficient, this disease can be divided into hemophilia A (factor VIII deficiency) and hemophilia B (factor IX deficiency). The former is the more common type and manifests in about 80% of all hemophiliacs. However, the symptoms are the same for both varieties, *i.e.*, a tendency to mild, moderate, or severe bleeding depending on the amount of factor deficiency. This most commonly leads to deforming arthritis caused by repeated bleeding into many joints (hemarthroses). Hematuria, intestinal obstruction, and respiratory obstruction may all occur with bleeding into the respective organs.

The Western medical treatment of this disease focuses on replacement of the deficient factor through plasma concentrates so as to control the bleeding. All drugs are given IV or orally. If pain from musculoskeletal complications is severe, non-steroidal anti-inflammatory drugs (NSAIDs) can be used in small amounts. However, the use of such drugs, especially aspirin, should be limited since they aggravate bleeding through their effect on platelet aggregation. Acetaminophen is the drug of choice for analgesia if pain is marked.

Chinese medical disease explanation:

In Chinese medicine, this disease corresponds to the disease categories of bleeding conditions (*xue zheng*), vacuity taxation (*xu lao*), and spontaneous bleeding of the flesh (*ji nu*). Because it is congenital, it is believed to be due to a former heaven natural endowment insufficiency with kidney essence vacuity and depletion. Because the former heaven qi is vacuous and because kidney qi is the root of all the body's qi, the source of warmth and nourishment is lacking, thus leading to an overall vacuity of bodily qi. If qi is vacuous, then the engenderment, movement, and containment of blood have no strength. Thus, A) blood is not engendered in sufficient quantity, B) it is not moved and

---

[1] This chapter only discusses the Western medical pathology of the hereditary coagulation factor deficiencies hemophilia A and hemophilia B. However, one should note that there are other types of hereditary bleeding disorders due to other factor deficiencies and factor pathologies. The most common hereditary factor pathology is Von Willebrand's disease (VWD). Von Willebrand's disease is an autosomal dominant disorder and thus presents in both girls and boys (not only in boys like in the sex-linked recessive hemophilias A and B). It also differs from the above discussed hemophilia A and hemophilia B in that it causes mucocutaneous bleeding rather than hemarthroses and deep muscle hemorrhage. In Chinese medicine, however, it is treated in the same way as hemophilia A/B.

may, therefore, become stagnant and static, and C) it cannot be contained within its vessels. This latter function is predominantly controlled by the spleen qi's function of containing or managing the blood. If spleen qi is too weak to do this duty, then blood spills over outside its vessels and bleeding may arise.

If spleen qi is weak and the kidney essence depleted, then defensive qi will also be weak and external evils easily invade the body. Heat evils may then damage the network vessels and cause frenetic movement due to hot blood with spilling of blood outside the vessels and into the surrounding tissues.

Heat evils entering the body may also consume yin blood and lead to yin vacuity with internal heat. Likewise, natural endowment insufficiency can give rise to congenital yin vacuity with internal fire. In either of these two cases, internal heat secondary to yin vacuity may cause detriment to the vessels and network vessels. If the blood becomes hot and moves frenetically, bleeding may ensue.

No matter what the cause, once blood leaves its normal pathways and spills over into the tissues, it gives rise to static or malign blood. Such stasis will then obstruct the vessels and network vessels and can also lead to transformative heat with subsequent frenetic movement of blood. Further, static blood may force the blood to move outside its vessels, creating yet another disease mechanism of bleeding. Because hemophilia's main symptom is bleeding, blood stasis accompanies every one of its patterns, and transformative heat causing frenetic movement secondary to blood stasis may arise even if the initial cause of bleeding was spleen qi vacuity.

Below, three distinct patterns of this disease are differentiated: 1) qi vacuity and blood depletion with impairment of ruling and containing, 2) qi vacuity and blood stagnation with stasis obstruction of the vessels and network vessels, and 3) frenetic movement of blood heat with stasis obstruction of the vessels and network vessels. However, all the prescriptions below contain at least some heat-clearing and bleeding stopping medicinals, even if they are primarily indicated for qi vacuity. In addition, the frenetic movement of blood heat is subdivided into replete and vacuity patterns.

Treatment based on pattern discrimination:

1. Qi vacuity & blood depletion with impairment of ruling & containing pattern

Main symptoms: Not very severe spontaneous bleeding, mild hematomas of the deep tissues and local stasis and stagnation, light-colored hematomas which are also small in size and not painful or hard to the touch, quick absorption of hematomas, a somber white or sallow yellow facial complexion, reduced appetite, and fatigued limbs with lack of strength of the body, a fat, enlarged, pale tongue with white fur, and a fine, forceless pulse

Treatment principles: Boost the qi and contain the blood, nourish the blood and stop bleeding

Chinese medicinal formula:

HUANG QI ZHI XUE TANG **(Astragalus Stop Bleeding Decoction)**
Radix Astragali Membranacei (*Huang Qi*), Radix Codonopsitis Pilosulae (*Dang Shen*), Rhizoma Atractylodis Macrocephalae (*Bai Zhu*), Sclerotium Poriae Cocos (*Fu Ling*), Gelatinum Corii Asini (*E Jiao*), Radix Rubiae Cordifoliae (*Qian Cao Gen*), uncooked Radix Rehmanniae (*Sheng Di*), carbonized Radix Sanguisorbae (*Di Yu*), uncooked Pollen Typhae (*Pu Huang*), Rhizoma Imperatae Cylindricae (*Bai Mao Gen*), Radix Glycyrrhizae (*Gan Cao*)

Additions & subtractions: For accompanying upper respiratory tract infections with fever, add Folium Daqingye (*Da Qing Ye*) and Fructus Forsythiae Suspensae (*Lian Qiao*). For slow absorption of hematomas, add Radix Salviae Miltiorrhizae (*Dan Shen*), Flos Carthami Tinctorii (*Hong Hua*), and Lumbricus (*Di Long*). For marked pain because of hematomas, add Rhizoma Corydalis Yanhusuo (*Yan Hu Suo*) and Herba Asari Cum Radice (*Xi Xin*).

2. Qi vacuity & blood stagnation with stasis obstruction of the vessels & network vessels pattern

Main symptoms: Recurrent bleeding, hard, painful hematomas which present like large tumors and are not absorbed readily. These blood swellings may further constrict blood vessels leading to necrosis, or they may press on nerves and lead to paralysis. If there is bleeding into a joint and hematoma forms inside the joint, there may be joint swelling which, if severe, can lead to malformation of the affected joint.

Note: The immediate treatment of this pattern is of great importance as prolonged obstruction of the vessels may easily lead to ulceration.

Treatment principles: Boost the qi and quicken blood, transform stasis and free the flow of the network vessels

Chinese medicinal formulas:

YI QI HUA YU TANG **(Boost the Qi & Transform Stasis Decoction)**
Semen Pruni Persicae (*Tao Ren*), Flos Carthami Tinctorii (*Hong Hua*), uncooked Radix Rehmanniae (*Sheng Di*), Radix Albus Paeoniae Lactiflorae (*Bai Shao*), Radix Ligustici Wallichii (*Chuan Xiong*), Radix Angelicae Sinensis (*Dang Gui*), Radix Pseudoginseng (*San Qi*), Radix Salviae Miltiorrhizae (*Dan Shen*), Gelatinum Corii Asini (*E Jiao*), Cortex Radicis Moutan (*Dan Pi*), Radix Astragali Membranacei (*Huang Qi*), Radix Codonopsitis Pilosulae (*Dang Shen*), Radix Glycyrrhizae (*Gan Cao*)

HUANG DAN TANG **(Astragalus & Salvia Decoction)**
Radix Astragali Membranacei (*Huang Qi*), Radix Ligustici Wallichii (*Chuan Xiong*), Radix Salviae Miltiorrhizae (*Dan Shen*), Radix Rubrus Paeoniae Lactiflorae (*Chi Shao*), uncooked Pollen Typhae (*Pu Huang*), Flos Carthami Tinctorii (*Hong Hua*), Semen Pruni Persicae (*Tao Ren*), Lumbricus (*Di Long*), blast-fried Squama Manitis Pentadactylis (*Chuan Shan Jia*), Radix Rubiae Cordifoliae (*Qian Cao Gen*), Herba Cephalanoploris Segeti (*Xiao Ji*), Radix Glycyrrhizae (*Gan Cao*)

Additions & subtractions: For abundant, hard, swollen hematomas on the upper limbs, add Fructus Gardeniae Jasminoidis (*Zhi Zi*) and Radix Platycodi Grandiflori (*Jie Geng*). If there are abundant, hard, and swollen hematomas distributed over all the body, also add Rhizoma Corydalis Yanhusuo (*Yan Hu Suo*) and Radix Achyrantis Bidentatae (*Niu Xi*). If hematomas are pressing on local nerves and causing numbness and tingling, add Scolopendra Subspinipes (*Wu Gong*) and Zaocys Dhumnades (*Wu Shao She*).

3. Frenetic movement due to hot blood with stasis obstruction of the vessels & network vessels pattern

A. Replete heat pattern

Main symptoms: The main symptoms are similar to the ones from the above two patterns with the addition of heat signs, such as a more acute onset of the bleeding, bright red-colored blood, a red, possibly dark tongue with yellow fur, and a rapid, forceful, possibly slippery pulse.

Treatment principles: Clear heat and cool the blood, stop bleeding and quicken the blood, transform stasis and free the network vessels

Chinese medicinal formula:

QING RE ZHI XUE TANG (**Clear Heat & Stop Bleeding Decoction**)
Rhizoma Coptidis Chinensis (*Huang Lian*), Radix Scutellariae Baicalensis (*Huang Qin*), Gypsum Fibrosum (*Shi Gao*), Rhizoma Imperatae Cylindricae (*Bai Mao Gen*), Rhizoma Anemarrhenae Asphodeloidis (*Zhi Mu*), Herba Agrimoniae Pilosae (*Xian He Cao*), Herba Dendrobii (*Shi Hu*), carbonized Radix Rubiae Cordifoliae (*Qian Cao Gen*), Radix Glycyrrhizae (*Gan Cao*)

Additions & subtractions: For accompanying qi and blood detriment and consumption, add Radix Codonopsitis Pilosulae (*Dang Shen*) and uncooked Radix Rehmaniae (*Sheng Di*). To strengthen the effect of clearing heat, add Radix Et Rhizoma Rhei (*Da Huang*), Fructus Gardeniae Jasminoidis (*Zhi Zi*), and Radix Sophorae Subprostratae (*Shan Dou Gen*).

B. Yin vacuity-vacuity heat pattern

Main symptoms: Similar symptoms as above plus signs and symptoms of yin vacuity, such as night sweats, malar flushing, afternoon tidal fever, vexatious heat in the five hearts, dizziness, tinnitus, lumbar aching, knee limpness, nocturia, a red tongue with scanty fur, and a fine, rapid pulse

Treatment principles: Enrich yin and clear heat, transform stasis and stop bleeding

Chinese medicinal formula:

QING RE LIANG XUE TANG (**Clear Heat & Cool the Blood Decoction**)
Uncooked Radix Rehmanniae (*Sheng Di*), Radix Scrophulariae Ningpoensis (*Xuan Shen*), Tuber Ophiopogonis Japonici (*Mai Men Dong*), Folium Daqingye (*Da Qing Ye*), Radix Lithospermi Seu Arnebiae (*Zi Cao*), Cortex Radicis Moutan (*Dan Pi*), Radix Rubrus Paeoniae Lactiflorae (*Chi Shao*), Radix Albus Paeoniae Lactiflorae (*Bai Shao*), Fructus Zizphi Jujubae (*Hong Zao*), Rhizoma Imperatae Cylindricae (*Bai Mao Gen*), Fructus Gardeniae Jasminoidis (*Zhi Zi*)

Additions & subtractions: For accompanying qi vacuity, add Radix Astragali Membranacei (*Huang Qi*). For severe blood vacuity, add Fructus Lycii Chinensis (*Gou Qi Zi*), processed Radix Polygoni Multiflori (*Shou Wu*), and Radix Salviae Miltiorrhizae (*Dan Shen*). For exuberant heat (*i.e.*, high fever), add Herba Viola Yedoensitis Cum Radice (*Zi Hua Di Ding*) and Herba Taraxaci Mongolici Cum Radice (*Pu Gong Ying*).

5 Purpura Simplex

Purpura simplex is the most common vascular bleeding disorder. It is seen most often in women. Increased vascular fragility leads to easy bruising which develops without a known cause on the thighs, buttocks, and upper arms. Other abnormal bleeding is uncommon. Furthermore, platelet counts and platelet function, blood coagulation, and fibrinolysis are all normal. A familial tendency to this disease can sometimes be established. There are no Western drugs which effectively limit or stop this bruising. Patients are advised to avoid aspirin and aspirin-containing drugs as they thin the blood. However, there is no evidence that such bruising is related to their use. This condition is not serious and patients should be reassured that they do not need to worry excessively about it.

Chinese medical disease explanation:

In Chinese medicine, this corresponds to the concept of purple macules (*zi ban*). In most cases, it is due to spleen vacuity not containing the blood. The other, less commonly seen pattern is yin depletion with internally engendered vacuity fire causing frenetic movement of the blood. Both frenetic movement due to hot blood and qi vacuity not containing the blood lead to the seeping of blood into the flesh and skin and, therefore, to the development of purple macules. Commonly used treatment principles are to fortify the spleen and nourish and contain the blood or to enrich yin and downbear fire, cool the blood and stop bleeding.

Treatment based on pattern discrimination:

1. Yin depletion with vacuity fire & frenetic movement of hot blood pattern

Main symptoms: Easy bruising, a red facial complexion, heat in the palms of the hands and soles of the feet, a dry mouth, dry nasal membranes with nasal bleeding (epistaxis), recurrent skin purpura, red tongue with scanty, possibly dry, possibly yellow fur, and a fine, rapid pulse

Note: This pattern is mostly seen in the elderly.

Treatment principles: Enrich yin and downbear fire, cool the blood and stop bleeding

Chinese medicinal formula:

LIANG XUE ZHI XUE XUAN SHEN TANG (Cool the Blood & Stop Bleeding Scrophularia Decoction)
Uncooked Radix Rehmanniae (*Sheng Di*), Radix Scrophulariae Ningpoensis (*Xuan Shen*), Rhizoma Anemarrhenae Asphodeloidis (*Zhi Mu*), Fructus Gardeniae Jasminoidis (*Zhi Zi*), Rhizoma Imperatae Cylindricae (*Bai Mao Gen*), Massa Medica Fermentata (*Shen Qu*), Radix Glycyrrhizae (*Gan Cao*)

Additions & subtractions: For lower abdominal menstrual pain in adolescent females, add Herba Leonuri Heterophylli (*Yi Mu Cao*) and Rhizoma Corydalis Yanhusuo (*Yan Hu Suo*). For an inflamed and sore throat, add Flos Lonicerae Japonicae (*Jin Yin Hua*), Fructus Forsythiae Suspensae (*Lian Qiao*), Folium Daqingye (*Da Qing Ye*), and Radix Platycodi Grandiflori (*Jie Geng*).

2. Spleen vacuity not containing the blood pattern

Main symptoms: Easy bruising, pale-colored purple macules, a bright white facial complexion, decreased food intake, loose stools, fatigue, lack of strength, an enlarged, pale tongue with teeth-marks on its edges, and a forceless and fine, weak, or soggy pulse

Note: This pattern is mostly seen in women.

Treatment principles: Fortify the spleen and nourish and contain the blood

Chinese medicinal formula:

GUI PI TANG (Return the Spleen Decoction)
Radix Astragali Membranacei (*Huang Qi*), Radix Panacis Ginseng (*Ren Shen*), Rhizoma Atractylodis Macrocephalae (*Bai Zhu*), Sclerotium Pararadicis Poriae Cocos (*Fu Shen*), Radix Angelicae Sinensis (*Dang Gui*), Semen Zizyphi Spinosae (*Suan Zao Ren*), Radix Polygalae Tenuifoliae (*Yuan Zhi*), Arillus Euphoriae Longanae (*Long Yan Rou*), Radix Auklandiae Lappae (*Mu Xiang*), Radix Glycyrrhizae (*Gan Cao*), uncooked Rhizoma Zingiberis (*Sheng Jiang*), Fructus Zizyphi Jujubae (*Da Zao*)

Book III:

Case Histories & Clinical Audits

Allergic Purpura

Case 1[1]

The patient was an eight year-old girl who was first examined on Feb. 7, 1997. This patient complained of recurrent abdominal pain for nearly one month and had a low-grade fever for one week prior to her first treatment. Purplish red patches were evenly distributed on her upper and lower limbs but were more severe on her lower limbs. Two days prior to treatment, her face had become edematous and her urine had turned reddish yellow. There was also lumbar pain, aching joints, and inability to freely move her joints. Examination found that she had a clear spirit, slight facial edema, a red throat, swollen kidney areas on both sides which were painful to the touch, and purplish red patches dispersed on her upper limbs and all over her lower limbs. The patient's joints were not obviously swollen, her abdomen was level (*i.e.,* not distended or tense), and the periumbilical region was sensitive to touch. The tongue was red with thin, yellow fur, and the pulse was rapid.

Laboratory blood examination revealed WBCs at $11,200/mm^3$, with a differentiation of 76% neutrophils and 34% leukocytes, and platelets at $170,000/mm^3$. Coagulation time was normal. Urine examination was positive one (+) for protein, and positive one (+) for red blood cells. Analysis of the stools was negative for blood but positive for roundworm eggs.

Thus, a modification of self-composed *Xiao Dian Jie Du Tang* (Spot-dispersing, Toxin-resolving Decoction) was prescribed: Radix Lithospermi Seu Arnebiae (*Zi Cao*), Radix Rubiae Cordifoliae (*Qian Cao Gen*), Radix Et Rhizoma Rhei (*Da Huang*), dried Lumbricus (*Gan Di Long*), Herba Agrimoniae Pilosae (*Xian He Cao*), 10g each, uncooked Radix Rehmanniae (*Sheng Di*) and Radix Salviae Miltiorrhizae (*Dan Shen*), 12g each, Periostracum Cicadae (*Chan Tui*), 15g, Rhizoma Imperatae Cylindricae (*Bai Mao Gen*), 12g, and Rhizoma Alismatis (*Ze Xie*), 9g. Five *ji*[2] were prescribed.

A second examination on February 13 revealed that the patient's facial swelling had dispersed, the lumbar pain had ceased, and her urine was clear. The color of the purple macules on her upper and lower limbs had turned dark purple and no new patches had formed. Therefore, another five *ji* were prescribed. Thereafter, urinalysis tested normal and, on follow-up after one year, there had been no recurrence.

---

[1] Zhang Yi, "The Treatment of 24 Cases of Allergic Purpura with *Xiao Dian Jie Du Tang* (Spot-dispersing & Toxin-resolving Decoction)," *Si Chuan Zhong Yi (Sichuan Chinese Medicine)*, #1, 1999, p. 18

[2] One *ji* means one packet of medicinals and usually refers to one day's dose. Thus five *ji* equals five day's worth of medicinals. The gram dosages listed in this and all subsequent formulas are for one *ji*.

Case 2[3]

The patient was a 13 year-old female who was first examined on Jan. 28, 1984. One month prior to treatment, this child contracted a cold and became sick. Initially, she itched all over her body, and then wind papules arose. Later, she developed abdominal pain, and she could not bear touch and could not eat. However, there was no fever, no nausea, and no vomiting, and her stools and urine were both normal. Three days later, dark red macules and papules appeared on both of the patient's lower legs and ankles. They were approximately the size of millet grains and scattered about. One day later, they slowly moved to the upper legs and the buttocks area. At the same time, a low-grade fever developed. Thus, the patient came to the hospital for diagnosis.

Examination revealed that the girl's body temperature was approximately normal and that macules and papules were dark red, circular, but not clearly demarcated. These were crowded on the upper and lower legs, and their color did not change upon pressure. Most of these macules and papules were distributed on the front and side of the lower limbs and around the knee joints. Their size varied between a millet grain and a mung bean. The abdomen was soft, but there was pain upon light pressure around the umbilicus. The patient's tongue was red with scanty fur, and her pulse was slightly rapid. Thus, diagnosis was allergic purpura. This disease was considered to be due to toxic evils entering the blood, transforming heat, and leading to frenetic movement of the blood.

Therefore, *Qing Ying Tang Jia Jian* (Construction-clearing Decoction with Additions & Subtractions) was prescribed: Flos Lonicerae Japonicae (*Jin Yin Hua*), 15g, Fructus Forsythiae Suspensae (*Lian Qiao*), 10g, Rhizoma Coptidis Chinensis (*Huang Lian*), 15g, Radix Scrophulariae Ningpoensis (*Xuan Shen*), 15g, uncooked Radix Rehmanniae (*Sheng Di*), 20g, Tuber Ophiopogonis Japonici (*Mai Men Dong*), 15g, Cortex Radicis Moutan (*Mu Dan Pi*), 5g, Radix Rubrus Paeoniae Lactiflorae (*Chi Shao*), 10g, Herba Mentha Haplocalycis (*Bo He*), 10g, Rhizoma Phragmitis Communis (*Lu Gen*), 5g, and Radix Glycyrrhizae (*Gan Cao*), 5g. One *ji* was taken every day.

Re-examination one week later revealed that the macules and papules had dispersed, the abdominal pain was greatly reduced, and the patient was able to eat again. The girl's tongue was still dark red with scanty fur and both bar pulses were floating and slippery. Thus, another four *ji* of the above formula were prescribed. Re-examination thereafter revealed that there was some remaining heat in the palms and soles but that the tongue was pale red and the pulse was slippery in the bar positions. Therefore, the therapeutic effect was consolidated by administering another eight *ji* of the same formula. On follow-up two years later, there had been no recurrence.

---

[3]   Zhang Guo-in, "The Cure of One Case of Allergic Purpura with *Qing Ying Tang* (Clear the Constructive Decoction) with Additions & Subtractions," *Zhong Xi Yi Jie He Za Zhi (Chinese Journal of Integrated Chinese-Western Medicine)*, #6, 1988, p. 329

Aplastic Anemia

Case 1[4]

The patient was a 20 year-old female who had been diagnosed with aplastic anemia one year prior to treatment when a bone marrow aspiration revealed pancytopenia. Her symptoms were prolonged and unabating fever, dizziness, lack of strength, recurrent bleeding of the mouth and skin, fear of cold, and profuse spontaneous perspiration. The tongue was pale with slimy, yellow fur, and the pulse was deep and fine. Thus, the pattern differentiation was spleen-kidney dual vacuity with qi vacuity fever, and spleen-fortifying and kidney-warming methods were used so as to eliminate heat with sweet and warm medicinals. In addition, blood transfusions were administered.

This treatment was given to the patient for four months. However, none of her symptoms improved. Upon re-examination, it was noted that that the palms of both the young woman's hands were hot and sweaty. Thus, his differentiation was yin vacuity with internal heat and qi and blood insufficiency. As for the treatment, he combined *Yi Guan Jian* (One Link Brew) with *Liu Wei Di Huang Wan* (Six Flavors Rehmannia Pills) in order to enrich the kidneys and supplement the liver; *Dang Gui Bu Xue Tang* (Dang Gui Blood-supplementing Decoction) and *Si Jun Zi Tang* (Four Gentlemen Decoction) in order to supplement and warm qi and blood; and *Bu Luo Bu Guan Tang* (Network-supplementing Bar-supplementing Decoction) and *Si Sheng Wan* (Four Uncooked [Ingredients] Pills) in order to supplement the qi, clear heat, and stop bleeding.

The ingredients of the formula were: Radix Astragali Membranacei (*Huang Qi*), 15g, Radix Angelicae Sinensis (*Dang Gui*), 15g, Radix Codonopsitis Pilosulae (*Dang Shen*), 15g, Sclerotium Poriae Cocos (*Fu Ling*), 15g, Rhizoma Atractylodis Macrocephalae (*Bai Zhu*), 15g, mix-fried Radix Glycyrrhizae (*Gan Cao*), 10g, cooked Radix Rehmanniae (*Shu Di*), 15g, Radix Albus Paeoniae Lactiflorae (*Bai Shao*), 10g, uncooked Radix Rehmanniae (*Sheng Di*), 15g, Tuber Ophiopogonis Japonici (*Mai Men Dong*), 15g, Fructus Lycii Chinensis (*Gou Qi Zi*), 15g, Radix Glehniae Littoralis (*Bei Sha Shen*), 15g, Fructus Corni Officinalis (*Shan Zhu Yu*), 15g, Cortex Radicis Moutan (*Dan Pi*), 10g, Arillus Euphoriae Longanae (*Long Yan Rou*), 9g, fresh Cacumen Biotae Orientalis (*Ce Bai Ye*), 30g, Folium Nelumbinis Nuciferae (*He Ye*), 15g, mix-fried Folium Artemesiae Vulgaris (*Ai Ye*), 10g, Os Draconis (*Long Gu*), 30g, Concha Ostreae (*Mu Li*), 30g, and Herba Taraxaci Mongolici Cum Radice (*Pu Gong Ying*), 15g. After 14 *ji*, all symptoms were reduced. After two months, the fever had abated and did not recur.

4   Qiu Zhong-quan & Hu Qi, "Wan Han-mang's Experience in the Treatment of Fevers in Blood Diseases," *Zhong Yi Za Zhi (Journal of Chinese Medicine)*, #8, 1999, p. 462-463

Case 2[5]

The patient was a 23 year old female. Because of a yellow facial complexion and lack of strength, the patient came to the hospital on October 12, 1992. Examination revealed the following: The patient's temperature was 36°C, her spirit was clear, there were signs of anemia, heart and lung sounds were normal, the spleen and liver were not enlarged, and everything else was normal. Blood examination revealed that the reticulocytes were 0.2%, the red blood cells were 1.9 million/mm^3, hemoglobin was 6 g/dL, WBCs at 3200/mm^3, with a differential count of 32% granulocytes and 68% lymphocytes, and the platelet count was 150 thousand/mm^3. Bone marrow aspiration revealed a low degree of hyperplasia with both the myeloid and erythroid systems depressed and the lymphocytes relatively increased. Plasma and reticulocytes were easily seen, and no megakaryocytes could be found. Other tests revealed normal functioning of the liver and spleen, and an abdominal ultrasound was normal. Therefore, the diagnosis was aplastic anemia. However, subsequent treatment for 13 months yielded no effect.

On November 28, 1993, the anemia signs had become more severe and hemoglobin was down to 3.2 g/dL. Thus a blood transfusion of 2400 mL of blood was administered for three days. This increased the hemoglobin level to 3.6 g/dL. At that point, there were no signs of bleeding. However, the patient's abdomen was distended and full and her urination was inhibited. Abdominal examination showed no signs of peritoneal irritation but was positive for shifting dullness. Ultrasound showed a large dark area in the abdominal cavity. Intestinal fluid wave signs were present. Thus, it was estimated that 1800mL of fluids had accumulated in her abdomen, and an abdominal puncture was given to extract 100mL of unsolidified blood. The diagnosis was therefore changed to aplastic anemia with large amounts of bleeding into the abdominal cavity.

Chinese medical examination revealed a somber white facial complexion, an abdomen as large as a drum, coolness of the four limbs, inhibited urination, and poor appetite. The tongue was dark yet pale with slimy, white fur. The pulse was deep, slippery, and rapid. The Chinese medical pattern discrimination was spleen vacuity with damp stagnation and static blood internally obstructing. The treatment principles, therefore, were to fortify the spleen and disinhibit dampness, quicken the blood and transform stasis. The formula selected was *Shi Pi Yin Jia Wei* (Spleen-firming Beverage with Added Flavors): Cortex Magnoliae Officinalis (*Chuan Po*), 15g, Rhizoma Atractylodis (*Cang Zhu*), 20g,

---

5   Li Da *et al.*, "The Integrated Chinese-Western Medical Treatment of One Case of Suffering from Abdominal Cavity Bleeding Secondary to Aplastic Anemia," *Zhong Guo Zhong Xi Yi Jie He Za Zhi (Chinese Journal of Integrated Chinese-Western Medicine)*, (issue unknown), during or after 1994, p. 492. A copy of this article was sent to the author by his teacher. At the time of publication, the teacher could not be reached to clarify the issue number and year of publication.

Pericarpium Arecae Catechu (*Da Fu Pi*), Sclerotium Poria Cocos (*Fu Ling*), Rhizoma Alismatis (*Ze Xie*), and Radix Salviae Miltiorrhizae (*Dan Shen*), 30g each, Ramulus Cinnamomi Cassiae (*Gui Zhi*) and Radix Ligustici Wallichii (*Chuan Xiong*), 10g each, Radix Et Rhizoma Rhei (*Da Huang*), 12g, and Radix Rubrus Paeoniae Lactiflorae (*Chi Shao*), 50g. One *ji*, brewed into a decoction, was administered every day. In addition, 10g of dicynone were administered intravenously every day as well as a platelet transfusion.

After six days of treatment, the abdominal distention was reduced, the urination was freely flowing, and the abdominal exam revealed a circumference of 68cm instead of 77cm. Shifting dullness was negative, and ultrasound did not pick up any abdominal water. Hemoglobin was back to 12.4 g/dL. Another five *ji* of the above formula were administered to consolidate the therapeutic effect. One month later, the illness had normalized and the abdominal exam was normal.

Case 3[6]

The patient was a 23 year old male. In January of 1966, this patient started having a nosebleed with pale-colored blood accompanied by dimming of vision in both eyes. He was then diagnosed at the local hospital with anemic conjunctivitis. Further blood and bone marrow exams revealed aplastic anemia. Upon examination, he presented with blood spots all over his body but most obvious on his chest, upper back, and lower back. He also suffered from heart throbbing which was aggravated when he walked for 10 minutes. The nose-bleeding stopped after one week of treatment with cortisone, penicillin, and testosterone propionate. However, when re-examined, he suffered from dizziness, heart palpitations, lack of strength of the entire body, dim and unclear vision, a somber white facial complexion, spontaneous perspiration, blood spots over his entire body, chilled limbs, testicular dampness, a pale tongue with no fur, and a vacuous, rapid pulse.

Based on the above signs and symptoms, the patient took *Yang Xin Tang* (Nourish the Heart Decoction), *Gui Pi Tang* (Return the Spleen Decoction), and *Ba Zhen Tang* (Eight Pearls Decoction) to no avail. Weekly blood transfusions were necessary so that he did not collapse. Laboratory examination of the blood revealed hemoglobin was 4.5 g/dL, red blood cells were 1.5 million/mm^3, white blood cells were 3500/mm^3, and platelets were 22,000/mm^3. The pattern discrimination was now changed to kidney yang vacuity. The selected formula was modified *Tu Si Zi Wan* (Cuscuta Pills) which consisted of: Semen Cuscutae Chinensis (*Tu Si Zi*), 25g, Rhizoma Alismatis (*Ze Xie*), 15g, Cortex Cinnamomi Cassiae (*Rou Gui*), 7.5g, Radix Lateralis Praeparatus Aconiti Carmichaeli

---

[6]   *Xue Zheng Zhuan Ji (A Collection of Experts on Bleeding Conditions)*, Shi Yu-guang & Shan Shu-jian, eds., Ancient Chinese Medical Books Press, Beijing, 1992, p. 241

(*Fu Zi*), 7.5g, Herba Dendrobii (*Shi Hu*), 9g, cooked Radix Rehmanniae (*Shu Di*), 25g, Sclerotium Poriae Cocos (*Fu Ling*), 20g, Radix Achyranthis Bidentatae (*Niu Xi*), 15g, Radix Dipsaci (*Xu Duan*), 15g, Fructus Corni Officinalis (*Shan Zhu Yu*), 20g, Herba Cistanchis Deserticolae (*Rou Cong Rong*), 20g, Fructus Psoraleae Corylifoliae (*Bu Gu Zhi*), 15g, Radix Morindae Officinalis (*Ba Ji Tian*), 20g, Lignum Aquilariae Agallochae (*Chen Xiang*), 5g, Fructus Schisandrae Chinensis (*Wu Wei Zi*), 10g, Radix Ligustici Wallichii (*Chuan Xiong*), 10g, Radix Panacis Ginseng (*Ren Shen*), 15g, Tuber Ophiopogonis Japonici (*Mai Men Dong*), 15g, Rhizoma Anemarrhenae Asphodeloidis (*Zhi Mu*), 15g, Radix Glycyrrhizae (*Gan Cao*), 7.5g, and Radix Angelicae Sinensis (*Dang Gui*), 20g.

The patient took the above formula with various modifications until March 28, 1968. At that time, all his symptoms had dispersed, and re-examination of his blood revealed hemoglobin at 15g/dL, red blood cells at 5 million/mm^3, white blood cells at 4200/mm^3, and platelets at 840,000/mm^3.

Case 4[7]

The patient was an 18 year old female. This patient had suffered from aplastic anemia for eight years and had presented with heart palpitations, dizziness, nose-bleeding, gum-bleeding, and subcutaneous bleeding for 10 days when she was admitted to the hospital. Blood laboratory examination revealed that her hemoglobin was 4 g/dL, red blood cells were 1.4 million/mm^3, white blood cells were 2400/mm^3, and platelets were 28,000/mm^3. Bone marrow examination revealed poor normoblast proliferation and other aplastic anemia marrow changes. Inspection and questioning revealed a bright white facial complexion, marked hair loss, somber white eyelids, nails, and lips, fatigue, lack of strength, amenorrhea, scanty nose and gum-bleeding, and purpura on her lower left limb. The patient's tongue was pale with scanty fur, and the pulse was fine, rapid, and forceless. The disease categories thus were vacuity taxation and bleeding condition, and the appropriate treatment was to supplement the qi and contain the blood, cool the blood and stop bleeding.

The formula used for these purposes was modified *Dang Gui Bu Xue Tang* (Dang Gui Blood-supplementing Decoction): Radix Codonopsitis Pilosulae (*Dang Shen*), 12g, Radix Astragali Membranacei (*Huang Qi*), 20g, Radix Angelicae Sinensis (*Dang Gui*), 6g, Rhizoma Atractylodis Macrocephalae (*Bai Zhu*), 9g, uncooked Radix Rehmanniae (*Sheng Di*), 12g, Rhizoma Imperatae Cylindricae (*Bai Mao Gen*), 12g, Rhizoma Nelumbinis Nuciferae (*Ou Jie*), 12g, Herbae Agrimoniae Pilosae (*Xian He Cao*), 9g,

---

[7]   *Ibid.*, p. 245

Radix Albus Paeoniae Lactiflorae (*Bai Shao*), 12g, Sclerotium Poriae Cocos (*Fu Ling*), 10g, and mix-fried Radix Glycyrrhizae (*Gan Cao*), 5g.

After taking these medicinals, the nose-bleeding stopped but the bodily strength did not return. Thus, the original formula was modified as follows: *Bai Mao Gen, Xian He Cao,* and *Ou Jie* were deleted, kidney-supplementing and blood-quickening medicinals, such as Cornu Cervi (*Lu Jiao*), 3g, Radix Morindae Officinalis (*Ba Ji Tian*), and Fructus Cornu Officinalis (*Shan Zhu Yu*), 9g each, Semen Cuscutae Chinensis (*Tu Si Zi*), Caulis Milletiae Seu Spatholobi (*Ji Xue Teng*), Radix Salviae Miltiorrhizae (*Dan Shen*), and Radix Rubrus Paeoniae Lactiflorae (*Chi Shao*), 12g each, were added. This formula, with possible slight modifications, was taken for 10 months. At that time, the disease was stable. Re-examination of the blood revealed hemoglobin at 6.5g/dL, red blood cells at 2.3 million/mm^3, white blood cells at 3800/mm^3, and platelets at 420,000/mm^3. Bone marrow examination revealed active proliferation.

Eosinophilia

Case history[8] A female patient presented with a leukocyte count of 5200/mm^3 and an eosinophil count of 1716/mm^3 (33%). The following formula was prescribed: Fructus Arctii Lappae (*Niu Bang Zi*), 10g, Cortex Radicis Mori Albi (*Sang Bai Pi*), 10g, Folium Mori Albi (*Sang Ye*), 11g, Rhizoma Anemarrhenae Asphodeloidis (*Zhi Mu*), 10g, Bulbus Fritillariae Thunbergii (*Zhe Bei Mu*), 10g, mix-fried Radix Stemonae (*Bai Bu*), 15g, Radix Peucedani (*Qian Hu*), 10g, Radix Glycyrrhizae (*Gan Cao*), 8g, Radix Platycodi Grandiflori (*Jie Geng*), 8g, Radix Adenophorae Strictae (*Nan Sha Shen*), 8g, Radix Glehniae Littoralis (*Bei Sha Shen*), 10g. After taking seven *ji* of this formula, the disease symptoms had obviously improved and a lab test revealed the leuckocyte count to be 6000/mm^3 and the eosinophil count at 765/mm^3 (13%).

Clinical audit[9] The following formula was used in the treatment of 25 cases suffering from eosinophilia: Concha Cyclinae Meretricis (*Hai Ge Ke*), 30g, Herba Houttuyniae Cordatae Cum Radice (*Yu Xing Cao*), 30g, Pulvis Indigonis (*Qing Dai*), 4.5g, Radix Scutellariae Baicalensis (*Huang Qin*), 9g, Cortex Radicis Mori Albi (*Sang Bai Pi*), 18g, Cortex Radicis Lycii Chinensis (*Di Gu Pi*), 12g, Radix Albus Paeoniae Lactiflorae (*Bai Shao*), 12g, and mix-fried Radix Glycyrrhizae (*Gan Cao*), 6g. Using this protocol, 18 of the 25 cases were cured. This meant that all their clinical symptoms

---

[8] "Hemotological Diseases," *Zhong Guo Zhong Yi Mi Fang Da Quan (Compendium of Chinese Medical Secret Formulas)*, Hu Xi-ming, ed., Literary Collection Publishing Company, Shanghai, 1997, p. 477-478

[9] *Ibid.*, p. 478

dispersed and that x-ray and peripheral blood values were normal. Seven cases had a turn for the better. This meant that the clinical symptoms had basically dispersed and that x-ray and peripheral blood values were near normal. The longest treatment course was 31 days, the shortest was three days, and the average was seven days.

Hemolytic Anemia

Case 1[10]

The patient was a 42 year old male who was first examined on March 15, 1990. Since his childhood, this patient had suffered from yellow eyes. In 1990, a laboratory test revealed that his icteric index was at 28U, hemoglobin at 9g/dL, red blood cells at 3.54 million/mm^3, and reticulocytes at 8%. A bone marrow examination showed erythroid hyperproliferation, among which orthochromatic normoblasts were dominating. An autologous serum hemolysis test was positive, and ATP and glucose were both normal. Glucose-6-phosphate dehydrogenase (G6PD) was at 0.53U. Therefore, diagnosis was congenital non-spherocytic hemolytic anemia, and only Chinese medicine was used for treatment.

The Chinese medical examination revealed a sallow yellow facial complexion, dark yellow eyes, decreased appetite, fear of cold, white tongue fur, and a moderate (*i.e.*, slightly slow), deep, and forceless pulse. Therefore, the man's pattern was categorized as spleen-kidney dual vacuity, and the formula prescribed was a modification of *Liu Wei Di Huang Tang* (Six Flavors Rehmannia Decoction): Radix Atractylodis Macrocephalae (*Bai Zhu*), 15g, processed Radix Polygoni Multiflori (*He Shou Wu*), 20g, Fructus Corni Officinalis (*Shan Zhu Yu*), 15g, Radix Dioscoreae Oppositae (*Shan Yao*), 15g, Fructus Lycii Chinensis (*Gou Qi Zi*), 25g, Ramulus Loranthi Seu Visci (*Sang Ji Sheng*), 15g, Fructus Mori Albi (*Sang Shen Zi*), 15g, Radix Albus Paeoniae Lactiflorae (*Bai Shao*), 15g, Sclerotium Poriae Cocos (*Fu Ling*), 15g, and Pericarpium Citri Reticulatae (*Chen Pi*), 10g. One *ji* was administered every day.

Re-examination after 18 days revealed that the icteric index had decreased to 12U. Thus, the formula was continued and ATP injections were administered at the same time (20mg per day). One month later, hemoglobin had increased to 12.2g/dL, red blood cells were at 4.01 million/mm^3, reticulocytes were reduced to 1.5%, and the icteric index was at 9U. Thus, the patient resumed work, and the ATP injections were discontinued. However, the

---

[10] Chen Po, "Clincial Experiences in the Treatment of Hemolytic Anemia," *Zhong Yi Za Zhi (Journal of Chinese Medicine)*, #10, 1999, p. 592-593

patient continued taking three *ji* of the above formula every week. He was further prescribed *Liu Wei Di Huang Wan* (Six Flavors Rehmannia Pills), 6g three times per day.

Re-examination on September 26, 1990 revealed that the jaundice had dispersed, hemoglobin was at 13.9g/dL, and reticulocytes were at 4.8%. The above treatment method was continued to consolidate the effect.

Case 2[11]

The patient was a 35 year old female who was first examined on May 18, 1997. During the same month, this patient began to suffer from dizziness, lack of strength, and yellow eyes. Examination revealed a somber white facial complexion, slightly yellow sclera, and puffy swelling on the lower limbs. Laboratory examination found hemoglobin at 8.1g/dL, red blood cells at 3.83 million/mm^3, reticulocytes at 1.8%, and a total serum bilirubin of 22mol/L, of which 7.65mol/L were direct and 14.35mol/L were indirect. Pyrimidine-5-nucleotidase activity was at 8.9. Bone marrow examination revealed anemic proliferation signs. The diagnosis was hemolytic anemia due to lack of pyrimidine-5-nucleotidase, and erythropoietinogen, vitamin E, and inosine (HXR) were administered for two weeks with no effect. Therefore, the patient was referred for Chinese medical treatment.

Chinese medical examination revealed a somber white facial complexion, slight swelling of the lower limbs, a red tongue tip, and a deep, fine, bowstring pulse. Therefore, the patient's pattern was categorized as qi and blood dual vacuity and the following formula was prescribed: Radix Astragali Membranacei (*Huang Qi*), 12g, Rhizoma Atractylodis Macrocephalae (*Bai Zhu*), 15g, Gelatinum Corii Asini (*E Jiao*), 10g, Semen Cuscutae Chinensis (*Tu Si Zi*), 10g, Frucuts Lycii Chinensis (*Gou Qi Zi*), 15g, Sclerotium Polypori Umbellati (*Zhu Ling*), 12g, Pericarpium Citri Reticulati (*Chen Pi*), 10g, Semen Plantaginis (*Che Qian Zi*), 8g, Massa Medica Fermentata (*Shen Qu*), 15g, Bulbus Lilii (*Bai He*), 10g, and Concha Ostreae (*Mu Li*), 15g. One *ji* was taken daily.

Re-examination 21 days later revealed that all the symptoms were reduced, hemoglobin was up to 12g/dL, red blood cells were still at 3.84 million/mm^3, reticulocytes were decreased to 1%, and pyrimidine-5-nucleotidase activity had increased to 12.5. Thus, the patient resumed work.

---

[11] *Ibid.*, p. 593

Hemophilia

Case 1[12]

The patient was a 14 year old male. After cutting himself eight years ago, the bleeding did not want to stop. Furthermore, the boy also experienced common nosebleeds and swelling and purpling of his joints which limited his activity. For half a month prior to coming for treatment, his left eyeball had been red, swollen, and protruding and his vision had decreased. His elbow and knee joints were also swollen and enlarged, and walking was cumbersome and difficult. After being admitted to the hospital, he was diagnosed with hemophilia. Examination revealed the patient's body in relatively good condition but with a bitter and oppressed essence spirit, difficulty walking, a large purple spot on the left side of his face, and cotton balls blocking both nostrils due to nosebleeds. The upper and lower left eyelids manifested static blood of a purple color, and the upper eyelid was distended and swollen. The left eyeball protruded about 10mm, and the left vision was reduced. The pupil was increased in size, and the light reaction was slow. Fundic bleeding was noticed, and there was conjunctival edema. The tongue was red with thin, yellow fur, and the pulse was deep, fine, and slightly rapid.

The selected formula was *Tiao Xue Si Wu Tang* (Blood-regulating Four Materials Decoction): Radix Angelicae Sinensis (*Dang Gui*), 9g, Radix Rubrus Paeoniae Lactiflorae (*Chi Shao*), 9g, cooked Radix Rehmanniae (*Shu Di*), 15g, Radix Ligustici Wallichii (*Chuan Xiong*), 6g, Tuber Asparagi Cochinensis (*Tian Men Dong*), 15g, Rhizoma Bletillae Striatae (*Bai Ji*), 9g, Radix Anemarrhenae Asphodeloidis (*Zhi Mu*), 12g, Gelatinum Corii Asini (*E Jiao*), 6g, Cortex Radicis Moutan (*Dan Pi*), 6g, Herba Dendrobii (*Shi Hu*), 6g, and powdered Radix Pseudoginseng (*San Qi*), 6g, swallowed with the decoction.

After taking three *ji* of this formula, the patient's symptoms took a turn for the better. He was able to walk without difficulty, the swelling of the joints was reduced, the subcutaneous bleeding into the left eyelid was dispersed, the conjunctival edema was lessened, papilloretinal edema was also reduced, and no new bleeding could be seen. The stools were a little dry. Therefore, Radix Et Rhizoma Rhei (*Da Huang*), 9g, and Cortex Phellodendri (*Huang Bai*), 9g, were added to the base formula. After taking another three *ji*, the patient was able to walk smoothly, the joint swelling was basically gone, and the condition of the left eye was also further improved. Folium Lonicerae (*Ren Dong*), 20g, and Flos Lonicerae Japonicae (*Lian Qiao*), 12g, were added to the formula and another

---

[12] *Qian Jia Miao Fang (A Thousand Master's Wondrous Formulas)*, Li Wen-liang *et al.*, ed., Liberation Army Publishing House, Beijing, 1985, p. 205-206

three *ji* were administered. After this, the joint swelling was completely cured, the bleeding of the fundic region had been absorbed, and all other symptoms were completely eliminated. Semen Celosiae Argenteae (*Qing Xiang Zi*), 20g, was added to the formula and the patient was advised to take this modification for another 20 *ji*. Thereafter, the illness was cured.

Case 2[13]

After this patient had cut himself with a knife, bleeding started and could not be stopped with either Western hemostatic medicines or local treatments. Therefore, the following formula was prescribed: Rhizoma Coptidis Chinensis (*Huang Lian*), 6g, Radix Scutellariae Baicalensis (*Huang Qin*), 6g, uncooked Gypsum Fibrosum (*Shi Gao*), 30g, Rhizoma Imperatae Cylindricae (*Bai Mao Gen*), 30g, Rhizoma Anemarrhenae Asphodeloidis (*Zhi Mu*), 15g, Herba Agrimoniae Pilosae (*Xian He Cao*), 15g, Herba Dendrobii (*Shi Hu*), 12g, carbonized Radix Rubiae Cordifoliae (*Qian Cao Gen*), 12g, and Radix Glycyrrhizae (*Gan Cao*), 9g. After taking one *ji* of this formula, the bleeding was markedly improved. After six *ji*, the bleeding stopped.

Case 3[14]

This 25 year old female patient suffered from recurrent bleeding under the skin and into the joints and was hospitalized six times within the last year. She also suffered from frequent joint aches. Bleeding was always controlled through large blood transfusions. After Chinese medical examination, the following formula was prescribed: Semen Pruni Persicae (*Tao Ren*), 9g, Flos Carthami Tinctorii (*Hong Hua*), 6g, uncooked Radix Rehmanniae (*Sheng Di*), 12g, Radix Albus Paeoniae Lactiflorae (*Bai Shao*), 9g, Radix Ligustici Wallichii (*Chuan Xiong*), 9g, Radix Angelicae Sinensis (*Dang Gui*), 9g, Radix Pseudoginseng (*San Qi*), 3g, Radix Salviae Miltiorrhizae (*Dan Shen*), 12g, Gelatinum Corii Asini (*E Jiao*), 9g, Cortex Radicis Moutan (*Dan Pi*), 9g, Radix Astragali Membranacei (*Huang Qi*), 15g, Radix Codonopsitis Pilosulae (*Dang Shen*), 12g, and Radix Glycyrrhizae (*Gan Cao*), 3g.

After taking this formula, the skin and joint bleeding dispersed and the condition took a turn for the better. Re-examination revealed a red and moist facial complexion, good appetite, and improvement in the withering of both lower limbs. Thus, she was able to return to work. On follow-up after two years, there had been no recurrence of the bleeding.

---

[13] *Zhong Guo Zhong Yi Mi Fang Da Quan, op. cit.*, p. 516-517

[14] *Ibid.*, p. 516-517

Hereditary Spherocytosis

Case history[15] The patient was a four year old female who was first examined in August 1972. This young girl presented with natural endowment insufficiency manifesting with a weak and emaciated body. For one year prior to treatment, her appetite often was not good. When she was hungry, she typically ate fatty and sweet foods. She also had a liking to lie down and lacked strength. After playing for only a very short period of time, she had to sit or lie down. She was also tense and agitated and easily cried and got angry. Her urine was yellow, and her stools were sometimes bound and sometimes loose. She had become thinner day by day, her facial complexion was dull, yellow, and lusterless, and her essence spirit was not roused. She was not bright-spirited, and her mouth, lips, nails, and eyelids were pale and her hair dry, desiccated, and yellowish in color. Three months before coming to the hospital, she had been treated in another hospital for "jaundice due to hepatitis." During the last month prior to treatment, she had suffered from slight fever and a disease condition which progressively worsened. Her pulse was soggy and fine and her tongue was pale with scanty fur and teeth-marks on its edges.

Half a month ago, she had been examined in a Shanghai hospital and her blood values were as follows: WBCs were 5800/mm^3, neutrophils were 54%, lymphocytes were 36%, eosinophils were 4%, monocytes were 5%, basophils were 1%, RBCs were 3 million/mm^3, hemoglobin was 6.5g/dL, and reticulocytes were 20%. The red blood cells were spherically shaped, and no light area could be seen in their center. Thus, she was diagnosed with hereditary spherocytosis.

In order to cure this illness more quickly, Chinese medicinals were administered along with Western medications. The treatment principles used were to boost the kidneys and fortify the spleen, nourish the liver, and promote the engenderment of qi and blood. *Qing Ling Wan* (Dragonfly Pills) were prescribed. These consisted of: Dragonfly (*Qing Ling*)[16], Fructus Psoraleae Corylifoliae (*Bu Gu Zhi*), Herba Cistanchis Deserticolae (*Rou Cong Rong*), Radix Panacis Ginseng (*Ren Shen*), Rhizoma Atractylodis Macrocephalae

---

[15] *Qian Jia Miao Fang, op. cit.*, p. 184-185

[16] Dragonfly (*Qing Ling*), also called *Ling Ting*, is slightly cold and non-toxic. It engenders water within and can store water. It strengthens yin and astringes the essence. However, because it is red like strong heat, it can also be used to reinforce yang.

(*Bai Zhu*), Radix Angelicae Sinensis (*Dang Gui*), Testa Arachidis (*Hua Sheng Ren Lian Yi*)[17], and Semen Phaseoli Calcarati (*Chi Dou*).

These medicinals were made into pills with honey. After taking this prescription for two months, the patient's qi and blood gradually became full, and the child's essence spirit and appetite improved. Hemoglobin increased to 9g/dL. Thus, the pills were taken for another four months, after which the illness was judged completely cured.

Idiopathic Thrombocytopenic Purpura

Case 1[18]

The patient was a 47 year old female teacher. In May 1991, this patient was diagnosed with chronic idiopathic thrombocytopenic purpura (ITP) after a bone marrow analysis in a Zhongshan hospital. However, a year of treatment with prednisone did not increase the platelet count to more than 30,000-40,000/mm^3 and she continued suffering from recurrent nosebleeds, gum-bleeding, cutaneous purpura, and profuse menstruation. Because the Western medication did not lead to an improvement, she came to the hematology department in the author of this case history's hospital in December 1992. Blood laboratory examination revealed a platelet count of 35,000/mm^3 which was positive for platelet antibodies. Thus, self-composed *Duo Zi He Ji* (Many Seeds Mixture) was prescribed: Radix Astragali Membranacei (*Huang Qi*), Fructus Psoraleae Corylifoliae (*Bu Gu Zhi*), Fructus Lycii Chinensis (*Gou Qi Zi*), Fructus Schisandrae Chinensis (*Wu Wei Zi*), Fructus Ligustri Lucidi (*Nu Zhen Zi*), and Fructus Rubi Chingii (*Fu Pen Zi*). While taking this formula, the amount of prednisone was slowly reduced and then discontinued. After the patient had taken the above formula for two courses of treatment (*i.e.*, six months), the bleeding symptoms gradually stopped and the platelets increased to 80,000/mm^3. The prescription was continued for another half year, after which the patient was considered recovered and resumed work.

---

[17] Testa Arachidis (*Hua Sheng Ren Lian Yi*) is the seed coat of peanuts. It is sweet and neutral and enters the spleen and lungs. It moistens the lungs and harmonizes the stomach. Modern research has found this medicinal to be particularly effective for any type of bleeding and chronic bronchitis. No dosage is specified in the *Zhong Yao Da Ci Dian*.

[18] Wan Li-chuan *et al.*, "Clinical Analysis of the Treatment of Difficult-to-Treat Idiopathic Thrombocytopenic Purpura by the Treatment Methods of Boosting the Qi & Replenishing the Essence," *Zhong Yi Za Zhi (Journal of Chinese Medicine)*, #8, 1995, p. 478-480

Case 2[19]

The patient was a 64 year old female. This patient had suffered from recurrent static spots and macules on the four limbs with accompanying lumbar pain and lack of strength for 16 years. Through prednisone treatments, the platelets increased from around 40,000/mm³ to 82,000/mm³, and all the cutaneous purpura dispersed. However, when prednisone was gradually reduced, the platelet count dropped again, and the continued use of many steroids did not yield an obvious treatment effect. Examination revealed that she suffered from lumbar pain, limp limbs, dizziness, lack of strength, heart vexation, thirst, easy waking, and static macules distributed over her four limbs. Her tongue was dark red with yellow fur, and her pulse was deep, fine, and rapid.

Laboratory blood examination revealed the platelet count at 38,000/mm³. Examination of the bone marrow found a total of 118 megakaryocytes per sample, of which 5.1% were megakaryoblasts, 20.3% were promegakaryocytes, 63.6% were granular megakaryocytes, 2.5% were sporogenic disc megakaryocytes, and 8.5% were naked nucleus megakaryocytes. The myeloid as well as the erythroid system did not show any abnormalities. Thus, diagnosis was idiopathic thrombocytopenic purpura (ITP). The patient's Chinese medical pattern discrimination was kidney yin depletion and vacuity with static blood damaging the network vessels. Therefore, treatment principles were to enrich yin and supplement the kidneys, quicken the blood and quiet the network vessels, and the following formula was prescribed: cooked Radix Rehmanniae (*Shu Di*), uncooked Radix Rehmanniae (*Sheng Di*), Fructus Ligustri Lucidi (*Nu Zhen Zi*), Herba Ecliptae Prostratae (*Han Lian Cao*), Radix Salviae Miltiorrhizae (*Dan Shen*), and Herba Agrimoniae Pilosae (*Xian He Cao*), 30g each, Cortex Radicis Moutan (*Dan Pi*), Sclerotium Poriae Cocos (*Fu Ling*), and Radix Angelicae Sinensis (*Dang Gui*), 15g each, Semen Cuscutae Chinensis (*Tu Si Zi*), Fructus Corni Officinalis (*Shan Zhu Yu*), Radix Rubrus Paeoniae Lactiflorae (*Chi Shao*), and Rhizoma Atractylodis Macrocephalae (*Bai Zhu*), 10g each, Fructus Citri Aurantii (*Zhi Ke*) and Radix Glycyrrhizae Uralensis (*Gan Cao*), 6g each, and Fructus Cardamomi (*Bai Kou Ren*), 3g. This formula was prepared as a water decoction and one *ji* was taken every day. Concurrently, the patient was advised to take eight pills three times daily of *Qi Ju Di Huang Wan* (Lycium & Chrysanthemum Rehmannia Pills).

After seven days, the purpura was reduced, and the lumbar pain had improved. Thus, a modification of the above formula was prescribed for another month, after which all symptoms had normalized and the platelet count was up to 78,000/mm³. Three months

---

[19] Zhou Yong-ming *et al.*, "Clinical Observation of the Treatment of Idiopathic Thrombocytopenic Purpura in the Elderly by the Treatment Methods of Supplementing the Kidneys & Quickening the Blood," *Zhong Yi Za Zhi (Journal of Chinese Medicine)*, #12, 1993, p. 730-732

later, the platelet count was at 108,000/mm^3 and bone marrow examination found 84 megakaryocytes per sample, of which 3.6% were megakaryoblasts, 15.5% were promegakaryocytes, 42.9% were granular megakaryocytes, 27.4% were sporogenic disc megakaryocytes, and 10.7% were naked nucleus megakaryocytes. Follow-up after two years revealed that the condition had remained stable.

Case 3[20]

The patient was a 23 year old female worker. This patient presented with purpura dispersed over both lower limbs accompanied by profuse menstruation like a flood for already one year. Laboratory examination of the blood revealed that the WBCs were 4600/mm^3, RBCs were 3.1 million/mm^3, and platelets were 54,000/mm^3. The diagnosis was thrombocytopenic purpura, and treatment with leucogen and vitamin B$_4$ led to a turn for the better but did not completely recover the situation. The examination at the time of presentation revealed a bright white facial complexion and a markedly emaciated body with relatively severe aversion to cold, scanty intake, and loose stools. The tongue was pale with thin, white fur, while the pulse was fine and soft.

Thus, the pattern discrimination was spleen-kidney yang vacuity with qi not containing the blood. The treatment principles were to bank the spleen and boost the kidneys, supplement the qi and contain the blood. The formula consisted of: mix-fried Radix Astragali Membranacei (*Huang Qi*), 15g, Herba Epimedii (*Xian Ling Pi*), 15g, Caulis Milletiae Seu Spatholobi (*Ji Xue Teng*), 15g, Fructus Lycii Chinensis (*Gou Qi Zi*), 12g, Rhizoma Drynariae (*Gu Sui Bu*), 12g, Radix Angelicae Sinensis (*Dang Gui*), 10g, Lignum Nodi Pini (*You Song Jie*), 10g, mix-fried Radix Glycyrrhizae (*Gan Cao*), 5g, and blast-fried till carbonized Rhizoma Zingiberis (*Pao Jiang*), 2g.

After 15 *ji* of the above decoction, the patient's essence spirit was relatively roused, the purpura was dispersed, and re-examination of the blood revealed the platelets at 100,000/mm^3. Thus, another six *ji* were prescribed. After that, in order to improve the therapeutic effect, the patient was advised to take *Ren Shen Yang Rong Wan* (Ginseng Construction-nourishing Pills)[21] and *Gui Pi Wan* (Return the Spleen Pills), six grams

---

[20] *Xue Zheng Zhuan Ji, op. cit.*, p. 216

[21] *Ren Shen Yang Rong Wan* (Ginseng Construction-nourishing Pills) consist of Radix Panacis Ginseng (*Ren Shen*), Radix Glycyrrhizae (*Gan Cao*), Radix Angelicae Sinensis (*Dang Gui*), Radix Albus Paeoniae Lactiflorae (*Bai Shao*), cooked Radix Rehmanniae (*Shu Di*), Cortex Cinnamomi Cassiae (*Rou Gui*), Fructus Zizyphi Jujubae (*Da Zao*), Radix Astragali Membranacei (*Huang Qi*), Rhizoma Atractylodis Macrocephalae (*Bai Zhu*), Sclerotium Poriae Cocos (*Fu Ling*), Fructus Schisandrae Chinensis (*Wu Wei Zi*), Radix Polygalae Tenuifoliae (*Yuan Zhi*), Pericarpium Citri Reticulatae (*Chen Pi*), and uncooked uncooked Rhizoma Zingiberis (*Sheng Jiang*).

each in the morning and evening. On follow-up after three years, there had been no recurrence.

Iron Deficiency Anemia

Case 1[22]

The patient was a 26 year old female. In the years preceding this patient's visit to the doctor, she started suffering from a sallow yellow facial complexion, flusteredness, shortness of breath, and low-grade fever. Upon examination, her tongue was pale with thin, white fur, and the pulse was fine, forceless, and rapid. When asked about her thin body, she said she ate three meals per day but disliked meat dishes. Laboratory examination revealed hemoglobin at 6g/dL, normal levels of WBCs and platelets, serum iron at 8.234mol/L, and bone marrow sideroblasts at 0.12%. Therefore, the patient was diagnosed with iron deficiency anemia.

The Chinese pattern discrimination was qi and blood dual depletion and yin vacuity with internal heat and *Ba Zheng Tang* (Eight Pearls Decoction) was prescribed: Radix Angelicae Sinensis (*Dang Gui*), Sclerotium Poriae Cocos (*Fu Ling*), Radix Albus Paeoniae Lactiflorae (*Bai Shao*), and Rhizoma Atractylodis Macrocephalae (*Bai Zhu*), 15g each, cooked Radix Rehmanniae (*Shu Di*), 18g, Radix Ligustici Wallichii (*Chuan Xiong*), 9g, Radix Codonopsitis Pilosulae (*Dang Shen*), 25g, and mix-fried Radix Glycyrrhizae (*Gan Cao*), 8g. One *ji* of these medicinals was taken every day. Advice on correct food and drink was also given. After treatment, all the patient's symptoms improved, her facial complexion became red and moist, and her low-grade fever abated. One month later, hemoglobin had increased to 10g/dL. Three months later, it was up to 13g/dL.

Case 2[23]

The patient was a 28 year old female. This patient came for examination on Oct. 13, 1997. She complained of dizziness, vertigo, profuse menstruation, loss of hair, dry skin, frigid nails, numbness in the fingers, heart palpitations, shortness of breath, and aversion

---

[22] Huang Chun-lin *et al.*, "Pattern Discrimination, Disease Differentiation and Food & Drink Regulation & Supplementation for Iron Deficiency Anemia," *Xin Zhong Yi (New Chinese Medicine)*, #1, 1999, p. 58-59

[23] Personal observation at the First Hospital Affiliated with the Heilongjiang University of Chinese Medicine, Oct. 17, 1997. The patient was treated by Dr. Sun Wei-zheng.

to cold. Her tongue was covered with thin, white fur, and her pulse was slippery. The patient's appetite was normal. Blood examination revealed iron deficiency anemia. The Western medical diagnosis thus was iron deficiency anemia. The Chinese disease diagnosis was dizziness, and her pattern was categorized as heart-spleen dual vacuity.

The formula prescribed was as follows: Radix Angelicae Sinensis (*Dang Gui*), 15g, Radix Pseudostellariae (*Tai Zi Shen*), 15g, Radix Astragali Membranacei (*Huang Qi*), 50g, Radix Atractylodis Macrocephalae (*Bai Zhu*), 15g, Radix Glycyrrhizae (*Gan Cao*), 15g, Sclerotium Pararadicis Poriae Cocos (*Fu Shen*), 15g, Radix Polygalae Tenuifoliae (*Yuan Zhi*), 15g, Semen Zizyphi Spinosae (*Suan Zao Ren*), 15g, Arillus Euphoriae Longanae (*Long Yan Rou*), 15g, Radix Auklandiae Lappae (*Mu Xiang*), 5g, Fructus Ligustri Lucidi (*Nu Zhen Zhi*), 25g, Semen Cuscutae Chinensis (*Tu Si Zi*), 25g, Radix Albus Paeoniae Lactiflorae (*Bai Shao*), 15g, and Fructus Zizyphi Jujubae (*Da Zao*), 10 pieces.

Re-examination one week later revealed that the duration and severity of the patient's dizziness as well as her heart palpitations were all improved. Therefore, the same prescription was administered for another 10 days, at which point the patient was judged cured.

Leukemia

Case 1[24]

The patient was a 48 year old male who had suffered from lack of strength for the past eight months. For the past four months, this was more severe. There was also emaciation, a lusterless, somber white facial complexion, sweating, low-grade fever, and puffy swelling of the lower limbs. The spleen was swollen and hard, and 2-3 soybean-sized lymph nodes could be palpated under both armpits. On the left leg, there was a 5×5cm old static macule. Laboratory blood examination revealed the white blood cells at 250,000/mm^3, with a differentiation as follows: 55% neutrophils, 25% myelocytes, 8% late stage myelocytes, 4% eosinophils, and 8% lymphocytes. Hemoglobin was at 9.8g/dL, and platelets were at 90,000/mm^3. Bone marrow examination revealed extreme normoblast proliferation and chronic myelocytic signs. The tongue was red with thin fur, and the pulse was bowstring and rapid. Thus, the patient's pattern was categorized as evil toxins entering the marrow and damaging the blood with qi and blood vacuity and simultaneous blood stasis.

---

[24] *Xue Zheng Zhuan Ji, op. cit.*, p. 246

Therefore, the appropriate treatment was to quickly clear heat and cool the blood to prevent exuberant heat from stirring the blood. The formula prescribed contained: Cornu Bubali (*Shui Niu Jiao*), 30g, Herba Senecionis Integrifolii (*Gou She Cao*), 30g, Herba Oldenlandiae Diffusae Cum Radice (*Bai Hua She She Cao*), 30g, stir-fried Fructus Gardeniae Jasminoidis (*Zhi Zi*), 6g, Radix Scutellariae Baicalensis (*Huang Qin*), 6g, Cortex Radicis Moutan (*Dan Pi*), 12g, Radix Codonopsitis Pilosulae (*Dan Shen*), 12g, Radix Rubrus Paeoniae Lactiflorae (*Chi Shao*), 12g, uncooked Radix Rehmanniae (*Sheng Di*), 12g, Radix Lithospermi Seu Arnebiae (*Zi Cao*), 9g, Radix Scrophulariae Ningpoensis (*Xuan Shen*), 9g, Herba Taraxaci Mongolici Cum Radice (*Pu Gong Ying*), 15g, Fructus Meliae Toosendan (*Chuan Lian Zi*), 9g, and Rhizoma Corydalis Yanhusuo (*Yan Hu Suo*), 9g.

The second examination revealed an improvement of the pain and distention under the rib-side and no new static spots. Thus, *Zhi Zi, Huang Qin, Zi Cao, Xuan Shen, Chuan Lian Zi,* and *Yan Hu Suo* were removed from the formula and Rhizoma Sparganii (*San Leng*), 6g, Rhizoma Curcumae Zedoariae (*E Zhu*), 9g, Carapax Amydae Sinensis (*Bie Jia*), 12g, Concha Ostreae (*Mu Li*), 15g, Radix Rubrus Paeoniae Lactiflorae (*Chi Shao*), 12g, Spica Prunellae Vulgaris (*Xia Ku Cao*), 9g, and Tuber Curcumae (*Yu Jin*), 9g, were added.

The third examination revealed that the disease condition had become stable, the sweating had stopped, the fever had abated, and the swollen lump underneath the rib-side was smaller. Laboratory blood examination also showed an improvement. The WBCs were already down to 130,000/mm³. Thus, *Sheng Di, Xia Ku Cao, Mu Li, Chuan Xiong, Yu Jin,* and *Dan Shen* were removed from the formula, and Radix Pseudostellariae Heterophyllae (*Tai Zi Shen*) and Tuber Ophiopogonis Japonici (*Mai Dong*), 12g each, Herba Dendrobii (*Shi Hu*), 10g, and Semen Pruni Persicae (*Tao Ren*), 9g, were added.

Some type of modification of the above formula was taken for another three months, after which the WBCs were down to 7100/mm³, no immature white blood cells were seen, and hemoglobin was back to 11.3g/dL. The spleen was also obviously reduced in size, and the axillary lymph nodes were dispersed. Bone marrow examination revealed remission phase leukemia.

Case 2[25]

The patient was a 32 year old female. Because of lack of strength and static macules over her entire body for a month, fever since a recent removal of an ovarian cyst, and vaginal

---

[25] Xiang Yang, "Huang Shi-lin's Experience in the Treatment of Acute Promyelocytic Leukemia (APL)," *Zhong Yi Za Zhi (Journal of Chinese Medicine)*, #11, 1999, p. 653-654

bleeding for eight days, this patient came to the hospital on Nov. 25, 1992. Upon examination, she complained of dizziness, lack of strength, fever, cough, shortness of breath, vaginal bleeding, and watery diarrhea 8-10 times daily. Her temperature was 38°C, her pulse rate was 80 beats per minute, her respiration rate was 18 respirations per minute, and her blood pressure was 120/70mmHg. Anemic signs were of medium severity, static macules and static spots were visible all over her body, her heart and lung sounds were normal, and neither her liver or her spleen were enlarged. The tongue was dark yet pale with slimy, yellow fur. The pulse was slippery.

Laboratory examination of the peripheral blood revealed that the WBCs were at 2750/mm^3, hemoglobin was at 6g/dL, and platelets were at 80,000/mm^3. Bone marrow aspiration revealed a M:E ratio of 96.5:1 and abnormal myeloid production with an abundance of pathological promyelocytes (92%). Erythroid production was seriously depressed, and the megakaryocyte production was hypoplastic, with only a few platelets. Therefore, the Western medical diagnosis was acute non-lymphatic leukemia type M3a (acute promyelocytic leukemia).

Fu Fang Huang Dai Pian (Compound Realgar & Indigo Tablets)[26] were administered three times daily, 10 tablets each time. At the same time, the patient received antibiotics, hemostatic medication, and medication to regulate the acid-base water metabolite balance. Further, she was also given pure platelet transfusions. Thereafter, the patient's condition gradually improved. Her body temperature normalized, the infection was controlled, and the bleeding was stopped.

Forty-one days later, re-examination of the bone marrow revealed that she was in remission. The patient kept coming to the hospital to receive Western and Chinese medicines to stabilize remission. In July 1997, treatment was stopped. Follow-up at the time of writing revealed that the patient had already been kept in complete remission for six years and six months.

Leukopenia

Clinical audit 1[27]

This clinical audit used the following formula in the treatment of leukopenia: Fructus Psoraleae Corylifoliae (*Bu Gu Zhi*), 30g, Herba Epimedii (*Yin Yang Huo*), 15g, powdered

---

[26] The ingredients of *Fu Fang Huang Dai Pian* are Calculus Bovis (*Niu Huang*), Indigo Pulvis (*Qing Dai*), Radix Salviae Miltiorrhizae (*Dan Shen*), Radix Pseudostellariae Heterophyllae (*Tai Zi Shen*).

[27] *Zhong Guo Zhong Yi Mi Fang Da Quan*, p. 468-469

Placenta Hominis (*Tai Pan*), 15g, Fructus Ligustri Lucidi (*Nu Zhen Zi*), 60g, Fructus Corni Officinalis (*Shan Zhu Yu*), 15g, Radix Astragali Membranacei (*Huang Qi*), 30g, Fructus Zizyphi Jujubae (*Da Zao*), 30g, Radix Angelicae Sinensis (*Dang Gui*), 15g, Radix Salviae Miltiorrhizae (*Dan Shen*), 15g, Caulis Milletiae Seu Spatholobi (*Ji Xue Teng*), 60g, powdered Radix Pseudoginseng (*San Qi*), 9g, Rhizoma Polygoni Cuspidati (*Hu Zhang*), 30g.

Out of the 288 patients in this study, 46 suffered from leukopenia secondary to chemotherapy, whereas the other 242 suffered from leukopenia due to some other disease. All presented a pattern of spleen-kidney yang vacuity and blood vacuity with blood stasis. The 288 cases were divided into two groups: a treatment group of 177 cases receiving the above formula and a control group of 111 cases receiving butyl alcohol. One treatment course lasted two weeks. The treatment principles for the Chinese medicinal treatment group were to supplement and boost the spleen and kidneys, nourish the blood and transform stasis. One to four treatment courses later, the medicine of both groups was stopped for two weeks and the patients were re-examined. At that time, 50% of the treatment group was cured, whereas only 15.4% of the control group experienced such a cure. (P<0.001)

Clinical audit 2[28]

Sixty-two patients undergoing radiation therapy for cervical cancer were divided into two groups: a treatment group receiving the Chinese medicinal formula below while undergoing radiation therapy and a control group receiving the same formula after having undergone radiation therapy totaling 2000-3000 roentgen. The radiation therapy consisted of 5-6 treatments per week of 250-300 roentgen to the local area each time. The Chinese medicinal formula consisted of: Radix Astragali Membranacei (*Huang Qi*), 14g, Radix Pseudostellariae Heterophyllae (*Tai Zi Shen*), 12g, Radix Angelicae Sinensis (*Dang Gui*), 12g, Rhizoma Alismatis (*Ze Xie*), 7g, (all of the above medicinals powdered), Radix Salviae Miltiorrhizae (*Dan Shen*), 20g, Caulis Milletiae Seu Spatholobi (*Ji Xue Teng*), 20g, Folium Pyrrosiae (*Shi Wei*), 12g, Pericarpium Citri Reticulatae (*Chen Pi*), 8g, (all these medicinals decocted and made into a paste). The paste and powder were mixed with honey and prepared into pills.

The 30 patients in the treatment group who took the medicinal formula at the same time as receiving radiation therapy did not experience obvious leukopenia. On the other hand, the control group, after having received a total of 2000-3000 roentgen of radiation therapy experienced leukopenia, with white blood cell counts anywhere between 2000-

---

[28] *Ibid.*, p. 473

4000/mm³. When radiation was continued and the patients started taking the above formula, the condition did not further deteriorate in 20 patients whose leukocyte count was at 3500/mm³. As a matter of fact, not only did the leukocyte decline stop, on the contrary, the white blood cell count clearly began to increase.

Clinical audit 3[29]

The following three formulas were prescribed according to pattern discrimination to 128 cases suffering from leukopenia. Three weeks equaled one course of treatment.

Formula #1 fortified the spleen and warmed the kidneys. It was prescribed for those patients presenting a spleen-kidney dual vacuity pattern. It consisted of: Caulis Milletiae Seu Spatholobi (*Ji Xue Teng*), 30g, blast-fried Squama Manitis Pentadactylis (*Chuan Shan Jia*), 10g, Sclerotium Poriae Cocos (*Fu Ling*), 10g, Fructus Psoraleae Corylifoliae (*Bu Gu Zhi*), 15g, Herba Epimedii (*Xian Ling Pi*), 15g, Radix Astragali Membranacei (*Huang Qi*), 15g, and Rhizoma Atractylodis Macrocephalae (*Bai Zhu*), 20g.

Formula #2 enriched and supplemented the liver and kidneys. Therefore, it was prescribed to those patients: exhibiting a liver-kidney yin vacuity pattern. It consisted of: Caulis Milletiae Seu Spatholobi (*Ji Xue Teng*), 30g, blast-fried Squama Manitis Pentadactylis (*Chuan Shan Jia*), 10g, Cortex Radicis Lycii Chinensis (*Di Gu Pi*), 10g, Fructus Lycii Chinensis (*Gou Qi Zi*), 15g, uncooked Radix Rehmanniae (*Sheng Di*), 15g, Fructus Corni Officinalis (*Shan Zhu Yu*), 15g, Cortex Radicis Moutan (*Dan Pi*), 15g, and Fructus Ligustri Lucidi (*Nu Zhen Zi*), 15g.

Formula #3 was designed to supplement and boost the qi and blood. It was prescribed to those patients presenting a qi and blood dual vacuity pattern. It consisted of: Caulis Milletiae Seu Spatholobi (*Ji Xue Teng*), 30g, blast-fried Squama Manitis Pentadactylis (*Chuan Shan Jia*), 10g, Fructus Corni Officinalis (*Shan Zhu Yu*), 30g, Radix Astragali Membranacei (*Huang Qi*), 15g, cooked Radix Rehmanniae (*Shu Di*), 15g, Radix Codonopsitis Pilosulae (*Dang Shen*), 15g, and Radix Angelicae Sinensis (*Dang Gui*), 10g.

Of the 128 cases, 102 experienced an obvious turn for the better. This meant that, after 1-3 courses of treatment, the leukocyte count was 5000/mm³ or higher. Sixteen cases experienced a turn for the better. This meant that, after 1-4 courses of treatment, the leukocyte count had increased by 500-1000 in comparison to before treatment but was still lower than 5000/mm³. Ten cases experienced no effect. This meant that the

---

[29] *Ibid.*, p. 475

leukocyte count had increased by 400-800 but was still lower than 4500/mm^3. Thus, the total amelioration rate was 92.2%.

Lymphoma

Clinical audit[30]   The following formula was used in the treatment of 10 cases suffering from malignant lymphoma: Radix Angelicae Sinensis (*Dang Gui*), 10g, Radix Ligustici Wallichii (*Chuan Xiong*), 10g, Radix Rubrus Paeoniae Lactiflorae (*Chi Shao*), 10g, uncooked Radix Rehmanniae (*Sheng Di*), 10g, Radix Scrophulariae Ningpoensis (*Xuan Shen*), 15g, Bulbus Shancigu (*Shan Ci Gu*), 15g, Rhizoma Dioscoreae Bulbiferae (*Huang Yao Zi*), 15g, Herba Sargassii (*Hai Zao*), 15g, Thallus Algae (*Kun Bu*), 15g, Spica Prunellae Vulgaris (*Xia Ku Cao*), 15g, Concha Ostreae (*Mu Li*), 30g, and Rhizoma Paridis Heterophyllae (*Zao Xiu*), 30g.

Among these 10 patients, cancer staging was as follows: 4 cases were in stage I, 2 cases in stage II, 1 case in stage III, and 3 cases in stage IV. Seven cases were treated only with Chinese medicine. The tumor dispersed in three out of these seven, basically dispersed in one case, was reduced to half its size or less in two cases and did not change at all in one case. Post-treatment observation was performed for half a year in one case, one year in another case, and two years in three cases. Three cases were treated with a combination of chemotherapy and Chinese medicine. Among these three, the tumor dispersed in two and basically dispersed in one.

Case history[31]   The following formula was used in the treatment of one case of widespread superficially metastasized lymphoma with a yin vacuity, toxin accumulation, and phlegm nodulation pattern: Herba Oldenlandiae Diffusae Cum Radice (*Bai Hua She She Cao*), 100g, Spica Prunellae Vulgaris (*Xia Ku Cao*), 60g, Fructus Crataegi (*Shan Zha*), 50g, Radix Polygoni Multiflori (*He Shou Wu*), 30g, Carapax Amydae Sinensis (*Bie Jia*), 30g, Cortex Radicis Moutan (*Dan Pi*), 30g, Radix Codonopsitis Pilosulae (*Dang Shen*), 30g, Herba Scutellariae Barbatae (*Ban Zhi Lian*), 30g, Herba Lobeliae Chinensis Cum Radice (*Ban Bian Lian*), 30g, Semen Coicis Lachryma-jobi (*Yi Yi Ren*), 25g, uncooked Radix Rehmanniae (*Sheng Di*), 20g, Rhizoma Atractylodis Macrocephalae (*Bai Zhu*), 20g, Radix Albus Paeoniae Lactiflorae (*Bai Shao*), 20g, and Fructus Ligustri Lucidi (*Nu Zhen Zi*), 20g.

---

[30] "Tumors," *Zhong Guo Zhong Yi Mi Fang Da Quan, op. cit.*, p. 772

[31] *Ibid.*, p. 776

After taking 120 *ji* of this formula, the superficial lymphoma all over the body had dispersed, the food intake and essence spirit improved, the facial complexion became red and moist, body weight increased, and the patient was able to go back to work.

Megaloblastic Anemia

Case history[32] This 69 year old female patient was diagnosed with megaloblastic anemia, and laboratory examination revealed that her hemoglobin was at 4.2g/dL and the RBC count at 1.02 million/mm^3. Thus, the following formula was prescribed based on the principles of boosting the essence and replenishing the marrow, boosting the qi and supplementing the blood: Herba Cistanchis Deserticolae (*Rou Cong Rong*), 10g, Semen Cuscutae Chinensis (*Tu Si Zi*), 10g, Fructus Lycii Chinensis (*Gou Qi Zi*), 10g, Fructus Tribuli Terrestris (*Bai Ji Li*), 10g, Radix Achyranthis Bidentatae (*Niu Xi*), 6g, Cortex Cinnamomi Cassiae (*Rou Gui*), 4g, Fructus Chaenomelis Lagenariae (*Mu Gua*), 4g, Radix Dioscoreae Oppositae (*Shan Yao*), 12g, and Rhizoma Atractylodis Macrocephalae (*Bai Zhu*), 8g. One month later, the symptoms had obviously improved, hemoglobin had increased to 11g/dL, and RBCs had increased to 3.38 million/mm^3. On follow-up after one year, the woman's state of health remained normal.

Paroxysmal Nocturnal Hemoglobinuria

Case 1[33]

The patient was a 64 year old male who had been suffering from recurrent, frequent soy sauce colored urine for about one year. Accompanying signs and symptoms were lack of bodily strength, dizziness, flusteredness, shortness of breath, reduced appetite, aching and pain of the abdomen and back, a cumbersome and fatigued essence spirit, a pale tongue, and a vacuous, weak pulse. The diagnosis after examination at a Shanghai hospital was paroxysmal nocturnal hemoglobinuria, and a variety of Chinese medicines were prescribed to no avail. In May 1978, he sought treatment at the author of this case's hospital. Examination revealed the following: a medium developed but insufficiently nourished body, a chronically sick look, signs of anemia, and an apathetic essence spirit. The heart rate was 100 beats per minute with a third degree systolic murmur which could be heard at the apex, and dry rales heard in both lungs. The liver extended 3cm below the ribs on the mid-clavicular line but was not obviously tender upon touch. It was

---

[32] *Ibid..*, p. 451

[33] *Xue Zheng Zhuan Ji, op. cit.*, p. 185-186

somewhat resistant in feel. On the left side, the spleen extended 2cm below the ribs on the mid-clavicular line and was soft in consistency. Hemoglobin was 4.5g/dL, and RBCs were at 2 million/mm³.

This patient's Chinese medical pattern discrimination was spleen-kidney dual vacuity with spleen vacuity not able to secure and contain as well as kidney yin vacuity leading to yin vacuity-fire effulgence with vacuity fire leading to frenetic stirring and hematuria. The treatment principles were, therefore, to fortify the spleen and boost the kidneys, cool the blood and stop bleeding. The formula administered was *Bu Yi Pi Shen Tang* (Spleen-supplementing, Kidney-boosting Decoction): Radix Astragali Membranacei (*Huang Qi*), 30g, Radix Panacis Ginseng (*Ren Shen*), 9g, Radix Polygalae Tenuifoliae (*Yuan Zhi*), 9g, Rhizoma Atractylodis Macrocephalae (*Bai Zhu*), 9g, Radix Angelicae Sinensis (*Dang Gui*), 12g, Gelatinum Corii Asini (*E Jiao*), 9g, Sclerotium Poriae Cocos (*Fu Ling*), 9g, Herba Agrimoniae Pilosae (*Xian He Cao*), 30g, cooked Radix Rehmanniae (*Shu Di*), 15g, Herba Cephalanoploris Segeti (*Xiao Ji*), 30g, Radix Glycyrrhizae (*Gan Cao*), 6g, and Fructus Zizyphi Jujubae (*Da Zao*), 5 pieces.

After taking two *ji* of this formula, the soy sauce colored urine turned pale yellow. Therefore, the formula was continued for another two months, after which the disease symptoms of hematuria, dizziness, flusteredness, lumbar aching and pain, and the cumbersome and fatigued essence spirit had all almost disappeared and the bodily strength had increased. Blood examination then revealed the hemoglobin to be at 10g/dL. Thus, the medicinal decoction was stopped and, on follow-up after half a year, there had been no recurrence.

Case 2[34]

The patient was a 38 year old male. For one week prior to coming for treatment, the patient had suffered from fever, aching and painful joints all over the body, lumbar pain, and soy sauce colored urine. Thus, he was diagnosed with paroxysmal nocturnal hemoglobinuria (PNH) and admitted to the hospital. Later, his condition was changed to aplastic anemia-PNH (AA-PNH). Examination upon hospitalization revealed the following: his temperature was at 38°C, his pulse rate was 96 bpm; his respiration rate was 22 rpm; and his blood pressure was 120/80mmHg. The patient's spirit was clear, signs of anemia were severe, and static macules and papules presented all over his body. The man's eyelids were sallow yellow, his sclera were yellowish, his throat was hyperemic, and his tonsils were swollen (first degree). Breathing sounds in both lungs were rough. A 3rd

---

[34] Ying Hui-bei, "A Clinical Audit of the Effects of Treating 11 Cases of Paroxysmal Nocturnal Hemoglobinuria Based on Pattern Discrimination," *Shang Hai Zhong Yi Yao Za Zhi (Shanghai Journal of Chinese Medicine & Medicinals)*, #4, 1996, p. 38-39

degree systolic murmur could be heard at the apex. The patient's abdomen was soft, and his liver extended 5cm below his ribs. It was soft in consistency, and there was no pressure pain. An enlarged spleen could be felt on the left side. Hemoglobin was at 3g/dL, RBCs at 1.6 million/mm^3, WBCs at 4800/mm^3, and the reticulocyte index was 1.4%. A test for blood in the urine was positive.

Chinese medical examination revealed a sallow yellow facial complexion, heart palpitations, shortness of breath, dizziness, lack of strength, bodily fatigue, lumbar aching and pain, yellowish eyes, urine the color of thick tea, constipation, a red tongue tip with slimy, slightly yellow fur, and a rapid pulse. Thus, the pattern discrimination was spleen-kidney dual depletion with cold dampness having intruded into the exterior and not been resolved. This cold dampness had transformed into heat and was now smoldering.

The treatment principles were to dispel wind and free the flow of the network vessels, clear heat and disinhibit dampness, assisted by regulating and supplementing the spleen and kidneys. Hence the following formula was administered: Radix Clematidis Chinensis (*Wei Ling Xian*), 20g, Ramulus Cinnamomi Cassiae (*Gui Zhi*), 6g, mix-fried Resina Myrrhae (*Mo Yao*), 6g, mix-fried Resina Olibani (*Ru Xiang*), 6g, uncooked Radix Et Rhizoma Rhei (*Da Huang*), 6g, Herba Artemesiae Capillaris (*Yin Chen Hao*), 30g, Rhizoma Alismatis (*Ze Xie*), 30g, Radix Codonopsitis Pilosulae (*Dang Shen*), 12g, Radix Astragali Membranacei (*Huang Qi*), 20g, Sclerotium Poriae Cocos (*Fu Ling*), 12g, stir-fried Rhizoma Atractylodis Macrocephalae (*Bai Zhu*), 12g, and Fructus Corni Officinalis (*Shan Zhu Yu*), 12g.

After five *ji,* the fever subsided, and all the joint aches around the body were resolved. The color of the urine also changed. However, due to the prolonged course of the disease, the body was still vacuous and there was spontaneous perspiration and night sweats which did not stop. Thus, *Wei Ling Xian, Mo Yao, Ru Xiang*, and *Gui Zhi* were removed from the above decoction, the dose of *Huang Qi* was increased to 30g, and Radix Ledebouriellae Divaricatae (*Fang Feng*), 6g, Concha Ostreae (*Mu Li*), 30g, and Radix Albus Paeoniae Lactiflorae (*Bai Shao*), 30g, were added so as to secure the exterior and constrain sweating.

After another five *ji*, the sweating stopped. Thus, the formula was changed to the following: Radix Rubrus Panacis Ginseng (*Hong Shen*), 10g, mix-fried Radix Astragalus Membranacei (*Huang Qi*), 20g, Sclerotium Poriae Cocos (*Fu Ling*), 12g, stir-fried Rhizoma Atractylodis Macrocephalae (*Bai Zhu*), 12g, Radix Angelicae Sinensis (*Dang Gui*), 12g, Radix Salviae Miltiorrhizae (*Dan Shen*), 20g, Radix Albus Paeoniae Lactiflorae (*Bai Shao*), 15g, Herba Artemisiae Capillaris (*Yin Chen Hao*), 15g, and Rhizoma Alismatis (*Ze Xie*), 15g.

After three weeks, all the disease symptoms had dispersed and there were no more major complaints. Hemoglobin was 9g/dL, and RBCs were 2.95 million/mm³. Therefore, the patient was discharged from the hospital. Follow-up revealed that hemoglobin stayed at 9g/dL or above and that normal work was resumed.

Case 3[35]

The following formula was administered to a male patient suffering from paroxysmal nocturnal hemoglobinuria: Radix Astragali Membranacei (*Huang Qi*), 50g, Rhizoma Atractylodis Macrocephalae (*Bai Zhu*), 15g, Arillus Euphoriae Longanae (*Long Yan Rou*), 15g, Radix Panacis Ginseng (*Hong Shen*), 15g, Radix Albus Paeoniae Lactiflorae (*Bai Shao*), 15g, uncooked Radix Rehmanniae (*Sheng Di*), 15g, Pericarpium Citri Reticulatae (*Chen Pi*), 15g, Radix Auklandiae Lappae (*Mu Xiang*), 10g, Radix Ligustici Wallichii (*Chuan Xiong*), 10g, Rhizoma Cimicifugae (*Sheng Ma*), 10g, Radix Angelicae Sinensis (*Dang Gui*), 20g, and Fructus Zizyphi Jujubae (*Da Zao*), 7 pieces.

After 13 *ji* of this formula, the patient reported that he felt his symptoms had taken a turn for the better. After another 10 *ji*, the yellowing of the sclera and skin dispersed, the jaundice index returned to normal levels, and the face became moist. Hemoglobin improved from 6g/dL prior to treatment to 7.7g/dL, and the patient felt that he was symptom free. Another 85 *ji* were taken, and, on follow-up after one year, there was no hemoglobin in his urine.

Polycythemia Vera

Case 1[36]

This male patient suffered from polycythemia vera with an erythrocyte count of 8.8 million/mm³. His hemoglobin was 23.6g/dL, and his WBC count was 18,000/mm³. His Chinese medical pattern discrimination was upward flaming of fire, heat in the blood, yin vacuity, and blood stasis, and the treatment principles were to clear heat and downbear fire, cool the blood and resolve toxins, engender fluids, foster yin, and quicken the blood. Thus, the following formula was prescribed: Caulis Polygoni Multiflori (*Ye Jiao Teng*), 30g, Fructus Corni Officinalis (*Shan Zhu Yu*), 12g, Radix Salviae Miltiorrhizae (*Dan Shen*), 15g, Tuber Ophiopogonis Japonici (*Mai Men Dong*), 15g, Radix Scrophulariae Ningpoensis (*Xuan Shen*), 15g, Herba Dendrobii (*Shi Hu*), 15g,

---

[35] *Zhong Guo Zhong Yi Mi Fang Da Quan, op. cit.*, p. 465

[36] *Ibid.*, p. 485-486

Fructus Gardeniae Jasminoidis (*Zhi Zi*), 12g, Rhizoma Coptidis Chinensis (*Huang Lian*), 12g, Radix Ligustici Wallichii (*Chuan Xiong*), 10g, and stir-fried Fructus Zizyphi Jujubae (*Da Zao*), 15g. This formula was prepared as a decoction and was combined with *Niu Huang Jie Du Wan* (Bezoar Toxin-resolving Pills). After taking this combination for five months, the static macules which were present prior to treatment were dispersed, erythrocytes were down to 4.5 million/mm^3, hemoglobin was at 12g/dL, and WBCs were at 8800/mm^3.

Case 2[37]

This male patient suffered from polycythemia vera with a hemoglobin level of 20g/dL, an erythrocyte count of 7 million/mm^3, and other blood and bone marrow signs positive for polycythemia. His pattern discrimination was spleen vacuity with phlegm damp accumulation, stirring of internal wind, and heat. The treatment principles were to fortify the spleen and supplement the qi, dispel dampness and transform phlegm, extinguish wind and clear heat. Thus, the following formula was prescribed: Rhizoma Pinelliae Ternatae (*Ban Xia*), 12g, Sclerotium Poriae Cocos (*Fu Ling*), 12g, Rhizoma Atractylodis Macrocephalae (*Bai Zhu*), 10g, Rhizoma Gastrodiae Elatae (*Tian Ma*), 10g, Pericarpium Citri Reticulatae (*Chen Pi*), 10g, Rhizoma Acori Graminei (*Shi Chang Pu*), 10g, Flos Chrysanthemi Morifolii (*Ju Hua*), 10g, Radix Scutellariae Baicalensis (*Huang Qin*), 10g, Bombyx Batryticatus (*Jiang Can*), 8g, Rhizoma Arisaematis (*Tian Nan Xing*), 8g, and Radix Glycyrrhizae (*Gan Cao*).

After taking this formula for half a month, the static macules and spots dispersed and all the other symptoms also normalized. Hemoglobin decreased to 14g/dL, erythrocytes decreased to 3.59 million/mm^3, and all other blood and marrow signs normalized. After taking the formula for another month, the disease was cured. On follow-up after two years, no Western medications had to be taken throughout the entire course of this patient's disease and the patient had not suffered from any recurrences.

Pure Red Cell Aplasia

Case 1[38]

This patient suffered from pure red cell aplasia and presented with dizziness, heart palpitations, lack of strength, and a low-grade fever. His Chinese medical pattern

---

[37] *Ibid.*, p. 485-486

[38] *Ibid.*, p. 446-447

discrimination was spleen-kidney vacuity with blood and essence insufficiency. Therefore, he was administered the following formula: Radix Astragali Membranacei (*Huang Qi*), 15g, Radix Codonopsitis Pilosulae (*Dang Shen*), 9g, Radix Angelicae Sinensis (*Dang Gui*), 9g, Gelatinum Cornu Cervi (*Lu Jiao Jiao*), 9g, Plastrum Testudinis (*Gui Ban*), 9g, Gelatinum Corii Asini (*E Jiao*), 9g, Radix Rubrus Paeoniae Lactiflorae (*Chi Shao*), 9g, Radix Albus Paeoniae Lactiflorae (*Bai Shao*), 9g, Pericarpium Citri Reticulatae (*Chen Pi*), 9g, Radix Polygoni Multiflori (*He Shou Wu*), 12g, Fructus Lycii Chinensis (*Gou Qi Zi*), 12g, uncooked Radix Rehmanniae (*Sheng Di*), 10g, Herba Epimedii (*Yin Yang Huo*), 10g, Placenta Hominis (*Zi He Che*), 6g, and Fructus Zizyphi Jujubae (*Hong Zao*), 10 pieces.

After two weeks of treatment, the patient's dizziness, heart palpitations, lack of strength, and low-grade fever all gradually lessened. After two months of treatment, bone marrow examination revealed erythrocyte proliferation and a myeloid:erythroid ratio of 0.98:1, thus indicating that the condition had normalized. Laboratory blood examination results after treatment was stopped were as follows: hemoglobin was 6.5g/dL, WBCs were 6800/mm³, and platelets were 160,000/mm³. On follow-up after two years, it was ascertained that the condition had remained stable.

Case 2[39]

The patient was a 33 year old female who suffered from pure red cell aplasia accompanied by frequent occurrences of left lobar pulmonary cysts, water accumulation in the right pyelonephritic area, hepatosplenomegaly, and severe anemic water swelling of the entire body. The following two formulas were prescribed to be taken alternately, formula #1 for one day and formula #2 for two days.

Formula #1: mix-fried Herba Ephedrae (*Ma Huang*), 6g, Gypsum Fibrosum (*Shi Gao*), 12g, uncooked Rhizoma Zingiberis (*Sheng Jiang*), 3g, Fructus Zizyphi Jujubae (*Da Zao*), 9 pieces, mix-fried Radix Glycyrrhizae (*Gan Cao*), 3g, stir-fried Rhizoma Atractylodis Macrocephalae (*Bai Zhu*), 30g, uncooked Radix Et Rhizoma Rhei (*Da Huang*), 9g

Formula #2: uncooked Radix Astragali Membranacei (*Huang Qi*), 60g, Radix Angelicae Sinensis (*Dang Gui*), 12g

After taking these formulas for five months, the patient's hemoglobin improved from 1.6g/dL prior to treatment to 10.5g/dL, all her other signs and symptoms normalized, and her bodily strength returned.

---

[39] *Ibid.*, p. 448

Sickle Cell Anemia

Case history[40]

The patient was a four year old African-American female who was first examined on March 20, 1989. This little girl cried unstoppably for no obvious reason. She also suffered from recurrent upper respiratory tract infections. Her mother reported that she had occasional swelling of both ankles which, when even lightly touched, led to very loud screaming by the little girl. After admitting her to the hospital, blood examination revealed sickled red blood cells. Thus she was diagnosed with sickle cell anemia. At the time of her visit to the author of this case, there had been wandering pain on the right lower limb for four days. This pain was especially severe around the right knee, and touching the right knee was not possible. Based on comparison with same-age standards of other females, the girl's development was retarded. She suffered from lack of strength and fell whenever she tried to stand up. Examination of both lower limbs revealed no abnormalities preventing her standing, but touching her knee joints caused loud screaming. Her food intake was normal, her stools were thin and loose, and her mouth, lips, and eyelids were somber white. The patient's tongue was pale with teeth-marks on its edges and it had thin, white fur. The pulse was deep and fine and both cubit positions were weak.

Treatment consisted of acupuncture at the following points: *Gan Shu* (Bl 18), *Ge Shu* (Bl 17), *Pi Shu* (Bl 20), *Zu San Li* (St 36), *Tai Chong* (Liv 3) and *a shi* points around the painful local areas. Chinese medicinals consisted of: *Ren Shen Lu Rong Wan* (Ginseng & Deer Antler Pills) and *Ren Shen Jian Pi Wan* (Ginseng Fortify the Spleen Pills).

Half an hour after the first acupuncture treatment, the pain was completely gone and re-examination the next day revealed that the pain had remained absent for eight hours before returning. Thus, the same treatment was administered and, after 10 minutes, the pain was dispersed. After five acupuncture treatments, the pain did not recur, and, after eight treatments, acupuncture sessions were discontinued. The Chinese medicinals were taken for another four weeks. On follow-up nine months after treatment stopped, there had been one recurrence of pain in the left lower limb. However, no treatment was administered and the pain resolved spontaneously in one day.

---

[40] Li Qing-jiang, "Experiences in the Clinical Treatmnet of Sickle Cell Anemia," *Zhong Yi Za Zhi (Journal of Chinese Medicine)*, #3, 1994, p. 161

Thalassemia

Case 1[41]

Upon examination, this patient presented with hemoglobin at 8g/dL, RBCs at 2.5 million/mm³, and WBCs at 3600/mm³. The patient was diagnosed as suffering from thalassemia. The Chinese medical pattern was qi and blood dual vacuity, and the treatment principles were to boost the qi and engender the blood. Therefore, they were prescribed the following formula: Radix Astragali Membranacei (*Huang Qi*), 30g, Radix Angelicae Sinensis (*Dang Gui*), 15g, Radix Codonopsitis Pilosulae (*Dang Shen*), 15g, Radix Pseudostellariae Heterophyllae (*Hong Hai Er*), 60g, processed Radix Polygoni Multiflori (*He Shou Wu*), 20g, mix-fried Radix Glycyrrhizae (*Gan Cao*), 10g. After 15 *ji*, the patients signs and symptoms had taken an obvious turn for the better. Hemoglobin improved to 9.8g/dL, RBCs to 3.9 millions/mm³, and WBCs to 4600/mm³. The treatment effect was stable.

Case 2[42]

The patient was a 32 year old female suffering from thalassemia. Her Chinese medical pattern discrimination was yin and yang dual vacuity with exterior evils assailing. Thus she was administered the following formula: Radix Codonopsitis Pilosulae (*Dang Shen*), Radix Astragali Membranacei (*Huang Qi*), Cortex Cinnamomi Cassiae (*Rou Gui*), Radix Angelicae Sinensis (*Dang Gui*), Radix Lateralis Praeparatus Aconiti Carmichaeli (*Fu Zi*), uncooked Radix Rehmanniae (*Sheng Di*), Radix Albus Paeoniae Lactiflorae (*Bai Shao*), Radix Ligustici Wallichii (*Chuan Xiong*), Radix Et Rhizoma Notopterygii (*Qiang Huo*), Radix Ledebouriellae Divaricatae (*Fang Feng*),   mix-fried Radix Glycyrrhizae (*Gan Cao*), Tuber Ophiopogonis Japonici (*Mai Men Dong*), Fructus Zizyphi Jujubae (*Da Zao*), and uncooked Rhizoma Zingiberis (*Sheng Jiang*). After 20 *ji* of this formula, all the patient's signs and symptoms had obviously improved, hemoglobin increased from 7g/dL prior to treatment to 10g/dL, and WBCs increased to 4800/mm³.

---

[41] *Ibid.*, p. 458

[42] *Ibid.*, p. 459

Thrombocythemia

Case 1[43]

This patient suffered from an abnormal proliferation of thrombocytes and a platelet count of 700,000-860,000/mm³. The patient's pattern discrimination was blood stasis with heat and qi vacuity, and the corresponding treatment principles were to quicken the blood and dispel stasis, boost the qi and clear heat. Thus the following formula was prescribed: Radix Salviae Miltiorrhizae (*Dan Shen*), 30g, Radix Rubrus Paeoniae Lactiflorae (*Chi Shao*), 10g, Semen Pruni Persicae (*Tao Ren*), 10g, Flos Carthami Tinctorii (*Hong Hua*), 10g, Radix Angelicae Sinensis (*Dang Gui*), 10g, Carapax Amydae Sinensis (*Bie Jia*), 30g, Rhizoma Sparganii (*San Leng*), 10g, Rhizoma Curcumae Zedoariae (*E Zhu*), 10g, Radix Et Rhizoma Rhei (*Da Huang*), 5g, Pericarpium Citri Reticulatae Viride (*Qing Pi*), 10g, Herba Lycopi Lucidi (*Ze Lan*), 10g, Radix Astragali Membranacei (*Huang Qi*), 15g, Herba Artemisiae Apiaceae (*Qing Hao*), 15g.

After taking 40 *ji* of this formula followed by a pill version of the same formula for another three months, the patient's platelets were reduced to 140,000-220,000/mm³ and their marrow did not show any abnormalities. On follow-up after one year, except for an enlarged spleen, the illness had completely recovered.

Case 2[44]

Twelve days after a splenectomy, this female patient presented with an increase in platelets to 625,000/mm³. Later on, her platelets even increased to 1.57 million/mm³. Her accompanying signs and symptoms included lack of strength, joint aching, headaches, and a red tongue with slimy, yellow fur, and static spots on the tongue tip and both sides. The Chinese medical pattern discrimination was yin vacuity, blood heat, and blood stasis. The corresponding treatment principles were to enrich yin and cool the blood, clear heat and dispel stasis. Thus, the following formula was prescribed: powdered Cornu Cervi (*Lu Jiao*), 1.7g, Cortex Radicis Moutan (*Dan Pi*), 9g, uncooked Radix Rehmanniae (*Sheng Di*), 30g, Radix Albus Paeoniae Lactiflorae (*Bai Shao*), 15g, Semen Pruni Persicae (*Tao Ren*), 12g, Stigma Croci Sativi (*Zang Hong Hua*)[45], 1.5g, Semen

---

[43] *Ibid.*, p. 485-486

[44] *Ibid.*. P. 485-486

[45] Stigma Croci Sativi (*Zang Hong Hua*) is sweet and cold and enters the heart and liver channels. It nourishes the blood and frees the flow of the channels, cools the blood and scatters toxins. It is similar to Flos Carthami Tinctorii (*Hong Hua*) but stronger.

Coicis Lachryma-jobi (*Yi Yi Ren*), 22g, and Radix Lithospermi Seu Arnebiae (*Zi Cao*), 15g. After taking 18 *ji* of this formula, the patient's symptoms had basically dispersed, and the platelets were down to 590,000.

Bibliography

Chinese language bibliography

"Advances in the Chinese Medical Treatment of Allergic Purpura," Li Xiu-mei, *Zhong Guo Zhong Xi Yi Jie He Za Zhi (Chinese Journal of Integrated Chinese-Western Medicine)*, 1994, #6, p. 379-380

"Advances in Chinese Medical Research on Idiopathic Thrombocytopenic Purpura," Yang Yu-fei *et al.*, *Zhong Guo Zhong Xi Yi Jie He Za Zhi (Chinese Journal of Integrated Chinese-Western Medicine)*, 1994, #11, p. 699-701

"An Analysis of the Therapeutic Efficacy of the Treatment According to Pattern Discrimination of 11 Cases with Paroxysmal Nocturnal Hemoglobinuria," Ying Hui-bei, *Shang Hai Zhong Yi Yao Za Zhi (Shanghai Journal of Chinese Medicine & Medicinals)*, 1996, #4, p. 38-39

"An Exploration of the Use of Chinese Medicinals in Acute Leukemia [Treated by] Chemotherapy," Li Hai-yan *et al.*, *Zhong Guo Zhong Xi Yi Jie He Za Zhi (Chinese Journal of Integrated Chinese-Western Medicine)*, 1995, #10, p. 628-629

"Anti-Viral Chinese Medicinals in the Treatment of 32 Cases of Pediatric Idiopathic Thrombocytopenic Purpura," Yan Feng-shu *et al.*, *Zhong Guo Zhong Xi Yi Jie He Za Zhi (Chinese Journal of Integrated Chinese-Western Medicine)*, 1993, #12, p. 745-746

"Bleeding Conditions," Deng Tie-tao, *Xin Zhong Yi (New Chinese Medicine)*, 1999, #3, p. 7

"Clinical Analysis of the Treatment of Difficult-to-Treat Idiopathic Thrombocytopenic Purpura with the Treatment Methods of Boosting the Qi & Replenishing Essence," Wan Li-juan, *Zhong Yi Za Zhi (Journal of Chinese Medicine)*, 1995, #8, p. 478-480

"Clinical Experiences in the Treatment of Hemolytic Anemia," Chen Po, *Zhong Yi Za Zhi (Journal of Chinese Medicine)*, 1999, #10, p. 592-593

"Clinical Experiences in the Treatment of Sickle Cell Anemia," Li Qing-jiang, *Zhong Yi Za Zhi (Journal of Chinese Medicine)*, 1994, #3, p. 161

"Clinical Observations on the Treatment of 30 Cases of Acute Leukemia with a Combination of Chinese & Western Medicine," Chen Yong-zhen *et al.*, *Zhong Guo Zhong Xi Yi Jie He Za Zhi (Chinese Journal of Integrated Chinese-Western Medicine)*, 1998, #1, p. 43-44

"Clinical Observations on the Treatment of 120 Cases of Pediatric Iron Deficiency Anemia with *Er Le Yi Xue Chong Ji* (Children's Blood-supplementing Mixture)," Huang Yan-jie *et al.*, *Xin Zhong Yi (New Chinese Medicine)*, 1998, #12, p. 14-16

"Clinical Observations on the Treatment of Myelodysplastic Syndrome with *Yi Sui Kang* (Boost Marrow Health [Capsules])," Guo Pei-jing *et al.*, *Zhong Guo Zhong Xi Yi Jie He Za Zhi (Chinese Journal of Integrated Chinese-Western Medicine)*, 1995, #2, p. 74-76

"Clinical Observations on the Treatment of Idiopathic Thrombocytopenic Purpura in the Elderly with the Treatment Methods of Supplementing the Kidneys & Quickening the Blood," Zhou

Yong-ming *et al.*, *Zhong Yi Za Zhi (Journal of Chinese Medicine)*, 1993, #12, p. 730-732

"Clinical Study of the Effect of *Fu Zheng Kang Bai He Ji* (Support the Righteous Anti-white [Blood Cell] Mixture) on Long-term Survival of Patients with Acute Leukemia," Ma Rou *et al.*, *Zhong Guo Zhong Xi Yi Jie He Za Zhi (Chinese Journal of Integratred Chinese-Western Medicine)*, 1998, #5, p. 276-278

"Hematologic Diseases." *Zhong Guo Zhong Yi Mi Fang Da Quan (Compendium of Chinese Medical Secret Formulas)*, 14th ed., Hu Xi-ming, ed., Literary Collection Publishing Company, Shanghai, 1997, p. 429-519

"Huang Shi-lin's Experience in the Treatment of Acute Promyelocytic Leukemia (APL)," Xiang Yang, *Zhong Yi Za Zhi (Journal of Chinese Medicine)*, 1999, #11, p. 653-654

"Jiao Zhong-hua's Experience in the Treatment of Aplastic Anemia," Li Rui, *Zhong Yi Za Zhi (Journal of Chinese Medicine)*, 1999, #8, p. 462-463

Lao Nian Chang Jiang Bing Zheng Fang Zhi Fa (The Prevention & Treatment of Common Geriatric Diseases), Wu Jun-xi, ed., Chinese National Medicine & Medicinals Publishing House, Beijing, 1998

Nan Zhi Bing De Liang Fang Miao Fa (Fine Formulas & Wondrous Methods for Difficult-to-Treat Diseases), Wu Da-zhen & Ke Xin-qiao, Chinese National Medicine & Medicinals Publishing House, Beijing, 1992

Ning Bing Zhong Yi Zhi Liao Ji Yan Jiu (Recent Research on the Chinese Medical Diagnosis & Treatment of Knotty Diseases), Bao Xue-quan & Jin Xiao-lin, People's Health & Hygiene Press, Beijing, 1995

"Observations on the Chinese Medical Understanding & Treatment of Polycythemia Vera," Hou Pi-hua & Liang Yi-jun, *Bei Jing Zhong Yi (Beijing Chinese Medicine)*, 1996, #4, p. 26-27

"Observations on the Therapeutic Efficacy of the Treatment of 38 Cases of Acute Leukemia with a Combination of Chinese medicinals & Chemotherapy," Xiao Qian, *Zhong Yi Za Zhi (Journal of Chinese Medicine)*, 1998, #5, p. 283-285

"Observations on the Therapeutic Efficacy of the Treatment of 20 Cases of Chronic Aplastic Anemia," Shi Sai-yang *et al.*, *Zhong Xi Yi Jie He Za Zhi (Journal of Integrated Chinese-Western Medicine)*, 1988, #6, p. 364-365

"Pattern Discrimination, Disease Differentiation and Food & Drink Regulation & Supplementation for Iron Deficiency Anemia," Huang Chun-lin *et al.*, *Xin Zhong Yi (New Chinese Medicine)*, 1999, #1, p. 58-59

"Preliminary Analysis of the Relationship between Immunological Changes & Chinese Medical Pattern Discrimination in the Prognosis of Chronic Idiopathic Thrombocytopenic Purpura," Yang Yu-fei *et al.*, *Zhong Guo Zhong Xi Yi Jie He Za Zhi (Chinese Journal of Integrated Chinese-Western Medicine)*, 1995, #7, p. 401-404

Qian Jia Miao Fang (Thousands of Masters' Wondrous Formulas), Vol.1., 3rd ed., Li Wen-liang *et al.*, ed., Liberation Army Press, Beijing, 1985

"Summary of the Fifth All-China Integrated Chinese-Western Medicine Symposium on Blood Diseases," Blood Disease Association of the China Institute of Integrated Chinese-Western Medicine, *Zhong Yi Za Zhi (Journal of Chinese Medicine)*, 1998, #12, p. 752-754

"The Cure of One Case of Allergic Purpura with *Qing Ying Tang Jia Jian* (Constructive-clearing Decoction with Additions & Subtractions)," Zhang Guo-jin, *Zhong Xi Yi Jie He Za Zhi (Journal of Integrated Chinese-Western Medicine)*, 1988, #6, p. 329

"The Pattern Discrimination Treatment of Blood Ejection," Tian Wei-jun, *Xin Zhong Yi (New Chinese Medicine)*, 1998, #12, p. 50-51

"The Treatment of 11 Cases of Polycythemia Vera with *Zheng Hong Huan Jie Tang* (Moderating & Resolving True Red Decoction)," Han Ji-chong *et al.*, *Zhong Guo Zhong Xi Yi Jie He Za Zhi (Chinese Journal of Integrated Chinese-Western Medicine)*, 1995, #9, p. 555-556

"The Treatment of 24 Cases of Alleric Purpura with *Xiao Dian Jie Du Tang* (Patch-dispersing, Toxin-resolving Decoction)," Zhang Yi, *Si Chuan Zhong Yi (Sichuan Chinese Medicine)*, 1999, #1, p. 18

"The Treatment of 42 Cases of Chronic Thrombocytopenic Purpura with Integrated Chinese-Western Medicine," Hu Yang-hong, *Zhong Guo Zhong Xi Yi Jie He Za Zhi (Chinese Journal of Integrated Chinese-Western Medicine)*, 1994, #8, p. 495-496

"The Treatment of 50 Cases of Acute Non-lymphocytic Leukemia with a Combination of Chinese Medicine Pattern Discrimination & the HA Program," Xu Rui-rong *et al.*, *Zhong Guo Zhong Xi Yi Jie He Za Zhi (Chinese Journal of Integrated Chinese-Western Medicine)*, 1995, #5, p. 302-303

"The Treatment of Chronic Idiopathic Thrombocytopenic Purpura with the Methods of Boosting the Qi & Quickening the Blood Method," Qian Gang, *Shanghai Zhong Yi Yao Za Zhi (Shanghai Journal of Chinese Medicine & Medicinals)*, 1999, #2, p. 17

"Wu Han-xiang's Experience in the Treatment of Fevers in Blood Diseases," Qiu Zhong-quan & Hu Qi, *Zhong Yi Za Zhi (Journal of Chinese Medicine)*, 1999, #5, p. 279-280

Xian Zai Nan Zhi Bing Zhong Yi Zhen Liao Xue (A Study of the Chinese Medical Diagnosis & Treatment of Modern Difficult-to-Treat Diseases), Wu Jun-yu & Bai Yang-bo, Chinese Medical Ancient Books Press, Beijing, 1993

Xin Xue Guan Xue Ye Bing Shi Yong Fang (Practical Formulas for Cardiovascular & Hematologic Diseases), 2nd ed., Zhao Guo-ping, ed., Jiangsu Science & Technology Press, Hangzhou, 1994

Xue Ye Bing MiaoYong Zhong Yao (Magically Effective Chinese Medicinals for Blood Diseases), Zhang Shen-bing *et al.*, ed., Jiangsu Science & Technology Press, Hangzhou,1997

Xue Zheng Zhuan Ji (A Collection of Experts on Bleeding Patterns), Shi Yu-guang & Shan Shu-jian, ed., Ancient Chinese Medical Books Press, Beijing, 1992

"*Zhi Zi Hua Tang* (Gardenia Flower Decoction) in the Prevention & Treatment of Epistaxis," Xu Chang-yan, *Xin Zhong Yi (New Chinese Medicine)*, 1999, #1, p. 59

Zhong Yao Da Ci Dian (A Great Dictionary of Chinese Medicinals), 6th ed., Jiangsu College of New Medicine, Shanghai Science & Technology Press, Shanghai, 1993

Zhong Yi Er Ke Xue Ye Ye Bing Zhen Liao Jing Yan (Experiences in the Diagnosis & Treatment of Pediatric Blood Diseases with Chinese Medicine), 3rd ed., Cai Hua-li *et al.*, ed., People's Health & Hygiene Press, Beijing, 1996

English language bibliography

A Compendium of TCM Patterns & Treatments, Bob Flaws & Daniel Finney, Blue Poppy Press, Boulder, CO, 1996

Aging and Blood Stasis: A New Approach to Geriatrics, Yan De-xin, trans. by Tang Guo-shun & Bob Flaws, Blue Poppy Press, Boulder, CO, 1995

A Practical Dictionary of Chinese Medicine, Nigel Wiseman & Feng Ye, Paradigm Publications, Brookline, MA, 1998

Chinese Herbal Medicine: Formulas & Strategies, Dan Bensky & Randall Barolet, Eastland Press, Seattle, 1990

Chinese Herbal Medicine: Materia Medica, Dan Bensky & Andrew Gamble, Eastland Press, Seattle,1993

Clinical Hematology and Fundamentals of Hemostasis, 3rd ed., Denise M. Harmening, ed., F.A. Davis Co., Philadelphia, 1997

English-Chinese Chinese-English Dictionary of Chinese Medicine, Nigel Wiseman, Hunan Science & Technology Press, Changsha, 1995

Essential Pathology, 2nd ed., Emanuel Rubin & John Farber, ed., J.B. Lippincott Co., Philadelphia, 1995

Fundamentals of Chinese Medicine, rev. ed., Nigel Wiseman & Andrew Ellis, Paradigm Pulbications, Brookline, MA, 1996

Golden Needle Wang Le-ting: A 20th Century Master's Approach to Acupuncture, Yu Hui-chan & Han Fu-ru, trans. by Shuai Xue-zhong, Blue Poppy Press, Boulder, CO, 1997

Human Anatomy and Physiology, 2nd ed., Elaine Marieb, Benjamin/Cummings Publishing, Redwood City, CA, 1992

Oriental Materia Medica: A Concise Guide, Hong-yen Hsu, Oriental Healing Arts Institute, Long Beach, CA, 1986

Practical Diagnosis in Traditional Chinese Medicine, Deng Tie-tao, trans. by Marnae Ergil & Yi Su-mei, Churchill Livingstone, Edinburgh, 1999

Statements of Fact in Traditional Chinese Medicine, Bob Flaws, Blue Poppy Press, Boulder, CO, 1994

Taber's Cyclopedic Medical Dictionary, 17th ed., F.A. Davis Co., Philadelphia, 1989

The Chinese Herb Selection Guide, Charles Belanger, Phytotech, Richmond, CA, 1997

The Merck Manual, 16th ed., Merck Research Laboratories, Rahway, NJ, 1992

"Treatment Principles as Funnels," Bob Flaws, www.bluepoppy.com, Free Articles,1998

General Index

stools, loose and/or black 205
stools, loose 69, 71, 82, 91, 92, 96, 97, 101, 103, 111, 138, 139, 141, 146, 147, 164, 172, 220, 237
stools, non-free flowing 164
stools, occult blood in the 201, 206
strength, lack of 69-71, 78, 79, 81, 86, 87, 89, 91, 95, 97, 99, 101, 103, 107, 108, 141, 147, 150, 155-157, 170, 172, 178, 182, 183, 189, 205, 215, 220, 225-228, 231, 236, 239-241, 247, 249-251, 253
stroke 117, 121, 127
Stuart factor 22
swallowing, difficulty 74
sweating, profuse 73, 75, 112
swelling, puffy 111, 205, 207, 231, 239

T

throat, swelling of the, with a hoarse voice 206
throat, swollen 133, 150
tongue, swollen, enlarged 205
talking nonsense 126
tapeworm 89
tendency to take deep breaths 74
testicular dampness 227
tetany 40, 49
thalassemia 20, 66, 67, 106, 107, 252
throbbing, fearful 145
thrombocythemia 17, 18, 195, 196, 253
thrombocytopenia 17, 20, 25, 26, 30, 37, 66, 67, 80, 89, 119, 132, 137, 153-155, 161, 170, 196
thrombocytopenic purpura 3, 17, 18, 35, 36, 40, 60, 185, 235-237
thrombotic angitis 124
thrombotic phlebitis 124
thrombus formation 48
tidal reddening 191
tinnitus 65, 83, 92, 96, 100, 102, 121, 123, 147, 148, 150, 178, 183, 191, 199, 204, 217
tonsils, engorged 133
tonsils, swollen, yellow-white secretion covering the 133
transferrin saturation 24, 25
trace minerals, lack of 45
tuberculosis 13, 29, 176

U

upper respiratory infections 33, 42, 191
uremia 20, 110
urinary bleeding, severe 48
urination, inhibited 226
urination, long, clear 71, 84, 108, 141
urination, profuse 69

urination, short, reddish 74, 83, 178
urine, bloody 48, 125
urine, soy sauce colored 82, 245, 246
urine the color of thick tea 247
urticaria 201, 206
uvula, engorged 133

V

vascular disorders 18
vascular thrombosis 25
vertigo 65, 238
vexation and agitation 40, 74, 88, 93, 101, 121, 122, 132, 134, 135, 140, 148, 150, 151, 159, 162, 164, 167, 178, 182, 198, 209, 210
vexatious heat in the five hearts 83, 102, 183, 204, 217
vision, dimness of 110
vision, flowery 96, 100, 147
visual disturbances 96, 119
vitamin k deficiency 23
voice, raspy 139
vomiting of yellow water 95
von Willebrand's disease (VWD) 213
voice, weak 74

W

Wang Le-Ting 55
weakness 41, 42, 65, 68, 90, 96, 97, 107, 116, 119, 126, 127, 144, 146, 154, 161, 195, 197, 199
Wei v, viii, 47, 54, 57, 60, 71, 73, 82, 83, 85, 92, 94, 95, 99-101, 103, 104, 109, 123, 124, 126, 127, 130, 134, 135, 139, 140, 145, 146, 167, 171, 172, 179, 181, 193, 194, 204, 209, 211, 225, 226, 228, 230, 231, 235, 237, 238, 242, 247
western medical diagnosis of blood diseases 9, 19
wind, aversion to 139, 140, 203
Wiseman's terminology, Nigel vii
worm eggs 103
worms, parasitic 13, 16, 137

Pinyin Formula Index